Pediatric Psychopharmacology in the 21st Century

Guest Editors

DONALD E. GREYDANUS, MD
DILIP R. PATEL, MD
CYNTHIA FEUCHT, PharmD, BCPS

PEDIATRIC CLINICS
OF NORTH AMERICA

www.pediatric.theclinics.com

February 2011 • Volume 58 • Number 1

SAUNDERS an imprint of ELSEVIER, Inc.

W.B. SAUNDERS COMPANY
A Division of Elsevier Inc.

1600 John F. Kennedy Boulevard • Suite 1800 • Philadelphia, Pennsylvania 19103-2899

http://www.theclinics.com

THE PEDIATRIC CLINICS OF NORTH AMERICA Volume 58, Number 1
February 2011 ISSN 0031-3955, ISBN-13: 978-1-4557-0482-8

Editor: Kerry Holland
Developmental Editor: Jessica Demetriou

The Pediatric Clinics of North America (ISSN 0031-3955) is published bimonthly by Elsevier Inc., 360 Park Avenue South, New York, NY 10010-1710. Months of issue are February, April, June, August, October, and December. Periodicals postage paid at New York, NY and additional mailing offices. Subscription prices are $179.00 per year (US individuals), $423.00 per year (US institutions), $243.00 per year (Canadian individuals), $563.00 per year (Canadian institutions), $289.00 per year (international individuals), $563.00 per year (international institutions), $87.00 per year (US students and residents), and $149.00 per year (international and Canadian residents and students). To receive students/resident rare, orders must be accompanied by name of affiliated institution, date of term, and the signature of program/residency coordinator on institution letterhead. Orders will be billed at individual rate until proof of status is received. Foreign air speed delivery is included in all *Clinics* subscription prices. All prices are subject to change without notice. **POSTMASTER:** Send address changes to *The Pediatric Clinics of North America*, Elsevier Health Sciences Division, Subscription Customer Service, 3251 Riverport Lane, Maryland Heights, MO 63043. **Customer Service: 1-800-654-2452 (US and Canada). From outside of the US and Canada: 1-314-447-8871. Fax: 1-314-447-8029. For print support, E-mail: JournalsCustomerService-usa@elsevier.com. For online support, E-mail: JournalsOnlineSupport-usa@elsevier.com.**

Reprints. For copies of 100 or more, of articles in this publication, please contact the Commercial Reprints Department, Elsevier Inc., 360 Park Avenue South, New York, NY 10010-1710. Tel.: 212-633-3812; Fax: 212-462-1935; E-mail: reprints@elsevier.com.

The Pediatric Clinics of North America is also published in Spanish by McGraw-Hill Inter-americana Editores S.A., Mexico City, Mexico; in Portuguese by Riechmann and Affonso Editores, Rua Comandante Coelho 1085, CEP 21250, Rio de Janeiro, Brazil; and in Greek by Althayia SA, Athens, Greece.

The Pediatric Clinics of North America is covered in *MEDLINE/PubMed (Index Medicus), Excerpta Medica, Current Contents, Current Contents/Clinical Medicine, Science Citation Index, ASCA, ISI/BIOMED,* and *BIOSIS.*

Printed and bound by CPI Group (UK) Ltd, Croydon, CR0 4YY

Transferred to Digital Print 2011

GOAL STATEMENT

The goal of the *Pediatric Clinics of North America* is to keep practicing physicians and residents up to date with current clinical practice in pediatrics by providing timely articles reviewing the state-of-the-art in patient care.

ACCREDITATION

The *Pediatric Clinics of North America* is planned and implemented in accordance with the Essential Areas and Policies of the Accreditation Council for Continuing Medical Education (ACCME) through the joint sponsorship of the University Of Virginia School Of Medicine and Elsevier. The University Of Virginia School of Medicine is accredited by the ACCME to provide continuing medical education for physicians.

The University of Virginia School of Medicine designates this educational activity for a maximum of 15 *AMA PRA Category 1 Credits*™ for each issue, 90 credits per year. Physicians should only claim credit commensurate with the extent of their participation in the activity.

The American Medical Association has determined that physicians not licensed in the US who participate in this CME activity are eligible for a maximum of 15 *AMA PRA Category 1 Credits*™ for each issue, 90 credits per year.

Credit can be earned by reading the text material, taking the CME examination online at http://www.theclinics.com/home/cme, and completing the evaluation. After taking the test, you will be required to review any and all incorrect answers. Following completion of the test and evaluation, your credit will be awarded and you may print your certificate.

FACULTY DISCLOSURE/CONFLICT OF INTEREST

The University of Virginia School of Medicine, as an ACCME accredited provider, endorses and strives to comply with the Accreditation Council for Continuing Medical Education (ACCME) Standards of Commercial Support, Commonwealth of Virginia statutes, University of Virginia policies and procedures, and associated federal and private regulations and guidelines on the need for disclosure and monitoring of proprietary and financial interests that may affect the scientific integrity and balance of content delivered in continuing medical education activities under our auspices.

The University of Virginia School of Medicine requires that all CME activities accredited through this institution be developed independently and be scientifically rigorous, balanced and objective in the presentation/discussion of its content, theories and practices.

All authors/editors participating in an accredited CME activity are expected to disclose to the readers relevant financial relationships with commercial entities occurring within the past 12 months (such as grants or research support, employee, consultant, stock holder, member of speakers bureau, etc.). The University of Virginia School of Medicine will employ appropriate mechanisms to resolve potential conflicts of interest to maintain the standards of fair and balanced education to the reader. Questions about specific strategies can be directed to the Office of Continuing Medical Education, University of Virginia School of Medicine, Charlottesville, Virginia.

The faculty and staff of the University of Virginia Office of Continuing Medical Education have no financial affiliations to disclose.

The authors/editors listed below have identified no financial or professional relationships for themselves or their spouse/partner:
Lee A Bricker, MD; Joseph L. Calles Jr, MD; L. Lee Carlisle, MD; Madeline A. Chadehumbe, MD; Bantu Chhangani, MD; Cynthia L. Feucht, PharmD, BCPS (Guest Editor); Neville H. Golden, MD; Donald E. Greydanus, MD, Dr HC (ATHENS) (Guest Editor); Carla Holloway, (Acquisitions Editor); Iliyan Ivanov, MD; Ian Kodish, MD, PhD; Jon McClellan, MD; Ahsan Nazeer, MD; Dilip R. Patel, MD, FAACPDM, FAAP, FSAM, FACSM (Guest Editor); Helen D. Pratt, PhD; Karen Rheuban, MD (Test Author); Ruqiya Shama Tareen, MD; Susan M. Smiga, MD; Libbie Stansifer, MD; and Tiffany Thomas, MD.

The authors/editors listed below identified the following professional or financial affiliations for themselves or their spouse/partner:
Evelyn Attia, MD is an industry funded research/investigator for Eli Lilly & Co.
Glen R. Elliott, PhD, MD is an industry funded research/investigator for BioMarin Pharmaceuticals.
Robert L. Findling, MD receives grant/research support, is a consultant, and is on the Speakers' Bureau for Bristol-Myers Squibb, Johnson & Johnson, and Shire; receives grant/research support and is a consultant for Abbott, Addrenex, Astra-Zeneca, Forest, GSK, Lilly, Otsuka, Pfizer, Schering-Plough, Supernus Pharmaceuticals, and Wyeth; is a consultant for Biovail, KemPharm, Lundbeck, Novartis, Noven, Organon, Sanofi-Aventis, Sepracore, Solvay, and Validus; and receives grant/research support from Neuropharm.
Manmohan K. Kamboj, MD is on the Speakers' Bureau for Pfizer.
Gabriel Kaplan, MD is on the Speakers' Bureau for Shire, is a consultant for Commonhealth Hoboken, and is employed by University Medical Center.
Jeffrey H. Newcorn, MD is an industry funded research/investigator for Shire, Ortho McNeil Janssen, and Eli Lilly, and is a consultant and is on the Advisory Committee/Board for Shire.
Carol Rockhill, MD, PhD, MPH is an industry funded research/investigator for Seaside Therapeutics.
Sheryl Ryan, MD is on the Speaker's Bureau for Merck Pharmaceuticals.
Chris Varley, MD is on the Speaker's Bureau for Novartis.

Disclosure of Discussion of Non-FDA Approved Uses for Pharmaceutical Products and/or Medical Devices
The University of Virginia School of Medicine, as an ACCME provider, requires that all faculty presenters identify and disclose any off-label uses for pharmaceutical and medical device products. The University of Virginia School of Medicine recommends that each physician fully review all the available data on new products or procedures prior to clinical use.

TO ENROLL

To enroll in the Pediatric Clinics of North America Continuing Medical Education program, call customer service at 1-800-654-2452 or visit us online at www.theclinics.com/home/cme. The CME program is available to subscribers for an additional fee of $223.00

Contributors

GUEST EDITORS

DONALD E. GREYDANUS, MD
Professor, Department of Pediatrics and Human Development, Michigan State University College of Human Medicine, East Lansing; Pediatrics Program Director, Michigan State University/Kalamazoo Center for Medical Studies, Kalamazoo, Michigan

DILIP R. PATEL, MD
Professor, Department of Pediatrics and Human Development, Michigan State University College of Human Medicine, East Lansing; Division of Developmental-Behavioral Pediatrics, Pediatric Residency Program, Kalamazoo Center for Medical Studies, Kalamazoo, Michigan

CYNTHIA FEUCHT, PharmD, BCPS
Adjunct Professor, Ferris State University School of Pharmacy, Big Rapids; Clinical Pharmacist, Borgess Ambulatory Care, Kalamazoo, Michigan

AUTHORS

EVELYN ATTIA, MD
Clinical Professor of Psychiatry, Columbia University Medical Center, Weill Cornell Medical College; New York State Psychiatric Institute, New York, New York

LEE A. BRICKER, MD
Michigan State University/Kalamazoo Center for Medical Studies, Kalamazoo; Professor, Department of Internal Medicine; Director, Clinics in Adult Endocrinology, Diabetes, and Metabolism, Michigan State University College of Human Medicine, East Lansing, Michigan

JOSEPH L. CALLES Jr, MD
Associate Professor, Department of Psychiatry, College of Human Medicine, Michigan State University, East Lansing; Director, Child and Adolescent Psychiatry, Psychiatry Residency Training Program, Michigan State University/Kalamazoo Center for Medical Studies, Kalamazoo, Michigan

L. LEE CARLISLE, MD
Assistant Professor, Division of Child and Adolescent Psychiatry, Department of Psychiatry and Behavioral Sciences, University of Washington School of Medicine, Seattle, Washington

MADELINE A. CHADEHUMBE, MD
Assistant Professor of Pediatrics, Division of Pediatric Neurology, Michigan State University, Helen DeVos Children's Hospital, Grand Rapids, Michigan

BANTU CHHANGANI, MD
Sleep Medicine, Saint Mary's Neuroscience Program, Saint Mary's Neuroscience Institute, Kalamazoo, Michigan

GLEN R. ELLIOTT, PhD, MD
Chief Psychiatrist and Medical Director, Children's Health Council, Palo Alto, California

CYNTHIA FEUCHT, PharmD, BCPS
Adjunct Professor, Ferris State University School of Pharmacy, Big Rapids; Clinical Pharmacist, Borgess Ambulatory Care, Kalamazoo, Michigan

ROBERT L. FINDLING, MD
Director, Division of Child and Adolescent Psychiatry, University Hospitals Case Medical Center, Cleveland, Ohio

NEVILLE H. GOLDEN, MD
Professor of Pediatrics and Chief, Division of Adolescent Medicine, Stanford University School of Medicine, Palo Alto, California

DONALD E. GREYDANUS, MD
Professor, Department of Pediatrics and Human Development, Michigan State University College of Human Medicine, East Lansing; Pediatrics Program Director, Michigan State University/Kalamazoo Center for Medical Studies, Kalamazoo, Michigan

ILIYAN IVANOV, MD
Assistant Professor of Psychiatry, Department of Psychiatry, Mount Sinai Medical School, New York, New York

MANMOHAN K. KAMBOJ, MD
Associate Professor, Section of Endocrinology, Metabolism and Diabetes, Nationwide Children's Hospital, Columbus, Ohio

GABRIEL KAPLAN, MD
Clinical Associate Professor, Department of Psychiatry, Department of Psychiatry, Hoboken University Medical Center, Hoboken; Department of Psychiatry, University of Medicine and Dentistry of New Jersey, Newark, New Jersey

IAN KODISH, MD, PhD
Acting Assistant Professor, Department of Psychiatry and Behavioral Sciences, University of Washington School of Medicine, Seattle Children's Hospital, Seattle, Washington

JON McCLELLAN, MD
Professor, Division of Child and Adolescent Psychiatry, Department of Psychiatry and Behavioral Sciences, University of Washington School of Medicine, Seattle, Washington

AHSAN NAZEER, MD
Assistant Professor, Child and Adolescent Psychiatry, Department of Psychiatry, College of Human Medicine, Michigan State University, Kalamazoo Center for Medical Studies, Kalamazoo, Michigan

JEFFREY H. NEWCORN, MD
Associate Professor of Psychiatry, Department of Psychiatry, Mount Sinai Medical School, New York, New York

DILIP R. PATEL, MD
Professor, Department of Pediatrics and Human Development, Michigan State University College of Human Medicine, East Lansing; Division of Developmental-Behavioral Pediatrics, Pediatric Residency Program, Kalamazoo Center for Medical Studies, Kalamazoo, Michigan

HELEN D. PRATT, PhD
Licensed Psychologist, Professor, Department of Pediatrics and Human Development, Department of Pediatrics and Human Development, College of Human Medicine, Michigan State University; Director, Behavioral and Developmental Pediatrics, Pediatrics Program, Michigan State University/Kalamazoo Center for Medical Studies, Kalamazoo, Michigan

CAROL ROCKHILL, MD, PhD, MPH
Acting Assistant Professor, Department of Psychiatry and Behavioral Sciences, University of Washington School of Medicine, Seattle, Washington

SHERYL RYAN, MD
Associate Professor, Department of Pediatrics, Yale University School of Medicine, New Haven, Connecticut

SUSAN M. SMIGA, MD
Associate Professor and Director, Pediatric-Psychiatry Collaborative Programs, Department of Psychiatry, Dartmouth Hitchcock Medical Center, Lebanon, New Hampshire

LIBBIE STANSIFER, MD
Post Pediatric Portal Project Fellow, Division of Child and Adolescent Psychiatry, University Hospitals Case Medical Center, Cleveland, Ohio

RUQIYA SHAMA TAREEN, MD
Associate Professor, Department of Psychiatry, Michigan State University College of Human Medicine, East Lansing; Psychiatry Residency Program, Kalamazoo Center for Medical Studies, Kalamazoo, Michigan

TIFFANY THOMAS, MD
Clinical Instructor, Division of Child and Adolescent Psychiatry, University Hospitals Case Medical Center, Cleveland, Ohio

CHRIS VARLEY, MD
Professor, Department of Psychiatry and Behavioral Sciences, University of Washington School of Medicine, Seattle Children's Hospital, Seattle, Washington

Contents

The long-held view that medicine or therapy is an "art" is quickly becoming obsolete. To procure referrals and reimbursement, clinicians are being forced to be accountable (ie, use empirically supported, effective, reproducible, and efficient treatment interventions) by insurance companies, professional credentialing bodies, and their consumers. This article focuses on reviews of treatment interventions by scholars, researchers, clinicians, and study groups who have examined multiple databases of published studies and ongoing treatment protocols. Behavioral and cognitive-behavioral therapies were most often identified as well-established treatments for specific mental and behavioral health disorders in children and adolescents. Psychotherapy alone or in conjunction with pharmacotherapy can be powerful tools in helping youth manage or eliminate negative outcomes of mental and behavioral disorders.

An understanding of the basic principles of pharmacokinetics and pharmacodynamics of drugs is important in appropriate therapeutic use of various drugs. In simple terms, the effects of the body on the drug once it has entered the body has been referred to as *pharmacokinetics,* and it aims to provide a quantitative assessment of the main processes involved in biodisposition of the drug, including absorption, distribution, metabolism, and elimination. *Pharmacodynamics* concerns itself with the effects of the drug on the body and the main processes involved are the action of the drug on specific sites, especially the receptors. In addition, pharmacogenetics and pharmacogenomics evaluates the influence of genetics on drug response. This article reviews basic concepts of pharmacology applicable to psychotherapeutic agents used for the treatment of mental disorders of children and adolescents.

An understanding of synaptic neurotransmission is fundamental to the understanding of various neuropsychiatric symptoms and disorders. It is also essential to the discovery of pharmacologic agents that modulate neurotransmission to alleviate such symptoms and conditions. Various aspects of the process of neurotransmission and the synthesis, release, reuptake, or destruction are all potential events for action of therapeutic drugs. This article reviews the basic aspects of relevant neuroanatomy, neurotransmission, and major neurotransmitter systems.

Research in the past 2 decades showed that attention-deficit/hyperactivity disorder (ADHD) is a frequently occurring psychiatric disorder that causes considerable suffering to patients and their families. This article outlines current pharmacologic ADHD treatment options and focuses on their safety profile and efficacy. In addition, it addresses treatment selection, guidelines for monitoring treatment, and recent controversies in the field.

Eating disorders are serious psychiatric illnesses that often present during adolescence and young adulthood. They are associated with medical as well as psychological disturbances, and pediatricians play an important role in their identification, diagnosis, and management. There has been a paucity of treatment research that specifically focuses on children and adolescents with eating disorders. This article reviews the scientific evidence for the use of psychotropic medication in the treatment of children and adolescents with eating disorders.

The pharmaceutical search to induce weight loss was precipitated by the United States Food and Drug Administration's (FDA) 1959 formal approval of phentermine for short-term weight loss despite limited research supporting its assertions of weight loss. In addition to sympathomimetic amine products like phentermine, other medications considered in this article include herbal products, sibutramine, orlistat, metformin, and rimonabant. The use of pharmacotherapy for morbidly obese adolescents should be part of a comprehensive weight-loss program that recommends diet, exercise, and behavioral modification. Side effects and the possibility of major adverse effects should be remembered when considering use of these products.

Although much debate continues about the prevalence of depressive disorders in prepubertal children, depression clearly is common in adolescents, increasing rapidly throughout the teen years. All physicians who work with young patients must to be able to recognize and treat these disorders. This article provides a brief overview of depressive disorders in children and adolescence, including their clinical presentation, prevalence, etiology, course, and prognosis. Psychopharmacological treatment options are reviewed in detail, including practical information for medication management including patient education, making the decision to treat with medication, selection of specific medications, strategies for nonresponsive patients, and decisions about stopping medication.

> Pediatric bipolar disorder (PBD) is a chronic and disabling illness often leading to serious disruption in the lives of children and adolescents with this condition. Until recently, methodologically stringent data to guide pharmacologic interventions in the youth were scarce. However, clinical trials conducted recently have expanded the existing evidence base, and new data are emerging rapidly. Recent studies have examined the use of lithium, anticonvulsants, and atypical antipsychotics for acute and long-term treatment of PBD. Despite these new advances, further placebo-controlled trials investigating the efficacy and safety of pharmacologic treatment strategies for young people with bipolar disorder are still needed.

> Cognitive-adaptive disabilities (CADs) are not frequently seen in the general pediatric setting. Yet, given the high rates of comorbidity in that population, they commonly demand a lot of time and effort on the part of clinicians. One aspect of comorbidity is the degree to which psychiatric disorders occur in children, adolescents, and young adults with CADs. This article reviews the epidemiology, associated psychopathology, and pharmacologic treatment of selected CADs.

> The past 5 five years have seen major advances in the diagnosis and treatment of schizophrenia in children and adolescents. This article, reviews the clinical and diagnostic characteristics of schizophrenia in youth with an eye toward recent findings. This article also provides a more extensive review and update of the psychopharmacology of early-onset schizophrenia.

> There is a significant dilemma when underlying medical disorders present as psychiatric conditions. It is important to identify the medical condition because treatment and management strategies need to be directed to the presenting symptoms and also to the underlying medical condition for successful treatment of the patient. Some systemic disorders present with psychiatric manifestations more often than others. The pattern of psychiatric disturbance seen may be specific for a particular medical disorder but may also be varied. Many drug formulations and medications also may produce psychiatric presentations. This article considers the management of nonpsychiatric medical conditions presenting with psychiatric manifestations.

> The public health effects of adolescent substance abuse disorders (SUD) reaches further than the immediate intoxicating effects. Medications play a limited role in the treatment of youth beyond addressing short-term symptoms but may improve longer-term outcomes for some patients. Given the potential devastating consequences of SUD, clinicians should become familiar with all available treatment options. This article reviews the pharmacotherapy for adolescent SUD to inform clinicians considering the use of this modality for selected groups of patients.

> Tics in children and adolescents are a common occurrence; however, a small proportion of these disorders require pharmacologic interventions. Several limitations exist with the use of pharmacologic interventions, and hence, a more ideal multidisciplinary approach is recommenced, with emphasis on nonpharmacologic management for improved functioning, adaptation, and comorbidities. Mutual and realistic goals ensure a trustful and successful relationship between the clinician and patient. An individualized plan is recommended with the goal of limiting side effects and managing comorbid conditions as a priority before addressing the tics specifically. This article reviews medications used to treat tic disorders in children and adolescents.

> There is a high prevalence of sleep disorders in children and an apparent increasing need for pharmacologic management. However, because of the paucity of data available with regards to dosing, efficacy, tolerability, and safety profiles of medications as well as a lack of adequate well-designed clinical trials, medications are currently not approved for the pediatric population by the US Food and Drug Administration. There are no pharmacologic guidelines for the specific sleep disorders or the different pediatric age ranges. Additional research is needed for evidence-based pediatric sleep pharmacotherapy. This article reviews pediatric sleep disorders and the pharmacologic therapeutic options.

FORTHCOMING ISSUES

April 2011
Sleep in Children and Adolescents
Judith Owens, MD, MPH
and Jodi A. Mindell, PhD,
Guest Editors

June 2011
Food Allergies in Children
Hemant P. Sharma, MD, MHS,
Robert Wood, MD, and
Max J Coppes, MD, PhD, MBA,
Guest Editors

RECENT ISSUES

December 2010
Pediatric Chest Pain
Guy D. Eslick, PhD, MMedSc(Clin Epi),
MMedStat and Steven M. Selbst, MD,
Guest Editors

October 2010
Birthmarks of Medical Significance
Beth A. Drolet, MD and
Maria C. Garzon, MD,
Guest Editors

August 2010
Spina Bifida: Health and Development Across the Life Course
Mark E. Swanson, MD, MPH and
Adrian Sandler, MD, *Guest Editors*

THE CLINICS ARE NOW AVAILABLE ONLINE!

Access your subscription at:
www.theclinics.com

Preface

Pediatric and Adolescent Psychopharmacology: The Past, the Present, and the Future

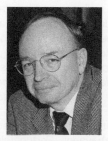 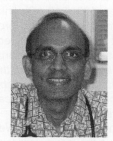 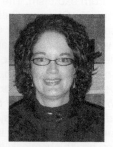

Donald E. Greydanus, MD   Dilip R. Patel, MD   Cynthia Feucht, PharmD, BCPS

Guest Editors

"An analysis of almost any scientific problem leads automatically to a study of its history."

(Mayr)[1]

The quest for ideal mental health chemicals has probably existed for the eons of time since hominoids evolved from other primates over 250,000 years ago and Homo sapiens emerged as the dominant hominoid species over 60,000 years ago.[1] Perhaps the first recorded official request for such a product was the forbidden fruit (erroneously referred to by folklore as an apple) consumed by Adam and Eve in the Fall of Humans in the Genesis 3:6 account.

The first classifier of medicinal herbs is noted by historians as the Chinese emperor Shen-Nung (2737 BC), and there is a classic painting of him holding leaves of *Ephedra* ("machuang").[2]

In additional to the thousands of years of medicinal product collection by the Chinese and Indian civilizations that resulted in extensive plant- and herbal-based pharmacopoeias, historians teach us about the 1550 BC Ebers Paprus of ancient Egypt that was a 110-page scroll containing over 700 formulas and remedies of animal, mineral, and vegetable origins.[3–5] Athletes have tried for thousands of years to "win the gold" from the Ancient Olympics (776 BC–393 AD) to the present by taking mushrooms, opioids (ie, amphetamines, strychnine, cocaine), figs, and other miscellaneous modern chemicals (ie, anabolic steroids, designer steroids), and others.[5] The search for medicines to optimize life has been long and often frustrating. Indeed, listen to

Pediatr Clin N Am 58 (2011) xv–xxiv
doi:10.1016/j.pcl.2010.11.005
0031-3955/11/$ — see front matter © 2011 Elsevier Inc. All rights reserved.

the somewhat skeptical words of the ancient and brilliant Greek philosopher, Aristotle (384–322 BC), who broadened his concern to medicine in general with his opine: "...the physician does not cure man, except in an incidental sense."[6]

Humans have turned to magic, mysticism, mantics, haruspex, and religion for thousands of years in attempts to cure illness—both medical and psychiatric—long before any such distinctions were made. The Gospel writer, Matthew, wrote in the first century about those who were cured from epilepsy (the "sacred" disease of Hippocrates of Cos: 460–377 BC) by Jesus of Nazareth in 28 AD (Matthew 4:24). Epilepsy and mental illness have long been identified with demon possession and the need for cure was not from chemicals but from exorcism. The famous Greek physician to Roman emperors and gladiator champions, Claudius Galen (130–210 AD), linked epilepsy and mental illness to adolescent and young adult masturbation and provided the best medical advice of his time with his concern that has unremittingly echoed down the halls of human history, lamenting about hebetic sexuality and its purported baneful effects:

Watch carefully over this young man, leave him alone neither day nor night; at least sleep in his chamber. When he has contracted this fatal habit (ie, masturbation), the most fatal to which a young man can be subject, he will carry its painful effects to the tomb—his mind and body will always be enervated.[7]

The fall of the Roman Empire issued in the Dark Ages in Western culture that placed this quest for utopian health chemicals in a thousand-year-long abeyance. Fortunately there were some experts that kept the flame of medical knowledge burning, such as Rhazes (Muhammad ibn Zakariya Razi [865–925 AD])—the famous physician of ancient Persia whose book on disorders of children remains a classic in pediatric medical writing. Gradually Western civilization awoke from its saturnine and sycophantic slumber with books dealing with medical problems of children, such as De Mylierum Passionibus by Trotula Platearius of Salerno, Italy (1050 AD) and The Boke of Chyldren by Thomas Phaer (1510–1560) of England in 1544 AD. The importance of the book by Dr Phaer was that it made a distinction between childhood and adulthood, encouraging further study into disorders of children. This encouragement led to a number of various books, including a 1776 textbook that was well-known in its time, and associated children's diseases to the idea that "the nerves of children are very irritable" (in contrast to that of adults) "and much more softened, and also covered with very thin membranes."[8]

The term, "biology," was initiated in the early 19th century and is a hallmark of attempts to discern diseases apart from ancient philosophical theories.[1] In 1869, Dr John Scudder, an Ohioan pathologist, wrote a pediatric textbook that taught "there are sufficient differences in the action of remedies upon the adult and child, to demand a careful study of the subject" (ie, the child).[9] He also wrote that children are capable of "receiving mental impressions and being pleasurably or painfully impressed by them....are more impressionable than the adult."[9] Concerns with drug abuse (ie, morphine and alcohol) were addressed by the most famous Western physician of the 19th and early 20th century, Dr William Osler.[10]

As scholars turned their attention to children, miscellaneous theories on child development were hypothesized in the 19th and 20th centuries including the landmark evolutionary model of Charles Darwin, the organismic model of G. Stanley Hall and Jean Piaget, the psychoanalytic model of Sigmond Freud, the contextualistic model of William James, and the mechanistic model of B.F. Skinner.[11] In 1877 Charles Darwin (1809–1882) published his observations on his first child as a study of behavioral development of humans. Heinrich Hoffman (1809–1894) was a German physician and writer/illustrator who wrote and drew the image of *Fidgety Phillip* (*Zappelphilipp*) that became the model for the classic picture of the 20th century's picture of aprosexia identified as attention deficit hyperactivity disorder (ADHD).[12]

As the 20th century progressed, research looked more carefully at biological and environmental factors in *child* development. The English physician, G. Still, linked children with what was later called ADHD with those having "defects of moral control"—a reflection of the classic tenebrous opinion of adults toward "unruly" minors.[13] However, the seeds of research and thought so carefully constructed by the brilliant scholars of the 19th and early 20th century gradually bore "fruit." This "fruit" did not promise one would become like a heavenly being, but firmly stated that children are not small adults and were important humans worthy of sincere as well as serious study by scholars and clinicians from a variety of disciplines.

Medical problems of children were finally appreciated in 1930 with the formation of the *American Academy of Pediatrics*. In 1937 Charles Bradley published his seminal paper on the benefit of benzedrine (racemic mixture of levoamphetamine and dextro-amphetamine) on 30 children in Providence, Rhode Island with various mental health issues including what would later be called ADHD that was based on the original Greek observation of aprosexia from the Greek words *a*- (un- or non-) and *prosexis* ("heedful-ness").[14] After eons of time, the race to find specific medications to improve *pediatric* mental health was stimulated just as the race toward immunization science was encouraged by the 1796 work of Edward Jenner in England 141 years earlier. Also, in 1937 Molitich and Eccles orchestrated what may be identified as the first placebo-control research study in child psychiatry, demonstrating positive effects of benzedrine on 93 males identified as juvenile delinquents—more work on children with Still's defects of moral control.[15] The field of modern psychopharmacology had begun in earnest and with credible scholars involved that adumbrated what was to come.

Prior to the 20th century, pediatric infections dominated the writings of earlier pediatric textbooks and the success of the fruit of the Jennerian-immunization science that reduced childhood infections and death allowed others to look more closely at mental health issues of children.[8,16–18] This inspired the development of child psychiatry in the 1920s and 1930s as well as behavior pediatrics later in the 20th century.[18] Family therapy was developed as a tool of therapy in the 1950s and psychopharmacology exploded in the latter part of the 20th century.

Chlorpromazine was introduced in 1950 as the first of many future antipsychotic medications to treat psychosis in adults. Also, in the 1950s, there was the introduction of two antidepressant classes, a monoamine-oxidase inhibitor (iproniazid) and a tricyclic antidepressant (imipramine).[19,20] Methylphenidate (MPH) was first Identified in 1959 by the Argentinean Knobel in Kansas, USA as a medication that would improve the behavior of children with "hyperkinesis and organicity," after MPH was first introduced to the market in 1957.[21] Lithium, antidepressants, and benzodiazepines were placed in the general market before 1965 and the use of psychopharmacology was then firmly placed in the available armamentarium by a coterie of adult psychiatrists valiantly struggling with adult mental disorders. Stimulating and recording such progress in the pediatric arena was the American Academy of Child Psychiatry, formed in 1953 and the establishment of *The Journal of the American Academy of Child and Adolescent Psychiatry* in 1962 to record research discoveries in mental health disorders of children and adolescents.[22]

The term "behavioral pediatrics" was first used in the early 1970s at the University of Rochester by Dr Robert Haggerty and colleagues to look at behavioral concerns of children from a pediatrician's perspective, not only from a child psychiatrist's perspective.[18] Behavioral pediatrics has also been defined as: "what the clinician does to diagnose, to treat, and most importantly, to *prevent* mental illness in children and adolescents."[18] Other groups became interested in mental health problems of children and adolescents; for example, the Society for Developmental and Behavioral

Pediatrics was founded in 1982.[23] Historically, the field of neurodevelopmental disabilities has evolved based on a firm foundation of basic and clinical neurosciences and
was founded by Dr Arnold J. Capute (1923–2003) as well as his fellows from the
Kennedy Krieger Institute at Johns Hopkins University.[24] Based on his observations
of youth in a boarding school in the earlier part of the 20th century, Dr J.R. Gallagher,
an internist, established the first adolescent medicine clinic in the early 1950s in
Boston, Massachusetts and also edited the first textbook of adolescent medicine
in 1960.[25] All this interest enthusiastically encouraged collaborative efforts by
a wide variety of professionals interested in significantly improving saturnine statistics
in pediatric mental health while avoiding the conclusion that this effort was a sisyphean
task of unremitting agony and futility.

Despite the seminal and inaugural work of Bradley[14] (1937) and Knobel et al[21]
(1959) formally launching the field of pediatric psychopharmacology, further work on
identifying drugs for *pediatric* mental illness was essentially placed in abeyance until
the 1990s. This state of suspended animation was influenced by a variety of complex
factors, including a belief that psychotherapy was best for children with mental illness
and the emphasis of pharmaceutical companies on developing medications for adults
with psychiatric illnesses. Interest in pediatric mental illness was rekindled in the late
1970s and was stimulated by the development of the selective serotonin reuptake
inhibitor (SSRI), fluoxetine, in the late 1980s.[19] Evidence of the growing science of
pediatric psychopharmacology can be seen in various ways, including the development of the *Journal of Child and Adolescent Psychopharmacology* in 1990 to record
the results of such Herculean efforts.[26]

Research trials, however, have remained limited and often under pharmaceutical
fiscal control in a era where these same companies heavily market their products to
physicians and consumers alike.[27–29] How do we deal with medical and ethical
concerns that arise when it may be difficult to find unbiased, double-blind, randomized
placebo control trials to guide what is best for children and adolescents with mental
illness? One answer to this potential dilemma has been the work of the United States
government agencies, such as that of the US National Institute of Mental Health
(NIMH)'s 1999 Multimodal Treatment study of MPH that validated the benefit of
MPH and behavioral interventions for children with ADHD[30] as well as the NIMH's
TADS (Treating Adolescent Depression Study) that validates the use of SSRIs (fluoxetine) along with cognitive-behavioral therapy.[31]

As we enter the second decade of the 21st century, the question remains, where do
we go from here with use of medications to manage mental illness of children and
adolescents? First of all, we need and will see more neutral research to more critically
identify the precise benefit of medication(s) in specific mental illnesses of pediatric
patients. There has been some research as well as articles in the lay press directly challenging the role of psychopharmacology in mental illness management.[32,33] Thus, there
will be more work looking at the role of medication versus therapy versus using both
forms of treatment.[34,35] Failure of some insurance plans to cover comprehensive
psychotherapy in the United States will encourage the use of medication even if
evidence-based research suggests therapy. Hopefully, such an oxymoronic and rapa-
cious approach can be curtailed and mollified in the future for the sake of our children.

Such concerns have been increased in light of research and worries about potentially severe adverse effects of mental health drugs, such as proposed suicidality
induced by many drugs,[36] addiction potential of stimulants,[37] and sudden death in
pediatric as well as adult patients on stimulants.[38] Thus, we can expect to see more
research in this regard to better determine specific benefit from such drugs, what
specific areas of the central nervous system (CNS) are involved in illnesses, what areas

of the CNS are directly as well as indirectly affected by medications, and what side effects are real versus mere minor opinion.

What are the long-term benefits of medication, such as establishing if stimulants are beneficial beyond their current benefit ceiling of 2 years?[39] More drugs will be approved for use in children and adolescents, although cautious use and careful observation for harm will always be in order in any century.[40] We will also see more clarifying research on the use of mono- versus poly-pharmacy for pediatric mental health management.[41] We can expect to see exciting research in this young decade that will identify new medications that are more specific to treat aggression, depression, ADHD, psychosis, and other mental health conditions.[42–48]

Clinicians and the lay public should expect to see improvement in the establishment of research studies not under the control of companies that profit from their drugs, pay researchers for work on these drugs, and vigorously market their products around the world to improve their profits. Safeguarding the rights of pediatric patients in this regard is critical and must be guarded or supervised by those not profiteering from such research and serving as an amicus curiae for the health of our children.[27,49] These companies are not intrinsically unethical but their conflict of interest must be recognized and morally monitored. The 1994 Dietary Supplement Health and Education Act of the US Congress allowed the production of dietary supplements with less restrictive guidelines and flooded the market with numerous products making great claims but with limited evidence-based underpinnings.[50] One solution is to encourage the continued entry of the government to fund important research, such as the *US NIMH Longitudinal Brain Scan Project* begun in 1989,[51,52] in addition to others already noted.[30,31] In fact, what we can expect and should see is an improved relationship between academicians, industry, and the government in improving the mental health treatment of our children and adolescents with mental health disorders.[53]

The emergence of sleep science as an accepted and valid area will continue to contribute to improvement in mental health understanding and management in this new decade. It has become clear that primary and secondary sleep disorders complicate the lives of Homo sapiens and contributes to their mental instability.[54–58] The effects of the Human Genome Project will be felt in this coming decade and for the rest of this century.[59] Our current myopic views of mental illness will be clarified as the science of psychogenetics and psychogenomics comes of age that will allow more individualized, precise, and improved methods of mental health treatments based on what specific brain parts are involved.[60–66]

Finally, all this new and exciting research potential will be limited unless we improve the global shortage of mental health specialists including the paucity of child and adolescent psychiatrists.[67–72] One assuaging effect in this crisis will be improved training of primary care clinicians (traditionally considered as being abecedarian in knowledge of psychiatry) in the management of pediatric mental health disorders to collaboratively and in an a fortiori conclusion to assist mental health experts in applying neoteric knowledge in pediatric psychopharmacology toward the improvement of their pediatric patients.[73–75]

This issue of *Pediatric Clinics of North America* celebrates the au courant progress in pediatric psychopharmacology after countless millennia of hope, hype, trial, and error. Psychopharmacology is no longer an arcane sesquipedalian term but an evidence-based treatment modality of paramount importance that will only augment as this century continues. The editors of this issue are very grateful to the many goluptious experts who provided us with their time and knowledge in this regard to alert the readers of this journal to the ad-hoc translational research of this field and provide us with an accurate accouterment of cognizance to help in the amaranthine agon against pediatric mental illness. The editors are appreciative of the opportunity to work with superb professionals at Elsevier—Kerry Holland, Peg Ennis, and Carla Holloway. DEG thanks Dilip Patel and Cynthia Feucht for their guidance and patience in developing this panoptic, perspicuous perlustration on pediatric psychopharmacology.

FINIS CORONAT OPUS

"Those having torches will pass them on to others."
(Plato, The Republic)

Donald E. Greydanus, MD
Department of Pediatrics and Human Development
Michigan State University College of Human Medicine
MSU/Kalamazoo Center for Medical Studies
1000 Oakland Drive
Kalamazoo, MI 49009-1284, USA

Dilip R. Patel, MD
Department of Pediatrics and Human Development
Michigan State University College of Human Medicine
MSU/Kalamazoo Center for Medical Studies
1000 Oakland Drive
Kalamazoo, MI 49009-1284, USA

Cynthia Feucht, PharmD, BCPS
Borgess Ambulatory Care, 1701 Gull Road, Kalamazoo, MI 49048, USA

Department of Pharmacy Practice, Ferris State University College of Pharmacy
Big Rapids, MI 49307, USA

E-mail addresses:
Greydanus@kcms.msu.edu (D.E. Greydanus)
Patel@kcms.msu.edu (D.R. Patel)
cynthia.feucht@gmail.com (C. Feucht)

REFERENCES

1. Magner LN. A history of the life sciences. 3rd edition. New York: Marcel Dekker, Inc; 2002. p. 502.
2. Greydanus DE, Patel DR. Sports doping in athletes. Pediatr Clin North Am 2010; 57(3):729–50.
3. Grollman AP. Alternative medicine: the importance of evidence in medicine and medical evidence. Is there wheat among the chaff? Acad Med 2001;76(3):221–3.
4. Porter R. The greatest benefit to mankind: a medical history of humanity. New York: WW Norton & Co; 1998.
5. Scholl R. Der Papyrus Ebers. Die grösste Buchrolle zur Heilkunde Altägyptens (Schriften aus der Universitätsbibliothek 7). Leipzig, Germany: Universitat von Leipzig; 2002.
6. Wheelwright P. Aristotle. New York: The Odyssey Press; 1951. p. 68.
7. Greydanus DE, Geller B. Masturbation: historical perspective. NY State Med 1980;80:1892–6.

8. Von Rosenstein R. The diseases of children and their remedies. London (England): T. Cadell; 1776. p. 31.
9. Scudder NJM. The eclectic practice of diseases of children. Cincinnati: American Publishing Co; 1869. p. 19.
10. Osler W. The principles and practice of medicine: designed for the use of practitioners and students of medicine. New York: D. Appleton and Company; 1892. p. 1079.
11. Pratt HD, Normal psychological development. In: Greydanus DE, Patel DR, Pratt HD, editors. Behaviorial pediatrics. 2nd edition. New York: iUniverse, Inc; 2006. p. 5–36, chapter 1.
12. Greydanus DE, Patel DR, Pratt HD. ADHD across the lifespan. Dis Mon 2007; 53(2):65–132.
13. Still G. The Coulstonian lectures on some abnormal physical conditions in children. Lecture 1. Lancet 1902;1:1008–12.
14. Bradley C. The behavior of children receiving Benzedrine. Am J Psychiatry 1937; 94:577–85.
15. Molitch M, Eccles AK. The effect of Benzedrine sulfate on the intelligence scores of children. Am J Psychiatry 1937;94:577–85.
16. Eberle J. Treatise on the diseases and physical education of children. Philadelphia: Grigg and Elliot; 1837. p. 489.
17. Radbill SX. The first treatise on pediatrics. Am J Dis Child 1971;122:369–76.
18. Haggerty R, Preface In: Greydanus DE, Wolraich M, editors. Behavioral pediatrics. New York: Springer-Verlag; 1992. p. 1–490.
19. López-Muñoz F, Alamo C. Monoaminergic neurotransmission: the history of the discovery of antidepressants from 1950s until today. Curr Pharm Des 2009;15: 1563–86.
20. Delini-Stula A. Discovery of the tricyclic antidepressants. Pharm Unserer Zeit 2008;37:194–7.
21. Knobel M, Wolman M, Mason A. Hyperkinesis and organicity in children. Arch Gen Psychiatry 1959;1(3):310–21.
22. Musto DF. History of child psychiatry. In: Lewis M, editor. Child and adolescent psychiatry. A comprehensive text. 3rd edition. Philadelphia: Lippincott Williams & Wilkins; 2002. p. 1448–9, chapter 133.
23. Friedman SB. Introduction: behavioral pediatrics. Pediatr Clin North Am 1975;22:55.
24. Accardo PJ. The father of developmental pediatrics: Arnold J. Capute, MD, MPH (1923–2003). J Child Neurol 2004;19(12):978-81.
25. Gallagher JR. Medical care of the adolescent. 1st edition. New York: Appleton-Century-Crofts; 1960.
26. Werry JS, Aman MG. Preface to the first edition. Practitioner's guide to psychoactive drugs for children and adolescents. New York: Plenum Medical Book Company; 1999. p. xi.
27. Greydanus DE, Patel DR. The role of pharmaceutical influence in education and research: the clinician's response. Asian J Paediatr Pract 2006;9:35–41.
28. Tan JO, Koeich M. The ethics of psychopharmacological research in legal minors. Child Adolesc Psychiatr Ment Health 2008;2:39–43.
29. Vitiello B, Heiligenstein JH, Riddle MA, et al. The interface between publicly funded and industry-funded research in pediatric psychopharmacology: opportunities for integration and collaboration. Biol Psychiatry 2004;56:3–9.
30. MTA Study Group. A 14-month randomized clinical trial of treatment strategies for attention-deficit/hyperactivity disorder. The MTA Cooperative Group. Multimodal Treatment Study of Children with ADHD. Arch Gen Psychiatry 1999;56:1073–86.

31. March J. Fluoxetine, cognitive-behavioral therapy, and their combination for adolescents with depression: Treatment for Adolescents with Depression Study (TADS) randomized controlled trial. JAMA 2004;292:807–20.
32. Fournier JC, DeRubeis RJ, Hollon SD, et al. Antidepressant drug effect and depression severity. A patient level metaanalysis. JAMA 2010;303:47–53.
33. Begley S. The depressing news about antidepressants. Newsweek February 8, 2010. p. 35–41.
34. Whalen CR, Henker B. Therapies for hyperactive children: comparisons, combinations, and compromises. J Consult Clin Psychol 1991;59:126–37.
35. Pelham W, Fabriano GA. Behavior modification. Child Adolesc Psychiatr Clin North Am 2000;9(3):671–88.
36. Fergusson D, Doucette S, Granley-Glass K, et al. The association between suicide attempts and SSRIs: a systemic review of 677 randomized controlled trials representing 85,470 participants. BMJ 2005;330:396–9.
37. Kadison R. Getting an edge—use of stimulants and antidepressants in college. N Engl J Med 2005;353:1089–91.
38. Nisson SE. ADHD drugs and cardiovascular risks. N Engl J Med 2006;354(14): 1445–8.
39. Hechtman L, Greenfield B. Long-term use of stimulant use in children with ADHD: safety, efficacy, and long-term outcome. Paediatr Drugs 2003;5(12):787–94.
40. MTA Study Group. FDA panel OKs 3 antipsychotic drugs for pediatric use, cautions against overuse. JAMA 2009;302:833–4.
41. Wilens TE. Combined pharmacotherapy in pediatric psychopharmacology: friend or foe? J Child Adolesc Psychopharmacol 2009;19(5):483–4.
42. Spencer TJ. Issues in the management of patients with complex attention-deficit hyperactivity disorder symptoms. CNS Drugs 2009;23(Suppl 1):9–20.
43. Spencer TJ. Toward a new understanding of attention-deficit hyperactivity disorder: advances in research and treatment. CNS Drugs 2009;23(Suppl 1):5–8.
44. Wink LK, Plawecki MH, Erickson CA, et al. Emerging drugs for the treatment of symptoms with autism spectrum disorder. Exp Opin Emerg Drugs 2010;15: 481–94.
45. Bassarath L. Medication strategies in childhood aggression: a review. Can J Psychiatry 2003;48(6):367–73.
46. Hamrin V, Lennaco JD. Psychopharmacology of pediatric bipolar disorder. Exp Rev Neurother 2010;10(7):1053–88.
47. Nevels RM, Dehon EE, Alexander K, et al. Psychopharmacology of aggression in children and adolescents with primary neuropsychiatric disorders: a review of current and potentially promising treatment options. Exp Clin Psychopharmacol 2010;18(2):184–201.
48. Steiner H, Karnik NS. Integrated treatment of aggression in the context of ADHD in children refractory to stimulant monotherapy: a window into the future of child psychopharmacology. Am J Psychiatry 2009;166(12):1315–7.
49. Kölch M, Ludolph AG, Plener PL, et al. Safeguarding children's rights in psycho-pharmacological research: ethical and legal issues. Curr Pharm Des 2010; 16(22):2398–406.
50. Greydanus DE, Feucht C. Performance-enhancing drugs and supplements. In: Pediatric practice: sports medicine. Patel DR, Greydanus DE, Baker RJ, editors. New York: McGraw-Hill Medical; 2009. p. 63–77, chapter 7.
51. Giedd JN. The teen brain: insights from neuroimaging. J Adolesc Health 2008; 42(4):335–43.

52. Waber DP. The NIH MRI study of normal brain development: performance of a population-based sample of healthy children aged 6 to 18 years on a neuropsychological battery. J Int Neuropsycholog Soc 2007;13:1–18.

53. DeVeaugh-Geiss J, March J, Shapiro M, et al. Child and adolescent psychopharmacology in the new millennium: a workshop for academia, industry, and government. J Am Acad Child Adolesc Psychiatry 2006;45: 261–70.

54. Schuen JN. Sleep disorders in the adolescent. In: Greydanus DE, Patel DR, Pratt HD, editors. Essential adolescent medicine. New York: McGraw-Hill Medical Publishing Div; 2006. p. 281–97, chapter 14.

55. Wolfson AR. Adolescents and emerging adults' sleep patterns: new developments. J Adolesc Health 2010;46:97–9.

56. McCrae CS, Taylor DJ, Smith MT, et al. The future of behavioral sleep medicine. Behav Sleep Med 2010;8(2):74–89.

57. Baldwin CM, Ervin AM, Mays MZ, et al. Sleep disturbances, quality of life, and ethnicity: the Sleep Heart Health Study. J Clin Sleep Med 2010;6(2):176–83.

58. Glickman G. Circadian rhythms and sleep in children with autism. Neurosci Biobehav Rev 2010;34(5):755–68.

59. Toriello J. The Human Genome Project. New York: Rosen Publishing Co; 2003. p. 64.

60. Dick DM, Riley B, Kendler MS. Nature and nurture in neuropsychiatric genetics: where do we stand? Dialogues Clin Neurosci 2010;12(4):7–23.

61. Duan J, Sanders AR, Gejman PV. Genome-wide approaches to schizophrenia. Brain Res Bull 2010;83:93–102.

62. Gunter TD, Vaughn MG, Philibert RA. Behavioral genetics in antisocial spectrum disorders and psychopathology: a review of the recent literature. Behav Sci Law 2010;28(2):148–73.

63. Purper-Ouakil D, Lepagnol-Bestel AM, Grosbellet E, et al. Neurobiology of attention deficit hyperactivity disorder. Med Sci (Paris) 2010;26:487–96.

64. Kendler KS. Genetic and environmental pathways to suicidal behavior: reflections of a genetic epidemiologist. Eur Psychiatry 2010;25(5):300–3.

65. Casey BJ, Soliman F, Bath KG, et al. Imaging genetics and development: challenges and promises. Hum Brain Mapp 2010;31(6):838–51.

66. Nestler EJ. Psychogenomics: opportunities to understand addiction. J Neuro Sci 2001;21:8324–7.

67. Kriechman A, Salvador M, Adelsheim S. Expanding the vision: the strengths-based, community-oriented child and adolescent psychiatrist working in schools. Child Adolesc Psychiatr Clin North Am 2010;19(1):149–62.

68. Staller JA. Service delivery in child psychiatry: provider shortage isn't the only problem. Clin Child Psychol Psychiatry 2008;13(1):171–8.

69. Kim W. Recruitment. Child Adolesc Psychiatr Clin North Am 2007;16(1):45–54.

70. Thomas CR. Holzer CE 3rd. The continuing shortage of child and adolescent psychiatrists. J Am Acad Child Adolesc Psychiatry 2006;45(9):1023–31.

71. Kim WJ. American Academy of Child and Adolescent Psychiatry Task Force on Workforce Needs. Child and adolescent psychiatry workforce: a critical shortage and national challenge. Acad Psychiatry 2003;27(4):277–82.

72. Berkovitz IH, Sinclair E. Training programs in school consultation. Child Adolesc Psychiatr Clin North Am 2001;10(1):83–92.

73. Paula CS, Nakamura E, Wissow L, et al. Primary care and children's mental health in Brazil. Acad Pediatr 2009;9(4):249–55.

74. Reeves G, Anthony B. Multimodal treatments versus pharmacotherapy alone in children with psychiatric disorders: implications of access, effectiveness, and contextual treatment. Paediatr Drugs 2009;11(3):165–9.
75. Sarvet BD, Wegner L. Developing effective child psychiatry collaboration with primary care: leadership and management strategies. Child Adolesc Psychiatr Clin North Am 2010;19(1):139–48.

Point-Counter-Point: Psychotherapy in the Age of Pharmacology

Helen D. Pratt, PhD[a,b],*

KEYWORDS

- Psychotherapy • Pharmacotherapy
- Evidenced-based and empirically supported treatments
- Children and adolescents

The long-held view that medicine or therapy is an "art" is quickly becoming obsolete. To procure referrals and reimbursement, clinicians are being forced to be accountable (ie, use empirically supported, effective, reproducible, and efficient treatment interventions) by insurance companies, professional credentialing bodies, and their consumers.[1–5] This article focuses on reviews of treatment interventions by scholars, researchers, clinicians, and study groups who have examined multiple databases of published studies, and ongoing treatment protocols. Evidence-based and empirically supported treatments (ESTs) for children and adolescents for treatment of mental and behavioral disorders are reviewed.

A LITERATURE REVIEW

Significant controversy continues to exist in the medical and psychological fields surrounding which therapies become designated as evidence based or empiric. Problems in methodology, subject selection, and measures plague most published studies.[6] Review articles were drawn from 9 major search engines: 4 where peer-reviewed articles on psychopharmacology versus psychotherapy with children and adolescents were the search criteria (First Search, Psych abstracts, Medline, EBSCO-host) and 5 research databases where reviewers had specified specific inclusion criteria, the topic, exclusion criteria, and identified treatment interventions. These databases included (1) National Registry of Evidence-based Programs and Practices (NREPP),[7] (2) The Office of Behavioral and Social Sciences Research (OBSSR),[8]

[a] Department of Pediatrics and Human Development, Michigan State University, College of Human Medicine, East Lansing, MI 48824-1317, USA
[b] Behavioral and Developmental Pediatrics, Pediatrics Program, Michigan State University/Kalamazoo Center for Medical Studies, 1000 Oakland Drive, Kalamazoo, MI 49008, USA
* Department of Pediatrics and Human Development, Michigan State University, College of Human Medicine, East Lansing, MI 48824-1317.
E-mail address: pratt@kcms.msu.edu

Pediatr Clin N Am 58 (2011) 1–9
doi:10.1016/j.pcl.2010.10.012   **pediatric.theclinics.com**

(3) Evidence-based Mental Health Treatment for Children and Adolescents,[8] (4) National Association of Cognitive-Behavioral Therapists (NACBT),[9] and (5) Cochrane Database of Systematic Reviews.[6]

Four of the 5 databases defined and described criteria for selection of articles and reviews from primarily behavioral and cognitive behavioral resources and were procured from a wide variety of search engines (**Box 1**).[6–10] Criteria for Cochrane Database of Systematic Reviews matched the 4 others but included articles and reviews from a variety of disciplines (eg, psychology, psychiatry, nursing, ambulatory medicine). Keywords used were psychopharmacology versus psychotherapy, mental health + psychotherapy, and psychotherapy + treatment interventions for children

---

Box 1
Major databases used for this review

Applied Social Sciences Index and Abstracts (ASSIA)

British Nursing Index (1994 to 2006)

Campbell Library (including SPECTR and CENTRAL)

Computer Retrieval of Information on Scientific Projects (CRISP)

Cumulative Index to Nursing and Allied Health Literature (CINAHL)

Cochrane Depression, Anxiety and Neurosis Trial Register

Cochrane Central Register of Controlled Trials

Cochrane Depression, Anxiety and Neurosis Group Register

Dissertation-Abstracts International

EBSCOhost

Education Resources Information Center (ERIC)

EMBASE is a biomedical database

OCLC First Search

Latin American and Caribbean Health Sciences Literature (LILACS)

MEDLINE

MetaRegister of Controlled Trials Ongoing and unpublished trials

National Research Register (NRR)

Pharmaceutical companies Ongoing and unpublished trials

PsycINFO

RCN database

System for Information on Gray Literature in Europe Archive (SIGLE)

Study Reference Lists

Sociofile Sociologic Abstracts

Sociologic Abstracts

Sportdiscus part of Sports Research Intelligence Supportive

Web of Science

World Health Organization (WHO) International Clinical Trials Registry Platform (ICTRP)

Note: most of these databases are fee for service.

and adolescents. Only empiric studies were included and details for the methodology are included on specific Web sites. These databases include a range of reviews and a variety of studies from several disciplines.

This search yielded 130 reviews; 22 reviews focused on children or adolescents and also reviews of treatment interventions for mental health disorders.[11-23] One review looked at pharmacologic versus psychological treatments for specific diseases and concluded that there were no significant differences between the two types of intervention, although both were effective. The Cochrane reviews also supported the findings from reviews conduced as part of the Evidence-Based Mental Health Treatment for Children and Adolescents group,[24-41] Evidence-based Therapy site, and the National Registry of Evidence-based Programs and Practices (NREPP) site.

PHARMACOTHERAPY

Empiric evidence supports that a combination of pharmacotherapy and psychotherapy is more beneficial to children and adolescents (attention deficit hyperactivity disorder [ADHD], body dysmorphic disorder, depression, oppositional defiant disorder, and substance abuse).[1-3,5,16] The Multimodal Treatment Study of Children with Attention Deficit and Hyperactivity Disorder study comparing pharmacology and psychotherapy in the treatment of children diagnosed with ADHD is the exception; however, these results are highly controversial and contested by several research psychologists.[2] For discussion of specific drugs effective in the treatment of mental health disorders outside the scope of practice and training of the current author, readers are referred to an excellent text written for clinicians and edited by Greydaus and colleagues[42] entitled *Pediatric and Adolescent Psychopharmacology: A Practical Manual for Pediatricians*.

PSYCHOTHERAPY

Psychotherapy can be a very effective tool for management of mental health disorders with children and adolescents, especially for parents and patients who may object to the use of pharmacotherapy. Some parents may not want their children medicated for a number of reasons. Some children and adolescents do not physiologically tolerate medications used to treat mental and behavioral health disorders. Additional obstacles to prescribing medication are the following: (1) some children reach the maximum dosage of a specific medication and can no longer be given higher dosages; (2) some youth are on multiple medications and are at the point where adding more medications or increasing dosages causes serious neurologic, gastrointestinal, or emotional side effects; and (3) many behavioral problems are not resolved with medication when there is an emotional component or environmental cause for the child's behavioral responses (eg, family conflict). **Table 1** contains a list of evidence- and empirically supported treatments.[24-41] Cognitive behavior therapy was the most researched form of psychotherapy and provided the most evidence to support its effectiveness in the treatment of depression, anxiety, disruptive behavior problems, posttraumatic stress disorder (PTSD), and substance abuse in adolescents.

Patient referrals for psychotherapy may result in the patient being denied access because of several issues that make access to psychotherapy difficult:

- Even with current changes in reimbursement rules, many insurance companies do not honor the concept of parity between clinicians who provide mental health and those who provide medical services. Those panels usually do not reimburse for services delivered based on diagnoses of behavioral disorders of childhood

Table 1
Evidence-based mental health treatment for children and adolescents

	Well-Established	Probably Efficacious
Anxiety, general symptoms		
School refusal behavior	None	I CBT
Child and adolescent OCD	None	I CBT individual CBT, plus sertraline (Zoloft)
Child and adolescent PTSD	CBT trauma focused CBT	CBT
Social phobia	None	CBT
Specific phobia	None	None
Children		CBT
Adolescents	IPT	Behavior therapy
	Individual IPT	
Child and adolescent ADHD	Behavior therapy	N/A
Disruptive behavior problems		
Oppositional defiant disorder	Behavior therapy	CBT
Conduct disorder		Behavior therapy
		Multisystemic therapy
Depression		
Children	CBT	CBT
Adolescents	CBT	CBT
	IPT	IPT

	CBT Group CBT Family therapy	Family therapy Multisystemic therapy
Adolescent Substance abuse		
Anorexia nervosa		
Adolescent anorexia nervosa	Family therapy	N/A
Bulimia nervosa		
Adolescent bulimia nervosa	N/A	N/A
Bipolar disorder		
Child and adolescent BPD	N/A	Family therapy N/A
Autism		
Early autism	Behavior therapy	N/A

Abbreviations: ADHD, attention deficit hyperactivity disorder; BPD, bipolar disorder; CBT, cognitive behavior therapy; IPT, interpersonal psychotherapy; N/A, not applicable; OCD, obsessive compulsive disorder; PTSD, posttraumatic stress disorder.

Adapted from the Web site of the Association for Behavioral and Cognitive Therapies and the Society of Clinical Child and Adolescent Psychology Evidence-based Mental Health Treatment for Children and Adolescents. Available at: http://www.abct.org/sccap/?m=sPro&fa=pro_ESToptions#sec2. Updated July 30, 2010. Accessed September 4, 2010.

Reprinted from Greydaus DE, Calles Jr JL, Patel DR, editors. Pediatric and adolescent psychopharmacology: a practical manual for pediatricians. Cambridge (NY): Cambridge Medical; 2008. p. 12–4; with permission.

and cap reimbursement for those mental health services they do provide. If services are covered, the reimbursements are at a lower rate than for medical services. These factors make the cost of mental/behavioral health services more burdensome for parents who are responsible for payment.

- Clinicians trained or credentialed in the treatment of mental/behavioral disorders with infants, children, and adolescents are not always available to provide care. Even fewer of these experts are trained to specifically treat youth with severe metal and behavioral disorders (ie, schizophrenia, or a combination of mental disorders and developmental disabilities, neurologic disorders, or severe mental disorders).
- Managed care panels limit the numbers of mental health clinicians they will add to their provider panels, thereby limiting their access to reimbursement from those panels for services provided.
- Parents and youth who are in psychological distress often want immediate relief but this is not generally possible whether the treatment is pharmacotherapy or psychotherapy. Both are time-consuming processes with medicines often advertised as faster acting. Pharmacotherapy requires supervision and sometimes assertiveness by parents to administer the prescribed medication to their child or adolescent. However, parents may falsely believe that they do not have to change to "fix" their child/adolescent because the "medicine" will "fix" the child's/adolescent's problem. Psychotherapy often requires daily and/or weekly involvement by the whole family (especially parents) who must devote time, energy, and effort to implementing treatment intervention; youth must be transported to the treating clinician and the process can be disruptive to the family routine. If a patient receives psychosocial treatment, his or her parents are also expected to change their behaviors to support their child's treatments gains.
- Referrals: Physicians must have knowledge of other clinicians and their treatment modalities to select appropriate referral resources. They must also maintain collegial relationships with those clinicians to ensure that their patients are receiving care and benefiting from that care. Although parents, teachers, and some adolescents will demand pharmacologic treatment, primary care physicians should consider the use of psychological and psychosocial treatments as a first line of treatment, or in combination with prescribing medicines.

Psychosocial treatments for emotional, behavioral, and mental disorders can be very effective and sufficient in resolving problems. However, in the case of severe or reoccurring emotional, behavioral, and mental disorders, a combination of pharmacotherapy and psychotherapy increases the positive effects of treatment.

SUMMARY

Behavioral and cognitive-behavioral therapies were most often identified as well-established treatments for specific mental and behavioral health disorders in children and adolescents. Psychotherapy alone or in conjunction with pharmacotherapy can be a powerful tool in helping youth manage or eliminate negative outcomes of mental and behavioral disorders. Youth should receive a comprehensive medical evaluation before being referred for psychosocial treatment. When referring patients for psychotherapy, it is important to maintain contact with the treating therapist and to remember to tell patients and their parents that the process for accessing treatment, evaluation, and the treatment process are often lengthy.

REFERENCES

1. Sava FA, Brian T, Yates BT, et al. Cost-effectiveness and cost-utility of cognitive therapy, rational emotive behavioral therapy, and Fluoxetine (Prozac) in treating depression: a randomized clinical trial. J Clin Psychol 2009;65(1):36–52.
2. Henggeler SW, Halliday-Boykins CA, Cunningham PB, et al. Juvenile drug court: enhancing outcomes by integrating evidence-based treatments. J Consult Clin Psychol 2006;74(1):42–54.
3. Hinshaw SP, Jensen PS, Kraemer HC, et al. ADHD comorbidity findings from the MTA study: comparing comorbid subgroups. J Am Acad Child Adolesc Psychiatry 2001;40:147–58.
4. Marsh EJ, Barkley RA. Treatment of childhood disorders. 3rd edition. New York (NY): Guilford; 2006. p. 314–5.
5. Clarke G, Debar L, Lynch F, et al. A randomized effectiveness trial of brief cognitive-behavioral therapy for depressed adolescents receiving antidepressant medication. J Am Acad Child Adolesc Psychiatry 2005;44(9):888–98.
6. Cochrane Database of Systematic Reviews. Available at: http://www.thecochranelibrary.com/. Accessed September 4, 2010.
7. SAMHSA's National Registry of Evidence-based Programs and Practices (NREPP). Substance Abuse and Mental Health Services Administration (SAMHSA). Available at: http://www.nrepp.samhsa.gov/. Accessed September 4, 2010.
8. The Office of Behavioral and Social Sciences Research (OBSSR). Available at: http://obssr.od.nih.gov/index.aspx. Accessed September 4, 2010.
9. National Association of Cognitive-Behavioral Therapists NACBT. Available at: http://nacbt.org/evidenced-based-therapy.htm. Accessed September 4, 2010.
10. The Association for Behavioral and Cognitive Therapies and the Society of Clinical Child and Adolescent Psychology. Evidence-based Mental Health Treatment for Children and Adolescents. Available at: http://www.abct.org/sccap/?m=sPro&fa=pro_ESToptions#sec2. Accessed September 4, 2010.
11. Bjornstad GJ, Ramchandani P, Montgomery P, et al. Child-focused cognitive behavioural therapy for children who have been physically abused. Cochrane Database Syst Rev 2009;2:CD007838.
12. Barlow J, Parsons J. Group-based parent-training programmes for improving emotional and behavioural adjustment in 0-3 year old children. Cochrane Database Syst Rev 2003;2:CD003680.
13. Barlow J, Johnston I, Kendrick D, et al. Individual and group-based parenting programmes for the treatment of physical child abuse and neglect. Cochrane Database Syst Rev 2006;3:CD005463.
14. Ekeland E, Jamtvedt G, Heian F, et al. Exercise for oppositional defiant disorder and conduct disorder in children and adolescents. Cochrane Database Syst Rev 2006;1:CD005651.
15. Gold C, Wigram T, Elefant C. Music therapy for autistic spectrum disorder. Cochrane Database Syst Rev 2006;2:CD004381.
16. Ipser JC, Sander C, Stein DJ. Pharmacotherapy and psychotherapy for body dysmorphic disorder. Cochrane Database Syst Rev 2009;1:CD005332.
17. James A, Soler A, Weatherall R. Cognitive behavioural therapy for anxiety disorders in children and adolescents. Cochrane Database Syst Rev 2005;4:CD004690.
18. Larun L, Nordheim LV, Ekeland E, et al. Exercise in prevention and treatment of anxiety and depression among children and young people. Cochrane Database Syst Rev 2006;3:CD004691.

19. Littell JH, Campbell M, Green S, et al. Multisystemic therapy for social, emotional, and behavioral problems in youth aged 10–17. Cochrane Database Syst Rev 2005;4:CD004797.
20. Littell JH, Winsvold A, Bjørndal A, et al. Functional family therapy for families of youth (age 11–18) with behaviour problems. Cochrane Database Syst Rev 2007;2:CD006561.
21. Macdonald G, Higgins JPT, Ramchandani P. Cognitive-behavioural interventions for children who have been sexually abused. Cochrane Database Syst Rev 2006; 4:CD001930.
22. Montgomery P, Bjornstad GJ, Dennis JA. Media-based behavioural treatments for behavioural problems in children. Cochrane Database Syst Rev 2006;1: CD002206.
23. O'Kearney RT, Anstey K, von Sanden C. Behavioural and cognitive behavioural therapy for obsessive compulsive disorder in children and adolescents. Cochrane Database Syst Rev 2006;4:CD004856.
24. Reeves G, Anthony B. Multimodal treatments versus pharmacotherapy alone in children with psychiatric disorders: implications of access, effectiveness, and contextual treatment. Paediatr Drugs 2009;11(3):165–9.
25. David-Ferdon C, Kaslow NJ. Evidence-based psychosocial treatments for child and adolescent depression. J Clin Child Adolesc Psychol 2008;37(1):62–104.
26. Lewinsohn PM, Clarke GN. Psychosocial treatments for adolescent depression. Clin Psychol Rev 1999;19(3):329–42.
27. Michael KD, Crowley SL. How effective are treatments for child and adolescent depression? A meta-analytic review. Clin Psychol Rev 2002;22(2):247–69.
28. Reinecke MA, Ryan NE, DuBois DL. Cognitive-behavioral therapy of depression and depressive symptoms during adolescence: a review and meta-analysis. J Am Acad Child Adolesc Psychiatry 1998;37(1):26–34.
29. Barrett PM, Farrell L, Pina AA, et al. Evidence-based psychosocial treatments for child and adolescent obsessive-compulsive disorder. J Clin Child Adolesc Psychol 2008;37(1):131–55.
30. Eyberg SM, Nelson MM, Boggs SR. Evidence-based psychosocial treatments for children and adolescents with disruptive behavior. J Clin Child Adolesc Psychol 2008;37:215–37.
31. Fristad MA, Verducci JS, Walters K, et al. Impact of multifamily psychoeducational psychotherapy in treating children aged 8 to 12 years with mood disorders. Arch Gen Psychiatry 2009;66(9):1013–21.
32. Goldstein TR, Axelson DA, Birmaher B, et al. Dialectical behavior therapy for adolescents with bipolar disorder: a 1-year open trial. J Am Acad Child Adolesc Psychiatry 2007;46(7):820–30.
33. Keel PK, Haedt A. Evidence-based psychosocial treatments for eating problems and eating disorders. J Clin Child Adolesc Psychol 2008;37:39–61.
34. Miklowitz DJ, Axelson DA, Birmaher B, et al. Family-focused treatment for adolescents with bipolar disorder: results of a 2-year randomized trial. Arch Gen Psychiatry 2008;65(9):1053–61.
35. Pelham WE, Fabiano GA. Evidence-based psychosocial treatments for attention-deficit/hyperactivity disorder. J Clin Child Adolesc Psychol 2008;37:184–214.
36. Rogers SJ, Vismara LA. Evidence-based comprehensive treatments for early autism. J Clin Child Adolesc Psychol 2008;37:8–38.
37. Silverman WK, Pina AA, Viswesvaran C. Evidence-based psychosocial treatments for phobic and anxiety disorders in children and adolescents: a review and meta-analyses. J Clin Child Adolesc Psychol 2008;37:105–30.

38. Silverman WK, Ortiz CD, Viswesvaran C, et al. Evidence-based psychosocial treatments for children and adolescents exposed to traumatic events: a review and meta-analysis. J Clin Child Adolesc Psychol 2008;37:156–83.
39. Waldron HB, Turner CW. Evidence-based psychosocial treatments for adolescent substance abuse. J Clin Child Adolesc Psychol 2008;37:238–61.
40. West AE, Jacobs RH, Westerholm R, et al. Child and family-focused cognitive behavioral therapy for pediatric bipolar disorder: pilot study of group treatment format. J Am Acad Child Adolesc Psychiatry 2009;18(3):239–46.
41. Young ME, Fristad MA. Evidence-based treatments for bipolar disorder in children and adolescents. J Contemp Psychother 2007;37:157–64.
42. Greydaus DE, Calles Jr JL, Patel DR, editors. Pediatric and adolescent psychopharmacology: a practical manual for pediatricians. Cambridge (NY): Cambridge Medical; 2008. p. 301.

Principles of Pharmacology

Cynthia Feucht, PharmD, BCPS[a,b,]*, Dilip R. Patel, MD, FSAM[c]

KEYWORDS

- Pharmacokinetics • Phamacodynamics • Pharmacogenomics
- Pharmacogenetics

An understanding of basic concepts is important when determining & evaluating drug dosing and providing individualized therapy. Knowledge of pharmacokinetics & pharmacodynamics as well pharmacogenetics & pharmacogenomics provides a solid foundation to maximize drug therapy within the pediatric population. These concepts will be discussed in further detail below.

PHARMACOKINETICS
Absorption

Drug can be administered via various routes and the specific route chosen largely depends on the urgency to achieve the desired effect in a given clinical circumstance. In our review of pediatric psychopharmacology, we are mainly concerned with the oral route. Once ingested, the drug is absorbed from the gastrointestinal tract. The extent of drug absorption is influenced by many factors (**Table 1**). Orally ingested drugs will undergo the first pass effect before reaching the circulation. The extent to which a drug is available at its site of action is referred to as the *bioavailability* of the drug.[1]

Controlled-release preparations have been available for several psychotropic drugs, especially the stimulants. The basis for such a preparation is to control the rate of dissolution of the solid form of the drug in the gastrointestinal tract. The advantages of such preparations include a steady therapeutic level of the drug owing to the elimination of peaks and troughs in drug concentrations and reduced frequency of administration (typically once daily). The interindividual variability of serum concentrations achieved is greater with controlled release preparations compared with immediate release forms; also failure of the dosage form may result in the release of the entire dose with consequent undesirable effects (dose dumping).[2] Generally, controlled release forms are more appropriate for drugs with short half-lives. Another

[a] Borgess Ambulatory Care, 1701 Gull Road, Kalamazoo, MI 49048, USA
[b] Department of Pharmacy Practice, Ferris State University College of Pharmacy, Big Rapids, MI 49307, USA
[c] Department of Pediatrics and Human Development, Michigan State University College of Human Medicine, MSU/Kalamazoo Center for Medical Studies, 1000 Oakland Drive, Kalamazoo, MI 49009-1284, USA
* Corresponding author. Borgess Ambulatory Care, 1701 Gull Road, Kalamazoo, MI 49048.
E-mail address: cynthia.feucht@gmail.com

Pediatr Clin N Am 58 (2011) 11–19
doi:10.1016/j.pcl.2010.10.005

Table 1 Factors that modulate gastrointestinal absorption of drugs	
Drug characteristics	Dosage form Local concentration of drug Polarity Water/lipid solubility Degree of ionization pKa
Intestinal factors	Surface area for absorption Local blood flow Motility Transit time Presence of food Presence of other agents
Gastric factors	Rate of dissolution Gastric pH Gastric enzyme activity

Data from Buxton I. Pharmacokinetics and pharmacodynamics: the dynamics of drug absorption, distribution, action, and elimination: introduction. In: Brunton K, Lazo J, Parker, editors. Goodman & Gilman's The Pharmacological Basis of Therapeutics. 11th edition. New York: McGraw-Hill; 2006. p. 1–39.

route that is developed for some psychopharmacologic agents is the transdermal route using a patch (eg, nicotine, methylphenidate, clonidine). The skin acts as lipid membrane and drug absorption depends on the surface area exposed to drug, duration of exposure, and its lipid solubility.[2]

For the drug to exert its effect, it has to reach a specific site of action and to do that the drug first needs to be transported across various cell membranes (**Table 2**). The molecular size and shape of the drug, degree of ionization, solubility at site of absorption, and protein binding are some of the factors that influence the drug's ability to cross cellular membranes and reach the target sites of action.[2] Crushing of the solid form and mixing it with food or liquids to make it more appropriate and palatable for children may also influence the absorption. Variation in transit time is of particular relevance for sustained release preparations.

Distribution

Once absorbed, the drug reaches the blood stream and is distributed to interstitial and intracellular fluids. In the blood, many psychopharmacologic agents circulate bound to

Table 2 Main mechanisms of cellular membrane transport	
Passive transport	The drug simply diffuses along a concentration gradient because of its lipid solubility properties
Active transport	The drug is transported by an energy-dependent carrier (ie, sodium-potassium ATPase mechanism)
Facilitated diffusion	Drug is transported by a non–energy-dependent carrier and in the direction of the concentration gradient

From Buxton I. Pharmacokinetics and pharmacodynamics: the dynamics of drug absorption, distribution, action, and elimination: introduction. In: Brunton K, Lazo J, Parker, editors. Goodman & Gilman's The Pharmacological Basis of Therapeutics. 11th edition. New York: McGraw-Hill; 2006. p. 1–39.

plasma protein (mainly albumin, alpha-1-glycoprotein, and lipoproteins). The extent of plasma protein binding is influenced by the concentration of drug in the blood, its affinity to the binding sites, and number of available binding sites.[2,3] Extensive protein binding has the potential to lead to decreased glomerular filtration but not tubular secretion or metabolism.[2] Such plasma protein binding is nonselective and another agent can potentially compete for the same binding sites and displace each other, changing the concentration of the unbound drug in the blood.[2,3] The unbound drug is the only one available for its action. A change in the concentration of the unbound drug could lead to an increase or decrease in the effect of that drug. This is more likely to be significant for drugs that have a narrow therapeutic window. Some drugs may also be stored in tissues, for example, the storage and accumulation of lipid soluble drugs in the adipose tissue.[3]

Unlike the distribution of the drug in various interstitial and intracellular fluids, the distribution of a drug into the central nervous system requires it to first cross the blood brain barrier. In the central nervous system, the capillary endothelial cells form continuous tight junctions and along with the pericapillary glial cells constitute the blood-brain barrier.[2] Thus, to reach the central nervous system, the drug must traverse across the endothelial cells and perivascular cell membranes.[2] Similarly at the choroid plexus, epithelial cells form tight junctions.[2] Therefore, lipid solubility or the lipophilic property of the drug is an important factor that facilitates its transport across the blood brain barrier.[2]

The *apparent volume of distribution* of a drug is defined as that volume of body fluid required to contain the entire amount of the drug in the body at the same measured concentration in the blood or the plasma.[2,4] In other words, it correlates the total amount of drug in the body to its concentration in the blood or plasma. The volume of drug distribution thus is a measure of its amount present in the extravascular tissues.

Volume of distribution value can be useful in determining the loading dose or dose needed to achieve the desired serum concentration of the drug (Loading dose = desired serum concentration of the drug [mg/L] × volume of distribution [L/kg] × patient's weight [kg]).[3,5] The volume of distribution of a given drug can vary significantly among children, adolescents, and adults, and between genders, because of differences in body composition.[2,5] Other factors that influence such variability include age-related differences in protein-binding capacity, cellular membrane permeability, hemodynamic factors, and concurrent disease states.[2,5]

Metabolism

Metabolism of a drug or its *biotransformation* generally converts it into a more water-soluble polar compound easy to excrete by the kidneys.[6] The drug is converted into its inactive or active metabolites. Although liver is the primary site for metabolism of drugs, biotransformation can also occur to a lesser extent at other sites including the skin, lungs, intestine, and kidneys.[7] Once ingested, some of the drug may be metabolized in the intestinal epithelium or the liver into its inactive metabolites, thereby reducing the amount of drug that reaches the circulation (*the first pass effect*).[5] *Bioavailability* of the drug refers to the drug that is available at its site of action and the fraction of the administered dose that is actually absorbed without undergoing the first pass effect.[5]

In the liver, various enzyme systems metabolize drugs by 2 major pathways. *Phase I biotransformation reactions* typically involve hydrolysis, oxidation, reduction, and hydroxylation by enzyme systems on the endoplasmic reticulum, whereas *phase II reactions* involve conjugation with glucuronic acid (or glutathione, sulfate, or acetate) by enzyme systems in the cytoplasm.[6,7] The cytochrome P450 (CYP450) enzymes, which are involved in Phase I oxidative reactions, play an important role in the biotransformation of drugs with wide-ranging therapeutic and drug interaction implications.[7] The genetic variability in CYP450 enzymes can account for clinically significant interindividual variability in drug effects.[4] Other factors affecting biotransformation include concurrent disease states, age, and the presence of other drugs.[2] These factors have the potential to increase the effect of a drug, decrease its efficacy, or increase its toxicity. Specific updated sources (http://www.medicine.iupui.edu/flockhart/; http://www.genetest.com/human_p450_database/index.html.p450+; www.mhc.com/Cytochromes/index.html) should be consulted to check for the possibility of such effects and drug-drug interactions related to CYP450 system. Manufacturer's product information should also be reviewed to check for drug-drug interactions (http://www.epocrates.com and http://www.pdr.net).

When there is saturation of the protein-binding sites, the capacity of the liver to further metabolize the drug or the capacity of the kidneys to excrete the drug follows the principles of *nonlinear pharmacokinetics*.[4] Overall, children metabolize drugs that use hepatic pathways more efficiently and therefore need a higher dose and more frequent daily dosing.

Excretion

Polar (hydrophilic) compounds are excreted more efficiently by the kidneys. Some drugs may be excreted unchanged, whereas others, particularly the lipid-soluble drugs, are first metabolized to more polar water-soluble compounds before being excreted by the kidneys.[2] Renal excretion may vary depending on the age of the patient and the efficiency of the renal function. Children have more efficient renal elimination of drugs compared with adults.

Clearance of a drug is a measure of body's efficiency in eliminating the drug.[1] A *steady state concentration of drug* is reached when the rate of drug elimination equals the rate of drug administration.[3] Thus, the dosing rate is the product of clearance and steady state concentration of the drug.[5] The rate of clearance of a given drug remains constant over a range of its measured blood (body fluid) concentrations.[5] When a constant fraction of drug in the body is eliminated per unit of time, it is said to follow *first-order kinetics*.[5] In first-order kinetics, the elimination rate is proportional to the concentration of the drug in the plasma.[2,3] When the metabolic system for drug elimination is saturated, a fixed amount of drug is eliminated per unit of time and it is said to follow *zero-order kinetics*.[2] In zero-order kinetics, clearance will vary with the drug concentration.[2,5]

The *half-life* of a drug is defined as the time it takes for the plasma concentration (or the amount of drug in the body) to be reduced by 50% and it varies depending on the clearance and volume of distribution of the drug.[3] Generally, half-life is a clinically useful indicator of the time required for the drug to reach steady state (~4 half-lives), the time that will be required to eliminate the drug from the body, and a mechanism by which to estimate the dosing interval.[3]

Drug Dosing and Therapeutic Drug Monitoring

The knowledge of the pharmacokinetic parameters of a drug is applied clinically in determining the appropriate dose and dose interval for a drug to achieve desired concentration and realize its therapeutic effect. For many drugs, a relationship exists between the measured level of the drug in the body fluid and its therapeutic effects; whereas, for many others such a relationship is not clear.[2,5] Some of the pharmacokinetic concepts useful in designing the optimum dosing regimen and therapeutic drug monitoring include clearance, apparent volume of distribution, elimination half-life, and bioavailability of the drug, reviewed previously.

A drug's concentration in the body that is within a range that provides optimal efficacy without undue side effects or toxicity, defines the *therapeutic window* for that drug.[2] The strategy for dosage determination of drug based on the relationship between its serum or plasma concentration and desired therapeutic effects (or toxic effects) is referred to as the *target concentration strategy*.[5]

To *maintain* a desired therapeutic level or the steady state concentration, the drug should be administered at a rate that equals its rate of elimination.[5] A drug dose and dosing interval can be calculated based on the desired concentration of the drug, its clearance, and bioavailability.[3] A *loading* dose is typically reserved for cases where a rapid action of the drug is desired.[2,5] A large loading dose may be associated with undesirable toxicity in some patients, and for drugs with long half-lives it will take a long time for the drug to clear from the body.[2]

It is important to understand that most recommended dosage ranges are designed for an average patient with a given disorder and there is considerable interindividual (genetic) variability in pharmacokinetics and pharmacodynamics; pharmacokinetics is also affected by any associated disease states. Because of lack of sufficient clinical trials and data, the drug dosage of many agents used in children and adolescents are extrapolated based on studies in adult subjects.[6] Therefore, individualization of the dosage is the most prudent approach starting with a low dose and gradually titrating up to achieve the desired effects.

Table 3			
Genetic polymorphisms associated with phase I and phase II reactions			
Enzyme	**Phase I or Phase II**	**Frequency of Poor Metabolizers**	**Medication Examples**
CYP2D6	Phase I	5%–10% Whites 1%–2% Asians 2%–7% Blacks	Codeine Dextromethorphan Paroxetine Fluoxetine Haloperidol Nortriptyline
CYP2C9	Phase I	1% Whites 0.4% Asians 0% Blacks	Phenytoin Warfarin Glipizide
CYP2C19	Phase I	2%–3% Whites 10%–25% Asians 4% Blacks	Proton pump inhibitors Fluoxetine Sertraline Nelfinavir
NAT 2	Phase II	52% Whites 17% Japanese	Isoniazid Hydralazine Procainamide
TMPT	Phase II	0.3% Whites 0.04% Asians	Mercaptopurine Azathioprine
UGT1A1	Phase II	10% Whites 4% Chinese 1% Japanese	Irinotecan
COMT	Phase II	25% Whites	Levodopa

Abbreviations: COMT, catechol O-methyltransferase; CYP, cytochrome; NAT2, N-acetyltransferase 2; TMPT, thiopurine s-methyltransferase; UGT1A1, UDP-glucuronosyl transferase 1A1.
Data from Refs.[11–13]

Not all drugs have a clear correlation between their measured concentration in blood (or body fluid) and the desired therapeutic effects; however, in many instances therapeutic drug monitoring can be useful to guide the treatment. The drug concentration just before the next dose is due (ie, the trough level) is the most useful to guide any adjustment of the dose during the initiation as well as the maintenance phase of therapy.[3] When the same dose of the drug is given at the same dosage intervals, a steady state is reached after 4 half-lives.[3] In cases when no loading dose is given and a drug has a narrow therapeutic window with concern for toxicity, the initial drug concentration should be measured after at least 2 half-lives so as to assess the need to adjust the dose.[2] Another level should then be measured after 2 more half-lives (that is after a total of 4 half-lives).[2] A pharmacokinetic consultation is valuable where available for appropriate individualization of the dosage regimen. Given the difficulties with therapeutic monitoring of drugs, it is neither necessary nor useful in all cases; rather individualization based on regular clinical assessment is more useful and desirable in most cases.

PHARMACODYNAMICS

Pharmacodynamics in simple terms refers to the effects of the drug on the body and in broad terms encompasses the concepts of sites of drug action, the structure activity relationship, various types of receptors, the drug-receptor interactions, concepts of specificity and selectivity of drug action, and mechanisms of drug action.[2,4] In our discussion of the psychopharmacological agents, these and other related concepts are reviewed in the context of chemical neurotransmission in a separate article in this issue (*see* Patel and Feucht: "Basic concepts of neurotransmission").

PHARMACOGENETICS AND PHARMACOGENOMICS

In addition to nongenetic factors (ie, age, organ function, dietary influence, and drug interactions) that can influence drug response, genetics has a strong influence on drug response and is an area of intense research.[8] Pharmacogenetics involves the relationship between individual gene variations and the resulting drug response, whereas pharmacogenomics evaluates drug response in relation to multiple gene variants.[9] By evaluating and understanding the genetic influence on drug response, it is anticipated that drug therapy can be individualized to select the appropriate patient and dose while avoiding drug toxicity.[9]

Common genetic variations are referred to as polymorphisms and may be seen in coding and noncoding regions and can be influenced by ethnicity.[9] The most common type of polymorphism is referred to as an SNP or single nucleotide polymorphism where one base pair is altered in the DNA sequence.[8] Reasons for individual differences in drug response can be attributed to polymorphisms in genes that encode for drug metabolism, drug transport, and targets of drug therapy.[10,11] Initial studies involving pharmacogenetics identified variations in single genes encoding drug metabolizing enzymes that lead to an alteration in drug response. An example of this involves the enzyme thiopurine methyltransferase (TPMT), which is responsible for the metabolism of azathioprine and 6-mercaptopurine.[8,9] Those patients who have 2 nonfunctional alleles for this enzyme are at high risk for severe hematological toxicity.[8,9] Often more than one gene may be involved in predicting clinical response or toxicity, which has led to evaluating the entire genome or genes involved in drug response pathways.[9] An example of this involves the use of warfarin where CYP2C9 is responsible for its metabolism and vitamin K epoxide reductase complex (VKORC1) is its primary site of action.[8,12] Polymorphisms in the genotypes (genetic makeup) of CYP2C9 and VKORC1 can lead to altered responses to warfarin therapy.[8,9,12]

Polymorphisms have been observed for both phase I and phase II metabolic reactions.[11] For metabolic reactions, patients are often described as either extensive or poor metabolizers based on their particular enzyme genotype. Genetic polymorphisms can vary by race and ethnicity.[12] CYP2D6 was the first cytochrome P450 enzyme identified to have genetic polymorphism and has been the most heavily studied.[11,12] Genetic polymorphisms of CYP2D6 are clinically important because of the number of drugs that undergo metabolism (eg, codeine, paroxetine, fluoxetine, haloperidol, venlafaxine) via this route and the potential for lack of efficacy in ultrarapid metabolizers and toxicity in poor metabolizers.[12] Genetic variations have also been observed for CYP2C9, CYP2C19, and CYP3A5.[11] Phase II genetic polymorphisms have been observed with the metabolism of isoniazid by N-acetyltransferase (NAT2), thiopurines metabolized by TMPT, and irinotecan by uridine diphosphate glucuronosyltransferase 1A1 (UGT1A1).[11] See **Table 3** for additional details.

Genetic polymorphisms have been observed with transport genes that play an important role in absorption, distribution, and excretion of certain medications.[10]

Table 4
Examples of currently available pharmacogenetic tests

Medication	Pharmacogenetic Test	Relevant Information
Abacavir	HLA-B*5701	Screening recommended before initiation so as to predict risk of hypersensitivity reaction.
Azathioprine 6-Mercaptopurine	TMPT	Recommended testing because of risk of myelotoxicity with decrease enzyme activity.
Warfarin	CYP2C9 VKORC1	Lower starting doses should be considered in those with certain genetic variations of CYP2C9 & VKORC1.
Carbamazepine	HLA-B*1502	Testing is recommended before start of therapy in those with ancestry that places them at risk for HLA-B*1502. Those who test positive should not start therapy unless benefits outweigh the risks.
Tetrabenazine	CYP2D6	Patients should undergo genotype testing before utilization of daily doses exceeding 50 mg. Those who are poor metabolizers should not exceed 50 mg per day.
Clozapine	HLA-DQB1	No recommendation in product label. Thought to be a contributing factor in the development of agranulocytosis. Association based on small studies.
Trastuzumab	HER2	Evaluation is necessary to determine patients appropriate for therapy because only these patients have demonstrated benefit in clinical studies.

Abbreviations: CYP, cytochrome; HER2, human epidermal growth factor receptor 2; TMPT, thiopurine s-methyltransferase; VKORC1, vitamin K epoxide reductase complex.
Reprinted by permission from Macmillan Publishers Ltd: Clinical Pharmacology & Therapeutics, Flockhart D, Skaar T, Berlin D, Klein T, Nguyen A. Clinically available pharmacogenomics tests. Clin Pharmacol Ther 2009;86(1):109–113; Ikediobi O, Shin J, Nussbaum R, Phillips K and UCSF Center for Translational and Policy Research on Personalized Medicine. Addressing the challenges of the clinical application of pharmacogenetic testing. Clin Pharmacol Ther 2009;86(1):28–31.

P-glycoprotein is one transport molecule that functions as a drug efflux transporter and genetic polymorphisms have led to variable drug responses.[9] Substrates that may be affected include digoxin, human immunodeficiency virus (HIV) protease inhibitors, glucocorticoids, and several anticancer drugs.[10] Genetic polymorphisms have also been observed with drug targets that influence the pharmacodynamic response of the drug. One genetic polymorphism previously discussed is VKORC1, which can lead to a decreased response to warfarin.[9] Other drug targets where genetic polymorphisms have been observed include angiotensin-converting enzyme (ACE), beta-2 adrenergic receptor, dopamine receptors, and serotonin transporter.[10]

Pharmacogenetic testing has expanded over the past decade with approximately 10% of drugs approved by the Food and Drug Administration (FDA) containing pharmacogenetic information within the label.[13] Pharmacogenetic testing is designed to optimize patient therapy and may provide information as to who would benefit from the medication, predict drug toxicity, and provide dosage guidance.[13] See **Table 4** for examples of currently available pharmacogenetic tests. The FDA has the ability to require pharmacogenetic testing so as to achieve efficacy and safety.[14] Although many product labels contain information regarding genetic testing, few require it as part of drug initiation. Utilization within clinical practice has been hampered by lack of dosage adjustment guidelines, limited information regarding clinical outcomes, insurance reimbursement, perception that other biomarkers are as suitable, and limited practitioner knowledge and experience.[15,16] The success of future pharmacogenetic tests will need to demonstrate clinical application, provide direction for alternative dosing where appropriate, evaluate for variations in different races and ethnicities, show benefit over other clinical biomarkers, and prove cost-effective so as to achieve insurance reimbursement.[14] It is also essential that clinicians expand their knowledge so as to successfully use pharmacogenetics within their practice.

SUMMARY

Important developmental differences exist between children and adults in terms of drug pharmacokinetics and pharmacodynamics that have significant implications for dosing, therapeutic effects, and toxicity. It is generally prudent to start at a low dosage and gradually titrating higher; however, the dosages required for therapeutic effects in children often are similar to those used in adults. Use of multiple drugs should generally be avoided but the presence of comorbid disorders is quite common necessitating the use of a combination of drugs. It is recognized that the immature or still maturing brain is more sensitive to the effects of a given drug and long-term implications are not clearly elucidated; at the same time, hepatic metabolism and renal excretion are relatively more efficient in children who eliminate the drug. The side effects between children and adults also vary; children tend to experience relatively more behavioral and cognitive side effects, whereas adults tend to experience more somatic side effects. It is hopeful that in the future, pharmacogenomics and pharmacogenetics may play a larger role in individualizing therapy to optimize efficacy while reducing adverse events.

ACKNOWLEDGMENTS

This article is partly adapted from the authors' previous work: Patel DR, Feucht C. The basics of pharmacology and neurotransmission. In: Greydanus DE, Calles JL Jr, Patel DR, editors. Pediatric and adolescent psychopharmacology. New York: Cambridge University Press; 2008. p. 25–48; with permission.

REFERENCES

1. Bauer L. Clinical pharmacokinetic and pharmacodynamic concepts: introduction. In: Applied Clinical Pharmacokinetics. 2nd edition. Chapter 1. Available at: http://0-www.accesspharmacy.com.libcat.ferris.edu/content.aspx?aid=3517000. Accessed September 28, 2010.
2. Buxton I. Pharmacokinetics and pharmacodynamics: the dynamics of drug absorption, distribution, action, and elimination: introduction. In: Brunton K, Lazo J, Parker, editors. Goodman & Gilman's the pharmacological basis of therapeutics. 11th edition. New York: McGraw-Hill; 2006. p. 1–39.
3. Winter M. Clinical pharmacokinetics. In: Young L, Koda-Kimble M, editors. Applied therapeutics, the clinical use of drugs. 6th edition. Vancouver (WA): Applied Therapeutics, Inc; 1995. p. 2(1)–2(21).
4. Bauer L. Clinical pharmacokinetics and pharmacodynamics. In: DiPiro J, Talbert R, Yee G, et al, editors. Pharmacotherapy, a pathophysiological approach. 7th edition. New York: McGraw-Hill; 2008. p. 9–30.
5. Holford N. Pharmacokinetics and pharmacodynamics: rationale dosing and the time course of drug action: introduction. Chapter 3. Available at: http://0-www.accesspharmacy.com.libcat.ferris.edu/content.aspx?aid=4513158. Accessed September 28, 2010.
6. Casavant M, Griffith J. Pediatric pharmacotherapy part 2: pediatric pharmacokinetics: why kids are not small adults. Pharmacology Update 8/30/10. Available at: http://0-www.accesspharmacy.com.libcat.ferris.edu/updatesContent.aspx?aid=1001655. Accessed September 28, 2010.
7. Gonzalez F, Tukey R. Drug metabolism. In: Brunton L, Lazo J, Parker K, editors. Goodman & Gilman's the pharmacological basis of therapeutics. 11th edition. New York: McGraw-Hill; 2006. p. 71–91.
8. Lanfear D, McLeod H. Pharmacogenetics: using DNA to optimize drug therapy. Am Fam Physician 2007;6:1179–82.
9. Roden D, Altman R, Benowitz N, et al. Pharmacogenomics: challenges and opportunities. Ann Intern Med 2006;145:749–57.
10. Evans W, McLeod H. Pharmacogenetics—drug disposition, drug targets, and side effects. N Engl J Med 2003;348:538–49.
11. Guttmacher A, Collins F. Inheritance and drug response. N Engl J Med 2003; 348(6):529–37.
12. Wilkinson G. Drug metabolism and variability among patients in drug response. N Engl J Med 2005;352(21):2211–21.
13. Food and Drug Administration US. U.S. Department of Health and Human Services. Drugs; table of valid genomic biomarkers in the context of approved labels. 2010. Available at: http://www.fda.gov/Drugs/ScienceResearch/ResearchAreas/Pharmacogenetics/ucm083378.htm. Accessed August 11, 2010.
14. Flockhart D, Skaar T, Berlin D, et al. Clinically available pharmacogenomics tests. Clin Pharmacol Ther 2009;86(1):109–13.
15. Kediobi O, Shin J, Nussbaum R, et al. Addressing the challenges of the clinical application of pharmacogenetic testing. Clin Pharmacol Ther 2009;86(1):28–31.
16. Belle D, Singh H. Genetic factors in drug metabolism. Am Fam Physician 2008; 77(11):1552–60.

Basic Concepts of Neurotransmission

Dilip R. Patel, MD, FSAM[a],*, Cynthia Feucht, PharmD, BCPS[b,c]

KEYWORDS

- Synapse • Neurotransmission • Neurotransmitter • Dopamine
- Serotonin • Glutamate • γ-Aminobutyric-acid

THE NEURON

The main components of a neuron or nerve cell are the cell body or soma, an axon, and the dendrites (**Fig. 1**). Each neuron is enclosed in a neuronal membrane. The nucleus, the rough endoplasmic reticulum, the smooth endoplasmic reticulum, the Golgi apparatus, and the mitochondria are contained within the cell body (**Fig. 2**).[1,2] The ribosomes on the rough endoplasmic reticulum and the free ribosomes are the major sites for protein synthesis directed by the messenger ribonucleic acid (mRNA).[3,4] The function of smooth endoplasmic reticulum varies depending on its location, and includes its role in finessing the protein structure and regulating concentration of certain intracellular chemicals. The Golgi apparatus plays a major role in chemical processing of the proteins. The mitochondrion is the site of cellular respiration and provides the chemical energy for the intracellular biochemical reactions. The neuronal cell membrane is a dynamic complex structure that wraps over the cytoskeleton of the cell consisting of microtubules, microfilaments, and neurofilaments. Specific genes are located on the deoxyribonucleic acid (DNA) in each chromosome inside the nucleus.

In addition to the structures of the cell body, the neuron is uniquely characterized by the axonal and dendritic processes. Each axon has 3 main parts, namely the axon hillock, the axon proper, and the axon terminal. The point of contact between the presynaptic axon terminal and the postsynaptic dendrite is called the *synapse* (**Fig. 3**).[5-7] The axon terminal may also end on the cell body of the postsynaptic neuron. The neurotransmitter is stored in the synaptic vesicles in the axon terminal.[2,3]

This article is partly adapted from authors' previous work: Patel DR, Feucht C. The basics of pharmacology and neurotransmission. In: Greydanus DE, Calles JL Jr, Patel DR Pediatric and adolescent psychopharmacology. New York: Cambridge University Press; 2008. p. 25–48.

[a] Department of Pediatrics and Human Development, Michigan State University College of Human Medicine, MSU/Kalamazoo Center for Medical Studies, 1000 Oakland Drive, Kalamazoo, MI 49009-1284, USA
[b] Borgess Ambulatory Care, 1701 Gull Road, Kalamazoo, MI 49048, USA
[c] Department of Pharmacy Practice, Ferris State University College of Pharmacy, Big Rapids, MI 49307, USA
* Corresponding author.
E-mail address: patel@kcms.msu.edu

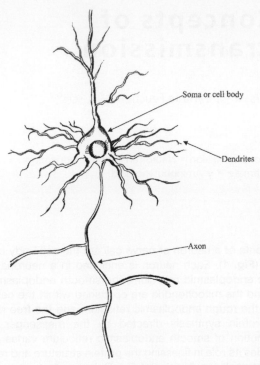

Fig. 1. Basic structure of a neuron. (*From* Patel DR, Feucht C. The basics of pharmacology and neurotransmission. In: Greydanus DE, Calles JL Jr, Patel DR, editors. Pediatric and adolescent psychopharmacology. New York: Cambridge University Press; 2008. p. 32; with permission.)

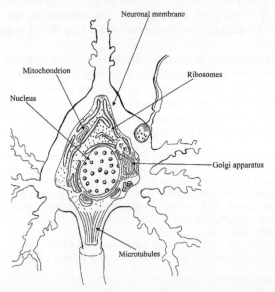

Fig. 2. Internal structure of a neuron. (*From* Patel DR, Feucht C. The basics of pharmacology and neurotransmission. In: Greydanus DE, Calles JL Jr, Patel DR, editors. Pediatric and adolescent psychopharmacology. New York: Cambridge University Press; 2008. p. 33; with permission.)

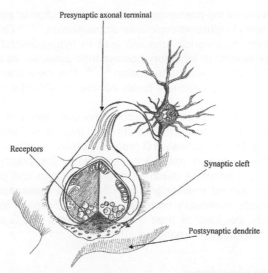

Presynaptic axonal terminal

Receptors

Synaptic cleft

Postsynaptic dendrite

Fig. 3. A chemical synapse. (*From* Patel DR, Feucht C. The basics of pharmacology and neuro-transmission. In: Greydanus DE, Calles JL Jr, Patel DR, editors. Pediatric and adolescent psycho-pharmacology. New York: Cambridge University Press; 2008. p. 34; with permission.)

Axons carry the neuronal impulse to various other neurons in the brain.[2,3] The informa-tion or input is carried to the cell body of the receiving neuron. On the receiving end, the information or impulse is received at the dendrites.[3]

THE SYNAPSE

At the synapse the electrical impulse from the presynaptic neuron is converted to a chemical signal that is carried to the postsynaptic receptors, where it is again con-verted to an electrical impulse in the postsynaptic neuron.[2–8] Synaptic plasticity is an important characteristic of neurons that allows for experience dependent adaptation and learning.[8–13]

There are 2 types of neuronal synapses: electrical and chemical. The electrical synapses are located at gap junctions and allow free bidirectional movement of ions across cell membranes.[3,7] Their function in the brain varies at different sites; they provide for fast transmission of impulses. Most of the synaptic transmission in the brain occurs at the chemical synapses.[3,6,7] Autoreceptors are membrane-bound receptors on the presynaptic membrane, which regulate the release and in some cases synthesis of the intrinsic neurotransmitter.[6,7] Certain other receptors on the presynaptic membrane can be modulated by neurotransmitters from nearby neurons and are called heteroreceptors.[6,7]

The membrane-bound postsynaptic neuroreceptors can generally be classified into 2 types: (1) Transmitter-gated (or ligand-gated) ion channels, and (2) G-protein–coupled receptors.[5,7,14–16] Transmitter- or ligand-gated ion channel receptor consists of 5 subunits that are arranged as columns in a circle, thus forming a pore or a channel in the middle.[7,16,17] The neurotransmitter binds to the specific site on the extracellular portion of the receptor, leading to opening of the channel. The effect on the postsyn-aptic neuron depends on which ion is preferentially passed through the channel into the postsynaptic neuron. Movement of *sodium* ions into the postsynaptic neuron results in depolarization of the postsynaptic cell and generation of excitatory postsynaptic potential, as seen in glutamatergic neurotransmission.[5,7,16] On the other hand, increased permeability to *chloride* ions will lead to hyperpolarization of the postsynaptic cell and generation of inhibitory postsynaptic potential, as seen in γ-aminobutyric acid (GABA)-ergic neurotransmission.[5,7,16] The neurotransmission at the ligand gated ion channels is relatively faster compared with that at the G-protein–coupled receptors.[3–5]

In the case of G-protein–coupled receptors, the occupancy of the extracellular receptor site by the neurotransmitter results in activation of intracellular receptor linked G proteins (**Fig. 4**).[7] The activated G proteins turn on the effector proteins, which in turn activates the G-protein gated ion channels in the postsynaptic neuronal membrane or activates enzymes (such as adenylyl cyclase and phospholipase C) to form intracellular second messengers.[3,6,7,16] Second messengers then lead to a biochemical cascade, eventually communicating the message to the DNA of the postsynaptic neuron. Because of their metabolic effects, the G-protein receptors are also known as metabotropic receptors.[7,13]

CHEMICAL NEUROTRANSMISSION

Chemical neurotransmission is mediated by specific neurotransmitters in the brain, and a large number of these have been identified. There are various classes of neurotransmitters in the central nervous system (CNS); amine and monoamines are of interest in a review of psychopharmacology.[3] Other classes of neurotransmitters, not reviewed here, use different pathways for synthesis, storage, release, and ways of communication. Still others follow nonsynaptic neurotransmission.

Synthesis of different neurotransmitters in the presynaptic neuron varies to some extent for specific neurotransmitters using specific amino acids and enzymes.[3–7] Neurotransmitter synthesis is directed by mRNA and occurs in the cytosol of the axon terminal. The amine and amino acid neurotransmitters are then taken into synaptic vesicles by specialized transporter proteins. The neurotransmitter is stored in the synaptic vesicles in the axonal terminal until it is released into the synaptic cleft.[1,3,7]

The peptide neurotransmitters are assembled from the amino acids in the rough endoplasmic reticulum and the active neurotransmitter segment is split in the Golgi apparatus.[16] The secretory granules containing the active peptide then are carried to the axon terminal.

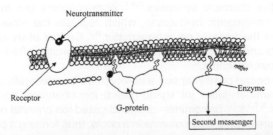

Fig. 4. Action of neurotransmitter at G-protein coupled receptors. (*From* Patel DR, Feucht C. The basics of pharmacology and neurotransmission. In: Greydanus DE, Calles JL Jr, Patel DR, editors. Pediatric and adolescent psychopharmacology. New York: Cambridge University Press; 2008. p. 36; with permission.)

A nerve impulse or action potential in the axon terminal triggers the release of specific neurotransmitter into the synaptic cleft.[6] Depolarization of the cell membrane results in activation of the voltage-gated calcium channels in the active zones to open, allowing influx of calcium ions into the presynaptic axon terminal.[6,7] The synaptic vesicle is anchored to the cell membrane and the neurotransmitter is spilled into the synaptic cleft, a process called exocytosis.[3,6] The process of recovery of the synaptic vesicle membrane after the neurotransmitter is released from the vesicle is called endocytosis.[7] Once released into the synaptic cleft, the neurotransmitters can be either destroyed by enzymes or transported back into the presynaptic axon terminal by membrane-bound neurotransmitter-specific transporters.

Postsynaptic receptor occupancy by the neurotransmitter initiates the postsynaptic neurotransmission process. It is thus understood that the electrical nerve impulse in the presynaptic neuron is converted by excitation-secretion coupling into a chemical signal.[7]

Postsynaptic receptor occupancy by the neurotransmitter (first messenger) results in the activation or formation of the second messenger in the postsynaptic neuron.[3,5] Cyclic adenosine monophosphate (cAMP) and phosphatidyl inositol are examples of second messengers. The second messenger triggers a biochemical cascade and synthesis of various elements, including the transcription factors.[3-7]

Each gene typically has a coding region and a regulatory region.[2,7] The regulatory region has an enhancer element and a promoter element. The coding region on the DNA has the template for the corresponding RNA.[2,7] Transcription factors activated by phosphorylation bind to the promoter region of the DNA, in turn activating the enzyme RNA polymerase.[3,7] The action of activated RNA polymerase on the coding region results in the formation of the messenger RNA. The process of mRNA formation from DNA template is called transcription and the mRNA is called the transcript. Certain noncoding regions (introns) on the DNA transcribed onto the initial mRNA are removed by the process of RNA splicing, leaving only the coding sequences (exons) in the mRNA. mRNA leaves the nucleus and reaches various sites in the neuron to initiate protein synthesis. The process of assembling various amino acids to create specific proteins as directed by the mRNA is called translation.[7]

These proteins are the building blocks for various elements in the postsynaptic neuron with specialized functions, including neurotransmitter receptors, the ion channels, various peptides and enzymes, transcription factors, neurotransmitter transporter, and neurotropic growth factors. The regulation of gene expression also affects the process of synaptogenesis.

Allosteric Modulation

When a neurotransmitter (primary) occupies its specific receptor site, it triggers the postsynaptic chemical neurotransmission. When a different neurotransmitter (secondary) occupies its receptor site and indirectly influences the primary neuroreceptor transmission, it is said to be modulating the primary neurotransmitter action allosterically.[2,3,7,16] The secondary neurotransmitter can only influence the primary neurotransmitter action when the primary neurotransmitter occupies its specific receptor site. Allosteric modulation can either amplify (positive allosteric interaction) or diminish or block (negative allosteric interaction) the actions of the primary neurotransmitter.[16] For example, the benzodiazepines are known to use positive allosteric modulation whereas antidepressants use negative allosteric modulation.

Nonsynaptic (Volume) Neurotransmission

In addition to the neurotransmission that occurs via the synapse, nonsynaptic or volume neurotransmission is also known to occur.[2,3,7,16] In this case a given neurotransmitter diffuses within a given radius and affects the various receptors with wide-ranging actions. This process is also the basis of single drug acting on different receptors with different actions.

Divergence and Convergence

A given neurotransmitter can activate multiple subtypes of receptors each mediating a different function. In fact, this ability of a neurotransmitter, referred to as divergence, is a common phenomenon, exemplified by glutamate.[7,15,16] On the other hand, different neurotransmitters acting on their specific receptors can activate a particular effector system, a phenomenon called convergence.[7,16] Neurons also have the ability to integrate both the divergent and convergent systems.

Agonists and Antagonists

Naturally occurring neurotransmitters stimulate the receptors on which they bind and are thus said to be *agonists*. Similarly, pharmacologic agents that stimulate specific receptors are also called agonists.[7] Antagonist agents block the actions of agonists. *Antagonists* do not have any intrinsic activity of their own, but in the presence of an agonist they block its activity.[7,16] Antagonists also will block the actions of inverse agonists and partial agonists as well. A pharmacologic agent that binds to a receptor, resulting in action that is opposite to that of agonist, is called an *inverse agonist*.[16] The action of an inverse agonist is not dependent on the presence of an agonist. *Partial agonist* binding to a specific receptor will have action that is similar to but relatively weaker than that of an agonist.[16]

MAJOR NEUROTRANSMITTER SYSTEMS
Cholinergic System

Acetylcholine (ACh) is the neurotransmitter used in the cholinergic system. Acetylcholine is synthesized in the cholinergic neurons by the interaction of choline and acetyl coenzyme A mediated by the enzyme choline acetyltransferase.[1,2] ACh is stored in the vesicles in the presynaptic neuron until it is released by appropriate nerve impulse into the synaptic cleft. From the synaptic cleft, ACh can either be transported back into the presynaptic neuron by the ACh transporter or destroyed by the enzyme acetylcholinesterase (AChE).[1,2] Because the ACh is destroyed by the AChE, it is mainly the choline that is transported back into the neuron and reused to synthesize ACh again. Another enzyme called pseudocholinesterase or butyrylcholinesterase can also inactivate ACh, especially in the glial cells. In addition to the cholinergic neurons, ACh is also present in various other sites in the body, including skeletal muscle and blood cells.[2]

Various types of muscarinic and nicotinic receptors are the major subtypes of cholinergic receptors; muscarinic receptors are G-protein linked whereas nicotinic receptors are ligand-gated ion channels.[2] The cell bodies of the cholinergic neurons are located between the septum and the nucleus basalis of Meynert in the basal forebrain with projections to hippocampus, amygdala, and cortex.[2,7] These pathways are believed to mediate memory, learning, problem-solving abilities, novelty seeking, sleep-wake cycles, and judgment. Drugs that inhibit AChE prevent the destruction of ACh and subsequently increase ACh concentration.

Dopaminergic System

The monoamine dopamine is the neurotransmitter of the dopaminergic system.[1,2] Dopamine is synthesized from its precursor amino acid tyrosine, which is converted to 3,4-dihydroxyphenylalanine (DOPA) by tyrosine hydroxylase. DOPA is converted to dopamine by DOPA decarboxylase. Once synthesized in the presynaptic nerve terminal, dopamine is packaged in the vesicles for storage. Presynaptic action potential triggers the release of dopamine from the vesicles into the synaptic cleft. Dopamine can be metabolized by the enzymes monoamine oxidase (MAO) or cate-chol-*ortho*-methyltransaminase (COMT). Dopamine is also transported back from the synaptic cleft into the presynaptic terminal by presynaptic dopamine-specific transporters, where it can be repackaged into vesicles and stored for future use. Dopamine transporter is a target for drug action (eg, stimulants).

Five subtypes of dopamine receptors have been described, namely D1 to D5, present both on the presynaptic neuron and the postsynaptic neuron.[1] Presynaptic receptors act as autoreceptors whereas dopamine occupation of the postsynaptic receptors acti-vates the second-messenger system and postsynaptic events. Different subtypes of dopamine receptors predominantly express themselves in specific regions or sites in the brain, thereby influencing specific functions. Postsynaptic receptors are targets for dopamine antagonist drugs (eg, antipsychotic agents).

Through various pathways dopamine is involved in numerous functions in the CNS.[3,18–24] Dopamine pathways from substantia nigra projecting to caudate and putamen modulate GABAergic neurons, and their imbalance leads to extrapyramidal symptoms (such as tremors).[1,2,7,18] Those from the ventral tegmental area projecting to mesolimbic system (amygdala, nucleus accumbens) are implicated in the develop-ment of addiction. The pathways from the ventral tegmental area to the mesocortical system are involved in "fine tuning" of cortical neurons, and their function is improved by stimulants. The projections from hypothalamus to pituitary play a role in prolactin release, and neuroleptic blockade leads to hyperprolactinemia.

GABAergic System

GABA is the main inhibitory neurotransmitter in the CNS.[2,25–30] The amino acid GABA is the neurotransmitter used in GABAergic neurotransmission. GABA is synthesized in the GABAergic neurons from its precursor glutamate by action of the enzyme gluta-mate decarboxylase.[1,2] GABA is stored in the presynaptic vesicles until released into the synaptic cleft following appropriate nerve impulse. The released GABA can be either destroyed by GABA transaminase or transported back into the presynaptic terminal by GABA-specific presynaptic transporter for repackaging and storage for reuse.

Two GABA receptor subtypes have been identified, namely GABA-A and GABA-B.[1–3] The role of GABA-B receptor is limited to its binding specifically with the muscle relaxant baclofen. Postsynaptic GABA-A receptors belong to the superfamily of ligand-gated ion-channel receptors. Receptor occupancy by GABA opens the ion channel and allows increased conductance of chloride ions into the neuron, leading to fast neuro-transmission and inhibitory action. The GABAergic system exerts inhibitory control over the glutamatergic system, and the balance between the 2 systems allows for normal neuronal function.

GABAergic neurons are widespread in the CNS and spinal cord, with interneurons in the cortex, and medium- to long-range projections, including: caudate nucleus and putamen to globus pallidus; globus pallidus to thalamus and substantia nigra; septum to hippocampus; and substantia nigra to superior colliculus.[1,2,30]

Benzodiazepine receptors are located at sites nearby the GABA-A receptors.[1,25] Different subtypes of benzodiazepine receptors are predominantly found at various locations in the CNS and are thought to mediate specific functions. Benzodiazepine receptors allosterically modulate the GABA-A receptors.[25] In addition to benzodiaze-pine receptors, various other receptors are located near GABA-A receptors. Thus, the interaction of these various receptors is involved in mediating the effects of benzodi-azepine agents.

Glutamatergic System

Glutamate is the predominant excitatory neurotransmitter in the CNS.[31–34] Glutamate is synthesized in the neuron by conversion of glutamine to glutamate by the enzyme glutaminase.[1] Glutamate is stored in the presynaptic vesicles until it is released into the synaptic cleft. Glial cells near the neuron also supply glutamine to the neuron for glutamate synthesis. Once glutamate is released into the synaptic cleft it binds to the postsynaptic receptors, initiating postsynaptic excitation. Glutamate is removed from the synaptic cleft by the presynaptic transporter back into the synaptic terminal, as well as by a glial transporter, into the nearby glial cell.[1,2]

The major glutamate receptor subtypes include N-methyl-D-aspartate (NMDA), α-amino-3-hydroxy-5-methyl-isoxazole-4-propionic acid (AMPA), and kainate, which are linked to ion channels; and a metabotropic glutamate receptor subtype that is G-protein linked, involved in long-term potentiation and memory formation.[1–3,13]

One of the receptors believed to mediate the excitotoxicity associated with glutama-tergic neurotransmission is the NMDA receptor.[1,2,17] Several other nearby receptors are believed to be involved in allosteric modulation of the NMDA receptor complex.[7,16] Stimulation of the NMDA receptor site allows increased conductance of calcium ions into the neuron and triggers postsynaptic excitatory neurotrans mission.[1,2,16] Glutama-tergic excitation represents the spectrum from normal excitation to too much excita-tion, resulting in neuronal damage.[16] Glutamatergic excitotoxicity is believed to play a major role in the pathophysiology of neurodegenerative diseases, seizures, and stroke. Decreased glutamate, on the other hand, can lead to psychosis.[16,31–36]

NMDA receptors in the hippocampus are associated with long-term memory. Glu-tamatergic neurons are widely distributed in the CNS and include various interconnec-tion pathways in the cerebral cortex, the extrapyramidal system, the pyramidal system, and the thalamocortical system.[1,2,37]

Noradrenergic System

Monoamine norepinephrine is the neurotransmitter for noradrenergic neurons.[1,2,35,36] Norepinephrine (NE) is synthesized from its precursor amino acid tyrosine in the cell body or axonal nerve terminal. Tyrosine is converted to DOPA by tyrosine hydroxylase. DOPA is then converted to dopamine by DOPA decarboxylase. Dopamine is con-verted to norepinephrine by dopamine β-hydroxylase.

Once synthesized, the NE is packaged into vesicles where it is stored until released into the synaptic cleft during noradrenergic transmission.[1,2,7] From the synaptic cleft the NE can be transported back into the presynaptic nerve terminal by NE-specific transporters. NE thus recovered is repackaged into storage vesicles for future use. NE is also destroyed by the enzyme MAO, predominantly located in the mitochondria, and COMT, predominantly located in the postsynaptic neuron.[2]

Once NE is released from the presynaptic neuron into the synaptic cleft, it occupies the NE-specific postsynaptic receptors. NE receptors are classified into α1, α2, β1, and β2 subtypes.[1,2] A 2-receptor subtype is present on the presynaptic axon terminal (terminal α2 receptor) and in the cell body and nearby dendrites (somatodendritic α2 receptor). The presynaptic α2 receptors regulate the release of NE and thus act as autoreceptors. α1, α2, β1, and β2 receptors are present on the postsynaptic membrane. Postsynaptic receptor occupation by NE triggers postsynaptic events, including second-messenger activation and gene expression.

The cell bodies for noradrenergic neurons are predominantly located in the locus coeruleus in the brainstem.[7] Different noradrenergic projections from the locus coeruleus are involved in specific effects of NE, including regulation of mood, attention, vigilance, cognition, emotions, information processing, working memory, energy, and movements.[1,2,35,36] NE deficiency syndrome is characterized by impaired attention, difficulty in concentrating, impaired working memory, decreased speed of information processing, depressed mood, fatigue, and psychomotor retardation.[16] Different functions are regulated by a different subtype of NE receptor in the CNS.

Actions of NE outside the CNS mediated via different pathways include regulation of blood pressure, heart rate, and bladder emptying.[7]

Serotonergic System

Serotonin, or 5-hydroxytryptamine (5HT) is synthesized in the presynaptic axon terminal from its precursor tryptophan.[1] Tryptophan is first converted to 5-hydroxytryptophan by the action of tryptophan hydroxylase. 5-Hydroxytryptophan is then converted to 5HT by the action of aromatic amino acid decarboxylase.

Serotonin is stored in the presynaptic vesicle until released by the presynaptic terminal into the synaptic cleft.[2] Serotonin can be destroyed by MAO and also transported back into the presynaptic terminal by serotonin transporters. There are several 5HT receptor subtypes.[1,2,7] Presynaptic receptors act as autoreceptors. In addition to 5HT autoreceptors, the presynaptic serotonergic terminal also has α2-noradrenergic heteroreceptors responsive to NE. Thus serotonin release can be blocked in part by NE via its action on the α2-noradrenergic heteroreceptors. On the other hand, the action of NE on the α1-adrenergic heteroreceptors present on the presynaptic cell body triggers the release of serotonin. Thus there is both an inhibitory and excitatory interaction between the noradrenergic and serotonergic systems.

The cell bodies of serotonergic neurons are located in the raphe nucleus in the brain stem. Various projections to different areas in the brain, brainstem, and spinal cord from raphe nucleus (including amygdala and hippocampus) are associated with various specific 5HT receptor subtypes and specific functions attributed to serotonin.[7,37–40] Deficiency of serotonin is clinically characterized by depressed mood, anxiety, panic attacks, phobias, obsessions, compulsions, and food craving.[16]

SUMMARY

Receptors, enzymes, and processes of neurotransmission are targets of drug action as well as causes of mental and neurologic disorders.[1,2,5,41–43] The various elements of the neurotransmission systems not only can be modulated by pharmacologic agents, but also are constantly changing because of the ongoing neuromaturation and experience (including psychotherapy) throughout childhood and adolescence.[4,9–12,28,41–43] Neuroplasticity of the synaptic system is an important consideration in the pathophysiology and recovery or treatment of mental and neurologic disorders in children and adolescents. Pharmacologic agents can have acute as well as long-term effects on the processes of neurotransmission. Some of the therapeutic effects as well as side effects can be explained by acute changes in the levels of neurotransmitter or the long-term alterations in responses of the postsynaptic neuron.

REFERENCES

1. Martin A, Oesterheld J, Konradi C, et al. Pediatric psychopharmacology I: pharmacokinetic and pharmacodynamic principles. In: Lewis M, editor. Child and

adolescent psychiatry: a comprehensive textbook. 3rd edition. Philadelphia: Lippincott Williams and Wilkins; 2002. p. 939–50.

2. Hecker S, Konradi C. Synaptic function and biochemical neuroanatomy. In: Martin A, Scahill L, Charney DS, et al, editors. Pediatric psychopharmacology. New York: Oxford University Press; 2003. p. 20–32.

3. Kandel ER, Siegelbaum SA. Overview of synaptic transmission. In: Kandel ER, Schwartz JH, Jessell TM, editors. Principles of neural science. 4th edition. New York: McGraw Hill; 2000. p. 175–86.

4. Kandel ER, Siegelbaum SA. Synaptic integration. In: Kandel ER, Schwartz JH, Jessell TM, editors. Principles of neural science. 4th edition. New York: McGraw Hill; 2000. p. 207–28.

5. Siegelbaum SA, Schwartz JH, Kandel ER. Modulation of synaptic transmission: second messenger. In: Kandel ER, Schwartz JH, Jessell TM, editors. Principles of neural science. 4th edition. New York: McGraw Hill; 2000. p. 229–52.

6. Kandel ER, Siegelbaum SA. Transmitter release. In: Kandel ER, Schwartz JH, Jessell TM, editors. Principles of neural science. 4th edition. New York: McGraw Hill; 2000. p. 253–79.

7. Bear MF, Connors BW, Paradiso MA. Neuroscience: exploring the brain. 3rd edition. Baltimore (MD): Lippincott Williams & Wilkins; 2007. p. 23–204.

8. Braithwaite SP, Paul S, Nairn AC, et al. Synaptic plasticity: one STEP at a time. Trends Neurosci 2006;29(8):452–8.

9. Centonze D, Gubellini P, Pisani A, et al. Dopamine, acetylcholine and nitric oxide systems interact to induce corticostriatal synaptic plasticity. Rev Neurosci 2003; 14(3):207–16.

10. Cooke SF, Bliss TV. Plasticity in the human central nervous system. Brain 2006; 129(Pt 7):1659–73.

11. Majewska AK, Sur M. Plasticity and specificity of cortical processing networks. Trends Neurosci 2006;29(6):323–9.

12. Mangina CA, Sokolov EN. Neuronal plasticity in memory and learning abilities: theoretical position and selective review. Int J Psychophysiol 2006;60(3):203–14.

13. Ferraguti F, Shigemoto R. Metabotropic glutamate receptors. Cell Tissue Res 2006;326(2):483–504.

14. Pinheiro P, Mulle C. Kainate receptors. Cell Tissue Res 2006;326(2):457–82.

15. Rollenhagen A, Lubke JH. The morphology of excitatory central synapses: from structure to function. Cell Tissue Res 2006;326(2):221–37.

16. Stahl DM. Essential psychopharmacology: neuroscientific basis and practical application. 2nd edition. Cambridge (UK): Cambridge University Press; 2000. p. 1–34.

17. Chen HS, Lipton SA. The chemical biology of clinically tolerated NMDA receptor antagonists. J Neurochem 2006;97(6):1611–26.

18. Damsa C, Bumb A, Bianchi-Demicheli F, et al. "Dopamine-dependent" side effects of selective serotonin reuptake inhibitors: a clinical review. J Clin Psychiatry 2004;65(8):1064–8.

19. Dujardin K, Laurent B. Dysfunction of the human memory systems: role of the dopaminergic transmission. Curr Opin Neurol 2003;16(Suppl 2):S11–6.

20. Greene JG. Gene expression profiles of brain dopamine neurons and relevance to neuropsychiatric disease. J Physiol 2006;575(Part 2):411–6.

21. Kienast T, Heinz A. Dopamine and the diseased brain. CNS Neurol Disord Drug Targets 2006;5(1):109–31.

22. Lee FJ, Wang YT, Liu F. Direct receptor cross-talk can mediate the modulation of excitatory and inhibitory neurotransmission by dopamine. J Mol Neurosci 2005; 26(2–3):245–52.

23. Sanger DJ. The search for novel antipsychotics: pharmacological and molecular targets. Expert Opin Ther Targets 2004;8(6):631–41.
24. Schmitz Y, Benoit-Marand M, Gonon F, et al. Presynaptic regulation of dopaminergic neurotransmission. J Neurochem 2003;87(2):273–89.
25. Allison C, Pratt JA. Neuroadaptive processes in GABAergic and glutamatergic systems in benzodiazepine dependence. Pharmacol Ther 2003;98(2):171–95.
26. Beleboni RO, Carolino RO, Pizzo AB, et al. Pharmacological and biochemical aspects of GABAergic neurotransmission: pathological and neuropsychobiological relationships. Cell Mol Neurobiol 2004;24(6):707–28.
27. Brambilla P, Perez J, Barale F, et al. GABAergic dysfunction in mood disorders. Mol Psychiatry 2003;8(8):721–37.
28. Fritschy JM, Brunig I. Formation and plasticity of GABAergic synapses: physiological mechanisms and pathophysiological implications. Pharmacol Ther 2003; 98(3):299–323.
29. Johnston GA. GABA(A) receptor channel pharmacology. Curr Pharm Des 2005; 11(15):1867–85.
30. Mody I, Pearce RA. Diversity of inhibitory neurotransmission through GABA(A) receptors. Trends Neurosci 2004;27(9):569–75.
31. HerescoLevy U. Glutamatergic neurotransmission modulators as emerging new drugs for schizophrenia. Expert Opin Emerg Drugs 2005;10(4):827–44.
32. Lujan R, Shigemoto R, Lopez-Bendito G. Glutamate and GABA receptor signaling in the developing brain. Neuroscience 2005;130(3):567–80.
33. Sem'yanov AV. Diffusional extrasynaptic neurotransmission via glutamate and GABA. Neurosci Behav Physiol 2005;35(3):253–66.
34. Wang SJ, Yang TT. Role of central glutamatergic neurotransmission in the pathogenesis of psychiatric and behavioral disorders. Drug News Perspect 2005; 18(9):561–6.
35. Berridge CW, Waterhouse BD. The locus coeruleus-noradrenergic system: modulation of behavioral state and state-dependent cognitive processes. Brain Res Brain Res Rev 2003;42(1):33–84.
36. Marien MR, Colpaert FC, Rosenquist AC. Noradrenergic mechanisms in neurodegenerative diseases: a theory. Brain Res Brain Res Rev 2004;45(1):38–78.
37. Celine F, Ouissame MF, Nasser H. Long-term adaptive changes induced by serotonergic antidepressant drugs. Expert Rev Neurother 2006;6(2):235–45.
38. Filip M, Frankowska M, Zaniewska M, et al. The serotonergic system and its role in cocaine addiction. Pharmacol Rep 2005;57(6):685–700.
39. Hensler JG. Serotonergic modulation of the limbic system. Neurosci Biobehav Rev 2006;30(2):203–14.
40. Middlemiss DN, Price GW, Watson JM. Serotonergic targets in depression. Curr Opin Pharmacol 2002;2(1):18–22.
41. Ziemann U, Meintzschel F, Korchounov A, et al. Pharmacological modulation of plasticity in the human motor cortex. Neurorehabil Neural Repair 2006;20(2):243–51.
42. Pallas SL, Wenner P, Gonzalez-Islas C, et al. Developmental plasticity of inhibitory circuitry. J Neurosci 2006;26(41):10358–61.
43. Greenhill LL, Tosyali MC. Child and adolescent psychopharmacology: Important developmental issues. Pediatr Clin North Am 1998;45(5):1021–36.

Herbal Medicines in Pediatric Neuropsychiatry

Cynthia Feucht, PharmD, BCPS[a,b,*], Dilip R. Patel, MD, FSAM[c]

KEYWORDS

• Herbal supplement • Neuropsychiatric • Pediatric • Adolescent
• Complementary medicine

Mainstream medicine in Western society is based on conventional medicine, also referred to as allopathic or biomedicine.[1] The National Center for Complementary and Alternative Medicine (NCCAM), a division of the National Institute of Health, was originally established in 1992 as the Office of Alternative Medicine and was promoted to a center in 1999.[2] The goal of the Center is to sponsor and support research in complementary and alternative medicine (CAM), with funding appropriations increasing from 2 million US dollars in 1992 to 128 million US dollars in 2010.[3] NCCAM has devised 4 domains for CAM therapy, recognizing that there is the potential for overlap as well as whole medical systems that may cover all 4 domains.[1] Whole medical systems are based on systems of theory and practice and within the United States most commonly include homeopathic and naturopathic medicine.[1] Mind-body medicine encompasses techniques including cognitive-behavioral therapy, meditation, and prayer, whereas biologically based practices include the use of herbal and dietary supplements.[1] Manipulative and body-based practices include massage and chiropractic or osteopathic manipulation.[1] Energy medicine revolves around the use of energy fields and includes Reiki, therapeutic touch, and use of electromagnetic fields.[1] This article focuses on the review of just one aspect of CAM therapy, herbal supplements, which have been used for pediatric and adolescent neuropsychiatric disorders, and includes a discussion of the various supplements and limited literature surrounding their use.

Herbal medicines have been used since the Greek and Roman era and gained popularity in the United States in the 1700s and 1800s.[4] As allopathic medicine became dominant in the twentieth century, use of herbal therapies diminished. In the 1990s the US Food and Drug Administration (FDA) proposed stringent regulations

[a] Borgess Ambulatory Care, 1701 Gull Road, Kalamazoo, MI 49048, USA
[b] Department of Pharmacy Practice, Ferris State University College of Pharmacy, Big Rapids, MI 49307, USA
[c] Department of Pediatrics and Human Development, Michigan State University College of Human Medicine, MSU/Kalamazoo Center for Medical Studies, 1000 Oakland Drive, Kalamazoo, MI 49009-1284, USA
* Corresponding author. Borgess Ambulatory Care, 1701 Gull Road, Kalamazoo, MI 49048.
E-mail address: Cynthia.feucht@gmail.com

Pediatr Clin N Am 58 (2011) 33–54
doi:10.1016/j.pcl.2010.10.006
0031-3955/11/$ – see front matter © 2011 Elsevier Inc. All rights reserved.

for the marketing of herbal supplements. Opposition by consumers and supplement manufacturers led to a compromise and passage of the Dietary Supplement Health and Education Act by Congress in 1994.[4] This Act led to the classification of herbal products as dietary supplements when manufacturers can make claims about health and nutrient content as well as about how the supplement affects structure and function of the body but cannot claim to cure, prevent, or treat specific diseases.[5] Herbal and dietary supplements are not subjected to the approval process that traditional medicines undergo by the FDA. The manufacturer should ensure safety and accurate labeling of the product but does not have to register the product or notify the FDA of its production unless a new dietary ingredient is used.[5] The FDA is responsible for post-marketing activities, including monitoring of adverse events via voluntary reporting and product information (eg, labels, claims, package inserts).[5]

HERBAL COMPONENTS

There are many different chemical constituents in herbal plants that can have therapeutic as well as toxic effects. Herbal supplements may come prepared as tablets/capsules, powders, tinctures, syrups, and brewed teas for oral consumption.[6] Other preparations for topical application include salves, ointments, and shampoos. Parts of the plant that may be used include the flower, leaves, stem, roots, seeds, and berries.[6] Bioflavonoids, one of the major herbal components, include flavonoids that can be found in flowers, citrus fruits, red wine, and tea and are believed to have antioxidant properties.[7] Essential oils give the characteristic odor of the plants and are often referred to as volatile oils or essences.[6,7] They have been used for treating skin and respiratory disorders and in aromatherapy.[7] Glycosides are derived from plant chemicals containing a carbohydrate residue attached to a noncarbohydrate residue. Common glycosides include digoxin (used in allopathic medicine for cardiovascular conditions), anthraquinones (laxatives), and isothiocyanates (alliin in garlic, used for food flavoring and cholesterol-lowering properties).[7] Resins are protective substances secreted by plants that when mixed with volative oils produce oleoresins and when mixed with cinnamic or benzoic acid produce a balsam.[7]

Other components include saponins (soaplike glycosides), which may be used for their mucolytic and expectorant properties, phytosterols (eg, soy), which claim to have antiinflammatory and antioxidant properties, and terpenes, which are the most common phytochemicals and are found in a variety of products including vegetables, soy, and grains.[7] Terpenes are varied in chemical structure and are promoted for their antioxidant properties. **Table 1** lists the various herbal components, examples, sources, and claimed benefits.

PRODUCT QUALITY ASSURANCE

Quality control of herbal supplements within the United States remains largely unregulated. There are no standard governmental regulations that ensure good manufacturing processes and product reliability. Standardization of herbal supplements is challenging because of the chemical complexity of botanicals, which may contain multiple active ingredients, and because of uncertainty about which ingredient is contributing to the therapeutic effect.[8] Laboratory analysis of multiple brands of a herbal supplement can reveal several-fold differences in the concentrations of the active components.[8] A variety of factors can also contribute to differences in the concentrations of the active constituents, including the part of the plant used, growing conditions, timing of harvest, geography and soil conditions, processing methods, and storage conditions.[6,8] Therefore, herbal supplements can vary in chemical composition,

Table 1
Chemical components of herbal supplements

Classification	Chemical	Source	Potential Benefit
Alkaloids			
Imidazole	Ephedrine	Ma Huang	Asthma, weight loss
Indole	Yohimbine	Yohimbe	Aphrodisiac, benign prostate hyperplasia
Purine	Caffeine	Coffee, tea	Stimulant
Bioflavonoids			
Flavonoid	Apigenin	Chamomile	Antiinflammatory
Isoflavonoids	Daidzein	Soy	Estrogenic, menopause
Flavonolignans	Silymarin	Milk thistle	Liver protection
Essential Oils			
Alcohols	Menthol	Mints	Antitussive
Phenols	Capsaicin	Capsicum	Counterirritant
Phenols	Thymol	Thyme	Antibacterial
Glycosides			
Saponins	Glycyrrhizin	Licorice	Peptic ulcer
Anthraquinones	Sennosides	Senna	Laxative
Isothiocyanates	Alliin	Garlic	Cholesterol-lowering
Coumarins	Dicumarol	Sweet clover	Anticoagulant
Resins			
Pure resins		Guaiac	Expectorant
Oleoresins		Turpentine	Expectorant
Balsams		Benzoin	Anesthetic
Saponins			
Steroidal	Digitoxin	Foxglove	Cardiovascular
Terpenoid	Cycloartanes	Black cohosh	Estrogenic
Sterols			
Phytosterol	β-Sitosterol	Soy	Cholesterol-lowering Antiinflammatory Benign prostate hyperplasia
Terpinoids			
Diterpenes	Capsianosides	Capsicum	Counterirritant
Diterpenes	Ginkoglides	Ginkgo	Antiinflammatory
Tetraterpenes	Carotene	Carrot	Antioxidant
Tetraterpenes	Lycopene	Tomato	Anticancer

Data from Chemistry of herbal medications. In: Rotblatt M, Ziment I, editors. Evidence-based herbal medicine. Philadelphia: Hanley & Belfus; 2002. p. 29–44.

concentrations of active ingredients, and overall quality, which give each brand its uniqueness.[8]

Contributing to the complexity of the problem is the potential for contamination or adulteration of herbal supplements. Production and harvesting of plants in contaminated soils or improper processing can lead to contamination, which if these substances are pharmacologically active can contribute to toxicity.[6,8] Contaminants and adulterants that have been found in supplements include heavy metals, bacteria, and fungi.[2,6,9–11] Chinese and Ayurvedic herbal medicines have been associated with contamination by heavy metals, with cases of lead poisoning being reported.[6,11] A review of 319 children in Taipei who tested positive for increased blood lead concentrations found a significant correlation with the use of Chinese herbal medicine (specifically *Ba-baw-san*).[12] Fungal contamination was observed in Croatia when 62 medicinal plant materials and 11 herbal tea samples were analyzed. The most common fungus species isolated included *Aspergillus* and *Penicillium*, with 18% of medicinal plants and 9% of herbal teas containing *Aspergillus flavus*.[13] Herbal supplements have also been found to be adulterated with other substances. In Taiwan, 2609 samples of Chinese medicines were collected over 1 year and analyzed. Of the medicines, 23.7% were found to be adulterated and 52.8% contained more than one adulterant.[14] The most common identified substances included acetaminophen, caffeine, indomethacin, hydrochlorothiazide, and prednisolone.[14] **Table 2** lists some of the contaminants and adulterants identified in herbal supplements.

Misidentification of the plant, whether intentionally or inadvertently, can lead to serious consequences.[10,11] A diet supplement that should have contained the Chinese supplement *Fangji* (*Stephania tetrandra*) may have contained *Fangchi* (*Aristolochia fangchi*), causing individuals in Brussels to develop interstitial nephritis.[15] In Colorado, 3 children who had taken large quantities of the Chinese supplement *Jin Bu Huan* developed bradycardia and respiratory and depression of the central nervous system (CNS). The reaction was attributed to large quantities of levo-tetrahydropalmatine,

Table 2
Contaminants and adulterants found in herbal supplements

Category	Examples
Heavy metals	Lead Aluminum Arsenic Cadmium Mercury
Bacteria	*Staphylococcus aureus* *Salmonella* *Shigella* *Pseudomonas aeruginosa*
Mycoses	*Aspergillus* *Penicillium* *Mucor*
Pesticides and herbicides	Chlorinated pesticides (eg, dichlorodiphenyltrichloroethane, dichlorodiphenyldichloroethylene, hexachlorobenzene) Organic phosphates Carbamate insecticides and herbicides Triazin herbicides
Other agents	Aspirin Caffeine Corticosteroids Diazepam Ephedrine Indomethacin Acetaminophen Theophylline Thiazide diuretics Chlorpheniramine

Data from Refs.[2,9,11]

which is found in the plant genus *Stephania* and not *Polygala* as noted in the package insert.[16] Numerous nomenclature systems of identifying plants contribute to the problem, with multiple names that can identify a single product, including common name, scientific name, foreign name, and brand name.[11]

In 2000, the World Health Organization published a report evaluating 8985 case reports of adverse events associated with herbal supplements from 1968 to 1997.[17] Of these adverse events, ~1% were noted to occur in children up to 9 years old and an additional 1% in those 10 to 19 years old.[17] Toxicity in children can occur because of the active ingredient itself, from contaminants or adulterants, and from interactions between the herbal supplement and other medications.[10] Although there is no standardization and little regulatory oversight of herbal supplements and the potential for contaminants and adulterants exists, there are manufacturers that produce high-quality products. Trying to identify those brands that choose to undergo more rigorous testing to ensure quality can be challenging, and the following recommendations have been put forth. These include use of specific herbal supplements that have shown efficacy in rigorous controlled trials.[8] If clinical trials do not exist, evaluate if the product has undergone independent laboratory quality-control testing.[8] These tests seek to determine if the correct plant has been identified, that there are minimum concentrations of major constituents, and that impurities do not exist.[8] One of the best sources for this is http://www.ConsumerLab.com, which performs product testing and provides supplement reviews and information regarding recalls and warnings; it requires a subscription for access to information.[8]

Additional quality control measures include the use of the United States Pharmacopeia (USP), which has established analytical standards (quality, purity, and potency) for a variety of botanic products.[8,18] Products that meet these standards may include a USP Verified Dietary Supplement symbol on the label.[18] The USP has a list of participating companies and verified products on their Web site (http://www.usp.org) and has also collaborated with the National Medicines Comprehensive Database and http://www.ConsumerReportsHealth.org in identifying USP-verified supplements alongside the drug information. Both of these systems require subscriptions for access to information. Currently all quality-assurance testing that manufacturers use for herbal supplements is on a voluntary basis. The other recommendations include use of herbal supplements that are manufactured by large pharmaceutical companies and researching manufacturers of herbal supplements.[8] For proper evaluation, product labeling should include detailed information regarding ingredients, batch number, expiration date, and manufacturer contact information.[8]

USE WITHIN THE GENERAL PEDIATRIC AND ADOLESCENT POPULATION

Use of CAM therapy continues to gain in popularity, with numerous studies trying to quantify the numbers and types of individuals using CAM therapy. CAM therapy has been well documented in the adult population, and an increasing number of studies have sought to evaluate use within the pediatric population. Studies have been limited by small sample sizes and restriction to a locale or region and specific illnesses. In regards to specific illnesses, CAM use has been reported in patients with cystic fibrosis, juvenile rheumatoid arthritis, cancer, and asthma, with rates ranging from 46% to 70%.[19]

One of the first national studies involved a cross-sectional analysis of the 1996 Medical Expenditure Panel Survey, which is a subsample of the 1995 National Health Interview Survey.[20] Of the 7371 children evaluated (age≤21 years), 2% reported having visited a CAM provider during the previous year, with only 12.3% reporting CAM use to their allopathic provider.[20] Herbal therapies were the most common office-based therapy provided (22.4%), followed by spiritual healing/prayer (19.4%), homeopathic treatments (14.1%), and massage therapy (13.2%).[20] The variable most highly associated with a child visiting a CAM provider was parents who visited a CAM provider. This study likely underestimates pediatric CAM use because there is no evaluation of self-administered CAM therapy and it relies on parental report.

A prevalence study in 1999 evaluated the use of CAM therapy within a pediatric emergency department. Of the 525 questionnaires returned, 10.9% of the families reported using one form of CAM therapy for their child.[19] Of those taking a herbal or homeopathic medicine, 40% reported using a prescription or over-the-counter product concurrently, 70.9% had informed their physician regarding the use of CAM therapy and only 35.8% noted that their physician had discussed the use of CAM therapy for treatment.[19] Limitations to this study include ~one-third of questionnaires were never returned, not all surveys were fully completed, the caregiver report was not reliable, and the study was limited to a single locale. Another survey in 2001 within an urban pediatric emergency department also sought to evaluate caregiver understanding and sources of information for herbal therapy in addition to patient use. Of the 142 families interviewed, 45% of caregivers noted use of herbal therapy within the past year.[21] Within the previous 3 months, 61% had used a herbal supplement in conjunction with a prescription medication.[21] Of all the caregivers interviewed, 77% did not believe that herbal supplements had side effects, or did not know if they had side effects, and 66% did not know if herbal supplements interacted with traditional medicines or believed that they did not interact with traditional medicines.[21] Of those who provided supplements to their children, 80% received their information from family and friends, and only 45% reported use to their primary care provider.[21] Although this study is limited by a small sample size and single location, it shows the prevalence of herbal use within the pediatric population and lack of knowledge on behalf of the caregivers, with underreporting to their primary care providers.

Unlike most of the other surveys, one performed in 2002 sought to evaluate CAM and use of dietary supplements within adolescents by self-report. Respondents were drawn from a national sample and included 1280 adolescents aged 14 to 19 years.[22] The study was conducted using an online self-administered survey, with incentives provided for completing the surveys. Of those surveyed, 46.2% reported using dietary supplements at least once in their lifetime, and 29.1% reported use within the past month.[22] The most common supplements for current users included zinc, echinacea, ginseng, herbal or green tea, *Gingko biloba*, and creatine.[22] Over their lifetime, 10.7% of the respondents had tried weight-loss supplements.[22] Higher prevalence was noted in female respondents, and similar to previous studies, CAM use by adolescents was associated with parental use.[22] This study indicates that adolescents are beginning to take an active role in their own health care and providers need to inquire about CAM use as well as provide education regarding risks and benefits.

The most recent national survey was conducted as part of the 2007 National Health Interview Survey. The survey had expanded from the 2002 survey to include data regarding CAM use in children aged 0 to 17 years, and expanded the types of CAM therapy as well as the list of supplement products listed.[23] Of the 9417 completed interviews of children, 3.9% reported use of supplements within the past 12 months.[23] CAM therapies were most often used for musculoskeletal pain, colds, anxiety or stress, and attention-deficit/hyperactivity disorder (ADHD)/attention-deficit disorder.[23] CAM use was more common among adolescents aged 12 to 17 years and White children, and increased with parental educational level.[23] CAM use had a positive correlation with the number of health conditions and health provider visits within the previous

12 months as well as parental use of CAM therapy.[23] CAM therapy was also more common when conventional care was unaffordable or worry about cost delayed conventional medical care.[23]

Unlike the other surveys, one study in 1997 sought out pediatricians' views regarding CAM therapy, whether patients used or discussed CAM therapy, personal use, and referral practices for CAM therapy. Surveys were sent to fellows of the Michigan article of the American Academy of Pediatrics, and 348 were completed (40.5% response rate).[24] Within the sample, 83.5% believed that their patients were using one form of CAM therapy but this comprised less than 10% of all their patients.[24] Fifty-three percent of the respondents reported talking about CAM therapy with their patients but most was initiated by patients and families (84.7%).[24] More than three-fourths (76.1%) believed that patients self-reported CAM use.[24] With regards to personal use, only 37% used any type of CAM therapy, and referrals were most often for relaxation (56%), self-help groups (54.3%), acupuncture (51.1%), hypnosis (50.3%), biofeedback (49.1%), and massage therapy (46.3%).[24]

The data from the various studies and surveys indicate that pediatric patients do use CAM therapy and that this has been strongly correlated with parental use of CAM therapy. Communication between patient and provider is often lacking, with patients underreporting use and providers not inquiring about patient use of such therapy. Family and friends often serve as a source of information for CAM therapy, and many providers may feel uncomfortable discussing alternative therapy. Education is a critical component for both patients and providers in promoting safe and effective use of CAM therapy.

HERBAL SUPPLEMENTS AND NEUROPSYCHIATRIC DISORDERS

It is not uncommon for patients to look to complementary therapy for the treatment of headaches, insomnia, depression, anxiety, and fatigue.[25] Many supplements are promoted for treating these symptoms and patients may often self-treat before seeking professional treatment. As seen in the general population, a few surveys indicate that pediatric patients with neuropsychiatric disorders also turn to complementary therapy for treating a variety of ailments, including the primary neuropsychiatric disorder.

A survey of adolescents with ADHD or depression in 5 community mental health centers in Texas found that 15% of the patients had taken herbal supplements within the past year.[26] Herbal supplements were most commonly used to treat the behavior problem and included Gingko biloba, echinacea, and St John's wort.[26] Most patients did not discuss therapy with their health care providers. A cross-sectional survey was administered to caregivers of patients seen in neurodevelopmental pediatrics clinic in Hong Kong.[27] Of the patients with autism spectrum disorder (ASD), 40.8% of patients had used CAM therapy in the past year, with acupuncture as the most common (47.5%) followed by sensory integration (42.5%) and Chinese medicine (30%).[27] Over three-fourths of those interviewed believed that CAM therapy augmented traditional medicine.[27]

There are limited studies documenting CAM therapy in pediatric patients with neuropsychiatric disorders and even fewer studies evaluating herbal supplement use in treating these disorders.[28] The following section reviews the most common herbal supplements (including St John's wort, melatonin, valerian, kava, eicosapentaenoic acid [EPA]/docosahexaenoic acid [DHA], and those for weight loss) used within this patient population and briefly discusses the limited literature evaluating their use within the pediatric population.

ST JOHN'S WORT

St John's wort is likely the most heavily researched supplement, with the major focus on the treatment of depression. Other indications in which St John's wort has been proposed to be beneficial but that lack sufficient supporting evidence include anxiety, obsessive-compulsive disorder (OCD), and seasonal affective disorder (SAD).[29] The primary active ingredients of St John's wort include naphthodianthrones (eg, hypericin), phloroglucinols (eg, hyperforin), flavonoids (eg, quercetin), proanthocyanidins (eg, catechin), and essential oils.[30] Most products are standardized to include hypericin at concentrations of 0.1% to 0.4% and hyperforin at 2% to 4%.[31]

The exact mechanism of St John's wort remains to be elucidated but it is believed to inhibit the reuptake of dopamine, serotonin, and norepinephrine.[31,32] Hypericin has been shown to inhibit monoamine oxidase (MAO) in vitro, but in vivo it does not reach sufficiently high concentrations to show an effect.[29,30] Studies of St John's wort in pediatric patients have been limited by study design, small sample sizes, and short duration. Simeon and colleagues[33] evaluated St John's wort (300 mg 3 times daily) in 26 adolescents with major depressive disorder for 8 weeks in an open-label pilot study. Eleven patients completed the study and 82% of those showed clinically beneficial effects based on clinical global improvement change.[33] Seven of the 15 who withdrew had persistent or worsening depression.[33] A study by Findling and colleagues[34] evaluated the use of St John's wort in 33 children aged 6 to 16 years in an open-label design for 8 weeks. The initial dose was 150 mg 3 times daily and could be titrated up to 300 mg 3 times daily.[34] Using the Children's Depression Rating Scale (CDRS), 76% of the patients clinically improved and 93% continued therapy at the end of the study.[34]

St John's wort has been fairly well tolerated in clinical studies, with the most common side effects reported as mild, including restlessness, insomnia, gastrointestinal (GI) upset, headache, fatigue, and dry mouth.[32,33] Hypericin is believed to contribute to a photosensitivity reaction that has been observed with higher than usual doses of St John's wort (2–4 g/d).[29] Individuals with light or fair skin should use protective measures with sun exposure.[29]

Drug interactions continue to be a limitation to the use of St John's wort. St John's wort has been shown to induce the metabolism of drugs metabolized by cytochrome (CYP) 3A4, 1A2, and 2C9 and can result in reduced drug concentrations. Examples of drugs affected include oral contraceptives, cyclosporine, warfarin, tacrolimus, and protease inhibitors.[29–31,35,36] In addition, St John's wort has been found to induce the intestinal P-glycoprotein transporter, which can result in decreased absorption of the drug. Some examples of drugs potentially affected include digoxin, antifungals (eg, ketoconazole, itraconazole), corticosteroids, and erythromycin.[29,30]

Because St John's wort increases serotonin, the risk of serotonin syndrome exists when combined with other agents that also increase serotonin.[29,30,35,37] Agents that should be avoided because of the potential risks include tricyclic antidepressants (TCAs), selective serotonin reuptake inhibitors (SSRIs), serotonin-norepinephrine reuptake inhibitors, tramadol, dextromethorphan, 5-HT$_1$ agonists (eg, sumatriptan), MAO inhibitors, and meperidine.[29,35] As seen with other antidepressants, St John's wort may take several weeks to determine the full clinical effect and may induce a withdrawal syndrome on sudden discontinuation.[30,31] Withdrawal symptoms may include GI upset, dizziness, confusion, insomnia, and fatigue.[30] To avoid these symptoms, patients should gradually taper the dose before discontinuation. **Table 3** gives a summary regarding St John's wort.

Table 3
Supplement information: St John's wort and melatonin

	St John's Wort	Melatonin
Scientific Name	*Hypericum perforatum*	*N*-Acetyl-5-methoxytryptamine
Active components	Hypericin Hyperforin	Melatonin
Possible indications	Depression Anxiety ADHD OCD SAD	Insomnia Circadian rhythm disorder Benzodiazepine and nicotine withdrawal Cancer

Mechanism of action	May inhibit reuptake of serotonin,
	  dopamine, and norepinephrine
	Inhibits GABA uptake
		Increase binding of GABA to
		  receptors

Dosage	300 mg daily	0.3–9 mg daily
Adverse effects	Insomnia Vivid dreams Restlessness Agitation GI upset Dizziness Headache Photodermatitis Paresthesias Serotonin syndrome	Nausea Headache Dizziness Fatigue

Drug interactions	Induces CYP 450 3A4, 2C9, and 1A2
	Induces *P*-glycoprotein/multidrug
	  resistance 1 (MDR-1) drug
	  transporter
		Substrate for CYP 1A2

Additional comments	Most supplements standardized to
	  contain 0.3% hypericin
	Increased risk of photosensitivity
	  with doses ≥2 gm/d (extract)
	Avoid abrupt discontinuation
	  because of risk of withdrawal
	  effects
	Avoid use with other agents that
	  increase serotonin (eg, SSRIs,
	  TCAs, tramadol,
	  dextromethorphan)
		Use synthetic preparations to
		  avoid risk of contamination with
		  animal-based products
		Avoid use in patients with immune
		  dysfunction or taking
		  immunosuppressive agents
		Start with 0.3–1 mg and titrate
		  accordingly

Data from Refs.[29–33,35–41]

Although St John's wort is one of the most commonly prescribed antidepressants in Germany, its use has been banned in France because of the potential for significant drug interactions.[29,31] St John's wort provides an alternative for treating depression in children and adolescents but still requires more well-designed studies to evaluate its benefits within the pediatric population. The side-effect profile and the potential for significant drug interactions should be considered before its initiation, and abrupt discontinuation should be avoided.

MELATONIN

Endogenous melatonin is secreted by the pineal gland, along with other organs, to maintain a normal circadian rhythm.[38] Production is regulated via a complex pathway, with stimulation occurring during periods of darkness and peak serum levels occurring before bedtime.[38] Because of its ability to regulate the circadian rhythm, melatonin has been evaluated for a variety of conditions, including jet lag, night-shift work, and neuropsychiatric disorders.[38] Melatonin is also believed to have immunomodulatory and antioxidant effects as well as antiproliferative properties.[38]

Melatonin is believed to exert its sedating effect by increasing binding of γ-aminobutyric acid (GABA) to its receptors.[38,39] Melatonin is rapidly absorbed on administration and undergoes extensive hepatic metabolism with a high first-pass effect.[40] Bioavailability of exogenous melatonin is poor (10%–56%) and has a short half-life of 12 to 48 minutes.[38] Evidence suggests that primary metabolism occurs via CYP1A2 and drugs that inhibit this isoenzyme (eg, fluvoxamine, cimetidine, ciprofloxacin) can lead to increased levels of melatonin.[38,39] Additional drug interactions include the potentiation of warfarin (mechanism unknown) and decreased production of endogenous melatonin by nonsteroidal antiinflammatory drugs.[38,39]

Melatonin is fairly well tolerated, with the most common side effects reported as fatigue, headache, dizziness, and nausea.[40,41] Melatonin lacks the hangover effect seen with other medications used to treat insomnia. Caution should be exercised when using melatonin in certain patient populations. Because of the immunostimulatory effects of melatonin, its use should be avoided in patients with immune dysfunction or who are taking immunosuppressive agents.[41] Exogenous melatonin is known to affect several hormones, including prolactin, progesterone, and estradiol, and high doses have been shown to inhibit ovarian function.[38,41] Use in patients with epilepsy has been controversial. A series of 6 patients with severe neurologic deficits received melatonin 5 mg nightly.[42] Five patients subsequently developed new or increased seizure activity, with return to baseline on discontinuation.[42] Three children were rechallenged with lower doses, and increased seizure activity was again noted.[42] In contrast, 6 children with severe intractable seizures received melatonin 3 mg nightly to evaluate its antiepileptic effects in addition to their current antiepileptic therapy.[43] Five of the 6 parents noted clinical improvement, and 2 of the 3 evaluated by polysomnography noted decreases in seizure activity.[43] Because of the conflicting data and lack of controlled clinical trials evaluating its use in this patient population, caution should be exercised and patients monitored appropriately.

Melatonin has been evaluated in children with primary and secondary sleep disorders. A meta-analysis by Buscemi and colleagues[44] included 2 studies that evaluated the use of melatonin in children with chronic idiopathic sleep-onset insomnia. Melatonin 5 mg nightly was found to significantly reduced sleep-onset latency compared with placebo (difference: 16.7 minutes).[40,44] Melatonin has also shown efficacy in treating insomnia in patients with developmental disabilities, ASD, and ADHD with or without concomitant stimulant medication.[40,45,46] Phillips and Appleton[45] performed a systematic review of exogenous melatonin in children with neurodevelopmental disabilities and sleep impairment. Only 3 randomized, double-blind, placebo-controlled studies were identified, which included a total of 35 children. The dosage of melatonin ranged from 0.5 to 7.5 mg daily across the 3 studies.[45] Overall, sleep latency was significantly reduced in 2 studies and not reported in the third study.[45] Total sleep time was increased in 4 of 6 patients in one study, with minimal effect in the other 2 studies, and no study reported an improvement in nighttime awakenings.[45] Bendz and Scates[46] performed a literature review and identified 4 studies evaluating exogenous melatonin in pediatric patients with ADHD. One open-label and 2 randomized, double-blind, placebo-controlled trials (sample size 24–105 patients each) found melatonin (3–6 mg daily) significantly reduced sleep latency, and one trial found an improvement in total sleep time.[46] Two of the 3 trials evaluated patients taking concurrent stimulant medications. The last trial was a follow-up to one of the previous trials and evaluated 94 stimulant-free patients who used melatonin (average 4 mg daily) for a mean duration of 18 months. Parent survey results noted a 90% efficacy for sleep-onset insomnia, 71% efficacy for behavior, and 61% efficacy for mood.[46] Studies evaluating melatonin have noted benefit, most significantly for a reduction in sleep onset but have been limited by small sample sizes, differing doses, and varying methodology.

Melatonin comes in a variety of formulations, including capsules, tablets, and liquid as well as immediate- and sustained-released products. Dosing guidelines have not been established within the pediatric population but if used, should begin with 0.3 to 1 mg and should be titrated accordingly.[41] Recommendations for administration have ranged from 30 minutes up to 1 to 2 hours before bedtime. Patients should use synthetic formulations and avoid products produced from animal pineal gland to avoid the risk of contamination.[39] See **Table 3** for an information summary.

VALERIAN

Valeriana officinalis is the most common species of the genus *Valeriana* that is used for medicinal properties.[47] The root of the plant has been used for centuries for its purported benefits as an anxiolytic and sedative hypnotic. Valerian is also considered to have antispasmodic, anticonvulsant, and antidepressant effects.[47] Volative oils and valepotriates may be the major components that contribute to the pharmacologic effects of valerian.[47] Volative oils contain monoterpenes and sesquiterpenes (eg, valerenic acid) as well as giving valerian its characteristic odor.[47–49] Valepotriates are unstable compounds and are quickly hydrolyzed in aqueous environments.[41,47] Concern has been raised about the potential for cytotoxic and carcinogenic effects of valerian because many valepotriates have epoxide groups that can alkylate DNA.[41] Although shown in vitro, these effects are unlikely to occur in vivo because of instability, minimal concentrations in marketed products, and poor absorption.[41,48] The effects of valerian are believed to be mediated via an interaction with GABA receptors and are unlikely to occur from one single component.[47–50] Other factors that can influence the effects of valerian and concentrations of active ingredients include species used, growing conditions of the plant, age of the herb, and method of extraction.[41,49]

The sedative and anxiolytic effects of valerian have been more extensively evaluated in adults than in pediatric patients. Most adult studies have used a valerian extract of 400 to 900 mg daily given 30 to 60 minutes before bedtime for the treatment of insomnia.[49] Most but not all studies have shown a mild hypnotic effect, with a reduction in sleep latency and an overall improvement in sleep quality.[41] A polysomnography study by Donath and colleagues[51] evaluated valerian extract in 16 adult patients with insomnia. Patients were randomized to receive valerian extract 600 mg or placebo nightly and were evaluated after a single dose and after 14 days.[51] Polysomnography results found no significant benefit after a single dose but after 14 days found a reduction in sleep latency (placebo 60 minutes vs valerian 45 minutes), onset to slow-wave sleep (SWS), and an increase in the duration of SWS.[51]

Only 2 studies have been conducted in pediatric patients: one evaluated its use for restlessness and dyssomnia, and the other for insomnia in children with intellectual deficits. For the treatment of restlessness and dyssomnia, 918 children (age<12 years) were given a combination product containing valerian and lemon balm.[52] The study was an open-label, multicenter trial, and each patient received 2 tablets twice daily for 30 days (each tablet contained 160 mg dried valerian root extract and 80 mg of lemon balm).[52] Analysis of the questionnaires revealed that symptoms changed from "moderate" and "severe" (66% at baseline) to "absent" and "mild" in 75% of those with restlessness at 4 weeks of treatment.[52] In those patients with dyssomnia, symptoms changed from "moderate" and "severe" (77.1% at baseline) to "absent" and "mild" in 76.6% of patients at the end of the study.[52] Investigators judged the tolerability to be "good" or "very good" in 96.7% of patients.[52] Overall, 157 discontinued treatment early, with the most frequent reasons cited as treatment no longer needed and parent's request.[52] The second study evaluated the effects of valerian in 5 children (aged 7–14 years) with intellectual difficulties (IQ<70) and sleep problems in a double-blind, cross-over fashion.[53] The children received valerian (dried and crushed whole root of *Valeriana edulis*) 20 mg/kg each night 1 hour before bedtime.[53] Sleep outcomes were measured at the end of each 2-week treatment period using diaries maintained by the parents. Valerian was found to significantly reduce time spent awake during the night, increase total sleep time, and improve parent-rated sleep quality.[53] Studies assessing valerian suffer from the same issues seen with other herbal supplements, including a variety of formulations and dosages, small sample sizes, varying methodology, and short duration.

Overall, valerian seems to be fairly well tolerated, with minimal side effects. Those side effects rarely reported include headache, GI discomfort, contact allergies, and vivid dreams.[49,54] Valerian does not seem to produce a hangover effect, as noted in one study of 91 patients comparing placebo and valerian 600 mg each evening after 2 weeks of treatment.[55] Four cases of acute hepatitis have been reported with valerian. Four women from England had been taking a herbal supplement believed to contain valerian and skullcap.[56] Each patient subsequently discontinued treatment, and tests of liver function eventually showed a return to normal.[56] Confirmation of ingredients in the 2 supplement products and evaluation for contaminants was not ascertained. No drug interactions with valerian have been noted in clinical trials.[47,48] Because of the sedative properties, theoretically patients should use caution or avoid other CNS depressants.[47,48]

Valerian is available in a variety of formulations, including tablets, capsules, liquid, teas, and tinctures. Products may contain whole herb and/or a proprietary blend or may also be combined with other herbal supplements (eg, lemon balm, hops, skullcap, kava, St John's wort). Some commercial products are standardized according to the content of valerenic acid but concentrations vary among products. **Table 4** gives an information summary.

Although evidence suggests some benefit in treating insomnia, conflicting data in the adult population and minimal studies in pediatrics warrant further investigation. Studies evaluating the benefit of valerian in treating anxiety are limited and need to be more clearly elucidated.

KAVA

Kava originates from the South Pacific Islands and is derived from the roots, rhizomes, and root stems of the shrub *Piper methysticum*.[57] In the South Pacific Islands it is used culturally as a social beverage as well as in ceremonial rituals.[57,58] It also has medicinal implications, which include treating anxiety, insomnia, premenstrual syndrome, and stress.[49] Kava is comprised of kavalactones (also known as kavapyrones), which are considered the pharmacologically active components. A variety of kavalactones exist, with most effect attributed to kavain (kawain), 5,6-dihydrokavain, methysticin, dihydromethysticin, yangonin, and desmethoxyyangonin.[58] Concentrations of kavalactones

Table 4
Supplement information: valerian and kava

	Valerian	Kava
Scientific Name	*Valeriana officinalis*	*Piper methysticum*
Active components	Monoterpenes Sesquiterpenes (valerenic acid) Valepotriates	Kavalactones: Kavain 5,6-Dihydrokavain Methysticin Dihydromethysticin Yangonin Desmethoxyyangonin
Possible indications	Insomnia Dyssomnia Anxiety Epilepsy Depression	Anxiety Insomnia Stress Premenstrual syndrome
Mechanism of action	Interaction with GABA receptors	Blockade of voltage-gated sodium channels Enhance GABA transmission

Dosage	Adult: 400–900 mg at bedtime
	Pediatric: 20 mg/kg at bedtime
	   (based on one study: see text)
		Adult: 70 mg (kavalactones)
		   3 times daily (most common
		   in Europe)

Adverse effects	Headache GI distress Contact allergies Vivid dreams	Headache Sedation GI upset Restlessness Tremor Allergic reactions Hepatotoxicity Kava dermopathy Extrapyramidal symptoms

Drug interactions	Avoid use with CNS depressants
	   and alcohol
		Potential inhibitor of CYP P-450
		Avoid use with dopamine-
		   blocking agents
		Avoid concurrent use with CNS
		   depressants and alcohol

Additional comments	Available in a wide variety of
	   formulations, dosages, and
	   combination products
	Commercial products may be
	   standardized to valerenic acid
		Use products with concentrations
		   standardized to kavalactones
		Avoid use in patients with
		   preexisting liver disease or at risk

Data from Refs.[47–50,53,54,58–64]

can vary considerably among the subspecies of kava as well as within the same subspecies.[57]

Kava is most widely used and evaluated for the treatment of anxiety. Its anxiolytic and sedative effects are believed to be caused by blockade of voltage-gated sodium channels and enhancement of GABA transmission.[58] Kavalactones have also been shown in vitro to inhibit MAO type B and block the reuptake of norepinephrine.[58] Multiple studies have assessed the effects of kava in treating anxiety, with no reported studies occurring in the pediatric/adolescent population. A Cochrane review of kava in treating anxiety was updated in 2010 and included 12 studies, with 7 of the studies included in the meta-analysis.[59] The 7 trials were randomized, double-blind, placebo-controlled clinical trials that used the Hamilton Anxiety Scale (HAM-A) to assess efficacy in treating anxiety.[59] A total of 380 patients were evaluated, with 6 of the studies occurring in Germany, and duration ranged from 4 to 24 weeks.[59] All except one trial used the same preparation, and dosages among the trials ranged from 105 mg to 280 mg kavalactones daily.[59] Results indicated a statistically significant reduction in HAM-A scores with kava compared with placebo, with a small effect size.[59] The other 5 studies not included in the meta-analysis found similar results. Six trials reported minor side effects, with no cases of hepatotoxicity noted.[59]

The most common side effects seen are mild and include GI upset, sedation, restlessness, headache, tremor, fatigue, and allergic reactions.[59,60] More concerning are the rare but potentially life-threatening reports of hepatotoxicity. Cases of hepatotoxicity, with most reports occurring in Europe, have ranged from increases found in liver-function tests and jaundice to severe hepatitis and liver necrosis, necessitating the need for liver transplantation.[58] At least 11 cases of liver failure requiring transplantation have been documented, with doses ranging from 60 to 240 mg of kavalactones daily. Most patients used kava that was prepared from either alcohol or acetone extraction.[60,61] Causality was not established in all cases because of concurrent use of other hepatotoxic medications and incomplete data. The FDA issued an advisory in March 2002 warning practitioners and consumers about the risk of hepatotoxicity associated with kava.[49,61] Additional countries at that time also issued advisories or suspended sales of kava products.[58] Given the risk for hepatic injury, it is recommended that patients with liver disease or at risk for liver disease avoid using kava-containing products.[49,61]

Kava dermopathy has been seen with higher than normal doses for prolonged periods.[57,62] The syndrome is characterized by a yellow discoloration of the skin, bloodshot eyes, and a scaly dermatitis that can be seen on the palms, soles of the feet, forearms, shins, and back.[57,62] Symptoms resolve with discontinuation of the kava-containing product.[57,62] Dyskinesias have been reported in 4 patients, including one patient with Parkinson disease who consumed kava.[60,63] Onset of symptoms ranged from 90 minutes after an initial dose to after 10 days of continual use, with symptom improvement after discontinuation of kava or initiation of biperiden.[60,63] Because of the potential ability of kava to antagonize dopamine, patients susceptible to extrapyramidal side effects or on dopamine-blocking medications should avoid using kava.[62]

There is the potential for drug interactions with kava because of its ability to inhibit CYP P-450 isoenzymes but there is limited clinical evidence.[62,64] Caution should be exercised if kava is used in conjunction with other medications or supplements. Patients should also avoid combining kava with alcohol or other CNS depressants because of the risk for additive effects.[62]

Because of variations in kavalactones among and within kava subspecies, products standardized to a kavalactone concentration are recommended over those containing raw ingredients.[57] Typical dosing in European studies was 70 mg 3 times daily, and the most common formulation used was standardized to 70% kavalactones.[62] Within the United States, most commercial kava products are standardized to 30% to 55% kavalactones and are available in capsule, tablet, and liquid formulation.[62] See **Table 4** for an information summary.

Clinical trials support a mild anxiolytic effect of kava within adults and most patients experience only minor side effects. There are no data within the pediatric population, and the potential for hepatotoxicity precludes the use of kava in pediatrics and adolescents. See **Table 4** for a summary.

DHA AND EPA

Omega-3 fatty acids (DHA and EPA) have been evaluated in several pediatric diseases, including asthma, Crohn disease, and eczema as well as ADHD, ASD, dyslexia, and juvenile bipolar disorder (JBD).[65,66] Omega-3 fatty acids (also referred to as long-chain polyunsaturated fatty acids) can be derived from their precursor α-lineolic acid (ALA) within the human body, but this process is not efficient.[65] ALA can be derived from plant sources, including green vegetables and some nuts, whereas omega-3 fatty acids are derived from fish and seafood.[67,68] Conversion of ALA to DHA and EPA from food sources is also insufficient, and therefore marine life is the primary source.[65,67] The Western diet has seen a shift, with a higher intake in lineolic acid and its derivative, omega-6 fatty acids, which are obtained from vegetable oils.[68] Omega-6 fatty acids are believed to have proinflammatory effects, whereas EPA and DHA are considered antiinflammatory.[65]

Omega-3 fatty acids are considered to be an essential component in brain development. DHA is an integral structural component of cell membranes, including neurons, and is found in phospholipids.[65] EPA is integrated into cholesterol esters, phospholipids, and triglycerides.[65] These essential fatty acids (EFAs) are considered important in regulating eicosanoids (EFA metabolites), which are involved in a wide array of activities, including vasodilation/vasoconstriction, inflammation, platelet aggregation, and adhesion.[67] EFAs are also considered important in regulating gene expression, affecting signaling pathways and synapse and nerve growth.[67] Neuropsychiatric disorders have been associated with abnormalities in cell membrane fatty acid content. Using red blood cell membranes as a substitute for brain cell membranes, a decrease in omega-3 fatty acids or an increase in omega-6 to omega-3 fatty acids ratio has been shown in patients with depression, bipolar disorder, schizophrenia, ADHD, and ASD.[68,69] In theory, the alteration in phospholipid content may alter neurotransmitter function, increasing the risk for neuropsychiatric disorders.[68] Physical signs associated with low EFA include increased thirst and urination and rough, dry skin and hair.[68] These symptoms have been reported in children with ADHD, dyslexia, and ASD, and studies in children with ADHD have suggested that physical signs correlated with low blood EFA concentrations.[68] There are no established guidelines as to what is considered normal EFA blood levels, and even though supplementation in trials has resulted in an increase in EFA blood levels, supplementation does not always correlate to clinical improvement.[68,69]

Most of the data using omega-3 fatty acids in pediatric neuropsychiatric disorders have been in children with ADHD. Several reviews have been published evaluating the efficacy of omega-3 fatty acids in ADHD; please refer to these studies for more detailed information than can be provided in this article.[65–68] Open-label trials have found omega-3 fatty acids to improve the behavioral aspects of ADHD as well as increase plasma EFA levels.[67] One of the trials included is the only one to use a weight-based approach (2.5g/d per 10 kg), whereas the others used a variety of formulations and varying concentrations of EPA and DHA.[66,67] The studies were also limited by small sample sizes, short duration, and lack of placebo effect. On the other hand, randomized, controlled clinical trials have produced mixed results. Overall, studies have had difficulty in substantiating an effect of omega-3 fatty acids in treating ADHD. Sample sizes were small (18–117 children) and treatment duration was short (4–18 weeks).[65–67] A variety of formulations and doses (including ratio of EPA and DHA) were used, and those studies evaluating only DHA failed to provide any benefit.[65–67] Studies also varied in their outcome measures, and benefit in more than one domain was not always found (eg, parent and teacher assessments).[65–67]

Studies that did show a benefit for omega-3 were studies that included children without a diagnosis of ADHD or who had symptoms of ADHD without a confirmed diagnosis.[65–67] Failure to find an overall benefit is limited by the varying methodologies, as noted earlier, as well as by high dropout rates in some studies.

One randomized, controlled trial assessed the efficacy of omega-3 fatty acids (400 mg EPA and 200 mg DHA daily) in treating a first episode of depression in children.[69] Twenty-eight children were randomized, with 20 completing at least 1 month of analysis.[69] A 50% reduction in the CDRS was seen in 7 of 10 children receiving active treatment compared with 0 of 10 in the placebo group.[69] Clinical global impression was also found to be significant for the group who received omega-3 fatty acids.[69] Two open-label trials have evaluated the benefit of omega-3 fatty acids in JBD. One trial evaluated the use of 360 mg EPA and 1560 mg DHA daily for 6 weeks in 18 patients.[70] Patients continued concomitant psychotropic medications throughout the study. Clinician rating of mania and depression significantly improved, and global functioning increased with treatment; 3 patients withdrew because of adverse effects.[70] Improvement in mania symptoms was believed to be clinically modest compared with the improvement in depressive symptoms.[70] The second study evaluated omega-3 fatty acids (1290–4300 mg/d EPA and DHA) in 20 children with JBD naive to therapy for 8 weeks.[71] A significant reduction in mania and depressive symptoms was seen but patients continued to have residual symptoms.[71] Four patients dropped out because of lack of efficacy.[71] These 2 studies provide the impetus for better-designed studies to evaluate the benefit of omega-3 fatty acids in JBD.

Two studies have been conducted in children with ASD and one study in children with dyslexia. The open-label trial evaluated omega-3 fatty acids in 9 children for 6 months.[65] An improvement was seen for general health, sleep patterns, cognition, concentration, and behavioral symptoms.[65] A randomized, controlled trial in 13 children evaluated 840 mg EPA and 700 mg DHA daily for 6 weeks.[65,66] No significant benefit was found for the active treatment.[65,66] The only study in dyslexia is an open-label trial evaluating 108 mg EPA and 480 mg DHA daily for 20 weeks.[66] An improvement was seen for reading speed, general schoolwork, and subjective evaluations completed by the parent and child.[66] Further studies are required to further elucidate the effect of omega-3 fatty acids in these conditions.

Overall, omega-3 fatty acids are fairly well tolerated. Common side effects include nausea, diarrhea, heartburn, belching, and flatulence.[72,73] Omega-3 fatty acids are also associated with a strong fishlike aftertaste.[72,73] These adverse effects can contribute to lack of adherence with therapy. Omega-3 fatty acids can interfere with platelet activation and can increase the risk for bleeding when given at high doses.[65,72,73] Patients receiving concomitant anticoagulants or antiplatelet therapy, as well as those with hematologic disorders, should use caution.[72,73]

Although omega-3 fatty acids are fairly well tolerated and have few drug/disease interactions, limited evidence exists (as shown by well-designed controlled clinical trials) regarding their efficacy in several neuropsychiatric disorders. Studies have been affected by the same limitations as discussed earlier with other herbal supplements. In addition, the varying ratios of EPA and DHA as well as high dropout rates in some studies provide additional limitations when evaluating the benefits of omega-3 fatty acids.

HERBAL SUPPLEMENTS FOR WEIGHT LOSS

A variety of herbal supplements exist for the treatment of obesity but no clinical trials have been performed in children or adolescents. **Table 5** lists supplements and

Table 5
Herbal supplements for weight loss

Herbal Supplement	Mechanism of Action	Common Side Effects
Guarana/caffeine	Stimulant	Insomnia Nervousness Restlessness Tachycardia Nausea/vomiting Headache
Citrus aurantium (bitter orange)	Stimulant	Tachycardia Headache Hypertension Photosensitivity Cardiovascular events
Chromium picolinate	Insulin sensitizer Stimulate thermogenesis Decrease insulin release	Headache Insomnia Irritability Mood changes
Garcinia cambogia (brindleberry)	Increase lipid oxidation Decrease carbohydrate use	Nausea GI upset Headache
Chitosan	Decrease absorption of dietary fats	Stomach upset Nausea Flatulence Constipation Increase stool bulk
Pyruvate	Increase fat oxidation	GI upset
Gingko biloba	Decrease glucocorticoid synthesis Antistress Neuroprotective	Stomach upset Headache Dizziness Palpitations Constipation Allergic skin reactions Spontaneous bleeding

Data from Refs.[75–81]

possible mechanisms of action. Many herbal supplements formerly contained ephedrine but because of its adverse effect profile, including sudden death, the FDA banned its use in 2004.[74] Since then, Citrus aurantium has been substituted for ephedrine because of its stimulant properties (α-adrenergic agonist) and/or caffeine, which can be derived from guarana, green tea, or the cola nut.[75] Many herbal products contain multiple ingredients, which increases the risk for toxicity as well as drug interactions. Herbal supplements should generally be avoided in the pediatric and adolescent population because of the risk of toxicity and lack of evidence for use.

SUMMARY

Complementary medicine, including the use of herbal supplements, continues to grow even within the pediatric population. The ease of use associated with supplements, including access and self-administration, patients' perceptions that herbals are safe, and consumer advertising, has led to an increased use in herbal supplements for prevention as well as treatment of chronic diseases. Parental use of CAM therapy is often associated with CAM use in pediatric patients, as noted in survey studies. Herbal supplements are not regulated by the FDA and it is up to the manufacturers to ensure safety and appropriate product labeling. Herbal supplements have been found to have been adulterated with medications, heavy metals, and bacteria/fungi. Manufacturers have the ability to undergo quality-assurance testing and it is recommended to use products from manufacturers who undergo this process. Herbal supplements have been evaluated for several pediatric neuropsychiatric diseases but the evaluation of data is limited because of methodological differences, small sample sizes, short duration, differences in dosage and formulation, and differences in outcome measures. Despite limited supporting evidence, it is likely that use will continue to increase. Because of increasing popularity and the potential for toxicity and drug interactions, practitioners should be knowledgeable regarding herbal supplements and inquire about patients' use to provide the most meaningful discussions.

REFERENCES

1. National Center for Complementary and Alternative Medicine. What is complementary and alternative medicine? Available at: http://nccam.nih.gov/health/whatiscam/. Accessed June 26, 2010.
2. Breuner C. Alternative and complementary therapies. Adolesc Med 2006;17: 521–46.
3. National Center for Complementary and Alternative Medicine. NCCAM Facts at a glance and mission. Available at: http://nccam.nih.gov/about/ataglance/. Accessed June 26, 2010.
4. Herbal practices in the US. In: Rotblatt M, Ziment I, editors. Evidence-based herbal medicine. Philadelphia: Hanley & Belfus; 2002. p. 6–16.
5. US Department of Health and Human Services, US Food and Drug Administration. Overview of dietary supplements. Available at: http://www.fda.gov/Food/DietarySupplements/ConsumerInformation/ucm110417.htm#regulate. Updated October 14, 2009. Accessed July 6, 2010.
6. Woolf A. Herbal remedies and children: do they work? Are they harmful? Pediatrics 2003;112:240–6.
7. Chemistry of herbal medications. In: Rotblatt M, Ziment I, editors. Evidence-based herbal medicine. Philadelphia: Hanley & Belfus; 2002. p. 29–44.
8. Quality assurance and choosing a brand or product. In: Rotblatt M, Ziment I, editors. Evidence-based herbal medicine. Philadelphia: Hanley & Belfus; 2002. p. 17–23.
9. Ernst E, Pittler M. Herbal medicine. Med Clin North Am 2002;86(1):149–61.
10. Ernest E. Serious adverse effects of unconventional therapies for children and adolescents: a systematic review of recent evidence. Eur J Pediatr 2003;162: 72–80.
11. Ernst E. Harmless herbs? A review of the recent literature. Am J Med 1998;104: 170–8.
12. Cheng T, Wong R, Lin Y, et al. Chinese herbal medicine, sibship, and blood lead in children. Occup Environ Med 1998;55:573–6.
13. Halt M. Moulds and mycotoxins in herb tea and medicinal plants. Eur J Epidemiol 1998;14:269–74.
14. Huang W, Wen K, Hsaio M. Adulteration by synthetic therapeutic substances of traditional Chinese medicines in Taiwan. J Clin Pharmacol 1997;37:334–50.
15. Vanherweghem J, Depierreux M, Tielmans C, et al. Rapidly progressive interstitial renal fibrosis in young women: association with a slimming regimen including Chinese herbs. Lancet 1993;341:387–91.

16. Horowitz R, Dart R, Gomez H, et al. Epidemiologic notes and reports. Jin Bu Huan toxicity in children – Colorado, 1993. Morb Mortal Wkly Rep 1993;42:633–6.

17. Farah M, Edwards R. International monitoring of adverse health effects associated with herbal medicines. Pharmacoepidemiol Drug Saf 2000;9:105–12.

18. US Pharmacopeia. USP verified. Available at: http://www.usp.org/USPVerified/. Accessed July 7, 2010.

19. Pitetti R, Singh S, Hornyak D, et al. Complementary and alternative use in children. Pediatr Emerg Care 2001;17(3):165–9.

20. Yussman S, Ryan S, Auinger P, et al. Visits to complementary and alternative medicine providers by children and adolescents in the United States. Ambul Pediatr 2004;4:429–35.

21. Lanski S, Greenwald M, Perkins A, et al. Herbal therapy use in a pediatric emergency department population: expect the unexpected. Pediatrics 2003;111: 981–5.

22. Wilson K, Klein J, Sesselberg T, et al. Use of complementary medicine and dietary supplements among U.S. adolescents. J Adolesc Health 2006;38:385–94.

23. Barnes P, Bloom B, Nahin R. Complementary and alternative medicine use among adults and children: United States, 2007. Natl Health Stat Report 2008; 12:1–23.

24. Sikand A, Laken M. Pediatricians' experience with and attitudes toward complementary/alternative medicine. Arch Pediatr Adolesc Med 1998;152:1059–64.

25. Yager J, Siegfried S, DiMatteo T. Use of alternative remedies by psychiatric patients: illustrative vignettes and a discussion of the issues. Am J Psychiatry 1999;156:1432–8.

26. Cala S, Crismon M, Baumgartner J. A survey of herbal use in children with attention-deficit-hyperactivity disorder or depression. Pharmacotherapy 2003;23(2): 222–30.

27. Wong VCN. Use of complementary and alternative medicine (CAM) in autism spectrum disorder (ASD): comparison of Chinese and western culture (part A). J Autism Dev Disord 2009;39:454–63.

28. Soh N, Walter G. Complementary medicine for psychiatric disorders in children and adolescents. Curr Opin Psychiatry 2008;21:350–5.

29. Natural Medicines Comprehensive Database. St. John's Wort. Available at: http:// 0-naturaldatabase.therapeuticresearch.com.libcat.ferris.edu/nd/Search.aspx? cs=mhsla~cp&s=ND&pt=9&Product=st.+john's+wort&btnSearch.x=0&btn Search.y=0. Accessed June 8, 2010.

30. St. John's Wort. In: Rotblatt M, Ziment I, editors. Evidence-based herbal medicine. Philadelphia: Hanley & Belfus; 2002. p. 315–21.

31. Lawvere S, Mahoney M. St. John's wort. Am Fam Physician 2005;72:2249–54.

32. Charrois T, Sadler C, Vohra S. Complementary, holistic and integrative medicine: St. John's wort. Pediatr Rev 2007;28(2):69–72.

33. Simeon J, Nixon M, Miulin R, et al. Open-label pilot study of St. John's wort in adolescent depression. J Child Adolesc Psychopharmacol 2005;15(2):293–301.

34. Findling R, McNamara N, O'Riordan M, et al. An open-label study of St. John's wort in juvenile depression. J Am Acad Child Adolesc Psychiatry 2003;42:908–14.

35. Izzo A, Ernst E. Interactions between herbal medicines and prescribed drugs, a systematic review. Drugs 2001;61(15):2163–75.

36. Yue Q-Y, Bergquist C, Gerden B. Safety of St. John's wort (*Hypericum perforatum*). Lancet 2000;355:576–7.

37. Lantz M, Buchalter E, Giambanco V. St. John's wort and antidepressant drug interactions in the elderly. J Geriatr Psychiatry Neurol 1999;12:7–10.

38. Melatonin. Altern Med Rev 2005;10(4):326–36.
39. Natural Medicines Comprehensive Database. Melatonin. Available at: http://0-naturaldatabase.therapeuticresearch.com.libcat.ferris.edu/nd/Search.aspx?cs=MHSLA~CP&s=ND&pt=9&Product=melatonin&btnSearch.x=0&btnSearch.y=0. Accessed August 30, 2010.
40. Shamseer L, Vohra S. Complementary, holistic and integrative medicine: melatonin. Pediatr Rev 2009;30(6):223–8.
41. Wagner J, Wagner M, Hening W. Beyond benzodiazepines: alternative pharmacologic agents for the treatment of insomnia. Ann Pharmacother 1998;32:680–91.
42. Sheldon S. Pro-convulsant effects of oral melatonin in neurologically disabled children. Lancet 1998;351:1254.
43. Peled N, Shorer Z, Peled E, et al. Melatonin effect on seizures in children with severe neurologic deficit disorders. Epilepsia 2001;42:1208–10.
44. Buscemi N, Vandermeer B, Hooton N, et al. The efficacy and safety of exogenous melatonin for primary sleep disorders. A meta-analysis. J Gen Intern Med 2005;20:1151–8.
45. Phillips L, Appleton R. Systematic review of melatonin treatment in children with neurodevelopmental disabilities and sleep impairment. Dev Med Child Neurol 2004;46:771–5.
46. Bendz L, Scates A. Melatonin treatment for insomnia in pediatric patients with attention-deficit/hyperactivity disorder. Ann Pharmacother 2010;44:185–91.
47. Plushner S. Valerian: Valeriana officinalis. Am J Health Syst Pharm 2000;57:333–5.
48. Valerian (Valeriana officinalis). In: Rotblatt M, Ziment I, editors. Evidence-based herbal medicine. Philadelphia: Hanley & Belfus; 2002. p. 355–9.
49. Meoli AM, Rosen C, Kristo D, et al. Oral nonprescription treatment for insomnia: an evaluation of products with limited evidence. J Clin Sleep Med 2005;1(2):173–87.
50. Hadley S, Petry J. Valerian. Am Fam Physician 2003;67(8):1755–8.
51. Donath F, Quispe S, Diefenbach K, et al. Critical evaluation of the effect of valerian extract on sleep structure and sleep quality. Pharmacopsychiatry 2000;33:47–53.
52. Muller S, Klement S. A combination of valerian and lemon balm is effective in the treatment of restlessness and dyssomnia in children. Phytomedicine 2006;13:383–7.
53. Francis A, Dempster R. Effect of valerian, Valeriana edulis, on sleep difficulties in children with intellectual deficits: randomized trial. Phytomedicine 2002;9:273–9.
54. Wheatley D. Medicinal plants for insomnia: a review of their pharmacology, efficacy and tolerability. J Psychopharmacol 2005;19(4):414–21.
55. Kuhlmann J, Berger W, Podzuweit H, et al. The influence of valerian treatment on "reaction time, alertness, and concentration" in volunteers. Pharmacopsychiatry 1999;32:235–41.
56. MacGregor F, Abernathy V, Dahabra S, et al. Hepatotoxicity of herbal remedies. Br Med J 1989;299:1156–7.
57. Pepping J. Kava: Piper methysticum. Am J Health Syst Pharm 1999;56:957–60.
58. Singh Y, Singh N. Therapeutic potential of kava in the treatment of anxiety disorders. CNS Drugs 2002;16(11):731–43.
59. Pittler M, Ernst E. Kava extract versus placebo for treating anxiety [review]. Cochrane Database Syst Rev 2010;6:CD003383.
60. Stevinson C, Huntley A, Ernst E. A systematic review of the safety of kava extract in the treatment of anxiety. Drug Saf 2002;25(4):251–61.

61. Hepatic toxicity possibly associated with kava-containing products–United States, Germany and Switzerland, 1999–2002. JAMA 2003;289(1):36–7.
62. Kava (*Piper methysticum*). In: Rotblatt M, Ziment I, editors. Evidence-based herbal medicine. Philadelphia: Hanley & Belfus; 2002. p. 244–7.
63. Schelosky L, Raffauf C, Jendroska K, et al. Kava and dopamine antagonism. J Neurol Neurosurg Psychiatry 1995;58:639–40.
64. Sayeed S, Bloch R, Antonacci D. Herbal and dietary supplements for treatment of anxiety disorders. Am Fam Physician 2007;76:549–56.
65. Clayton E, Hanstock T, Garg M, et al. Long chain omega-3 polyunsaturated fatty acids in the treatment of psychiatric illnesses in children and adolescents. Acta Neuropsychiatr 2007;19:92–103.
66. Burlotte J, Bukutu C, Vohra S. Complementary, holistic, and integrative medicine: fish oils and neurodevelopmental disorders. Pediatr Rev 2009;30(4):e29–33.
67. Raz R, Gabis L. Essential fatty acids and attention-deficit-hyperactivity disorder: a systematic review. Dev Med Child Neurol 2009;51:580–92.
68. Richardson A. Omega-3 fatty acids in ADHD and related neurodevelopmental disorders. Int Rev Psychiatry 2006;18(2):155–72.
69. Nemets H, Nemets B, Apter A, et al. Omega-3 treatment of childhood depression: a controlled, double-blind pilot study. Am J Psychiatry 2006;163:1098–100.
70. Clayton E, Hanstock T, Hirneth S, et al. Reduced mania and depression in juvenile bipolar disorder associated with long-chain omega-3 polyunsaturated fatty acid supplementation. Eur J Clin Nutr 2009;63:1037–40.
71. Wozniak J, Biederman J, Mick E, et al. Omega-3 fatty acid monotherapy for pediatric bipolar disorder: a prospective open-label trial. Eur Neuropsychopharmacol 2007;17:440–7.
72. Natural Medicines Comprehensive Database. EPA (Eicosapentaenoic acid). Available at: http://0-naturaldatabase.therapeuticresearch.com.libcat.ferris.edu/nd/Search.aspx?cs=MHSLA~CP&s=ND&pt=9&Product=epa&btnSearch.x=0&btnSearch.y=0. Accessed August 30, 2010.
73. Natural Medicines Comprehensive Database. DHA (Docosahexaenoic acid). Available at: http://0-naturaldatabase.therapeuticresearch.com.libcat.ferris.edu/nd/Search.aspx?cs=MHSLA~CP&s=ND&pt=9&Product=dha&btnSearch.x=0&btnSearch.y=0. Accessed August 30, 2010.
74. Seamon M, Clauson K. Ephedra: yesterday, DSHEA, and tomorrow–a ten year perspective on the dietary supplement health and education act of 1994. J Herb Pharmacother 2005;5:67–86.
75. Natural Medicines Comprehensive Database. Guarana. Available at: http://0-naturaldatabase.therapeuticresearch.com.libcat.ferris.edu/nd/Search.aspx?cs=MHSLA~CP&s=ND&pt=9&Product=guaran&btnSearch.x=0&btnSearch.y=0. Accessed September 14, 2010.
76. Natural Medicines Comprehensive Database. Citrus aurantium. Available at: http://0-naturaldatabase.therapeuticresearch.com.libcat.ferris.edu/nd/Search.aspx?cs=MHSLA~CP&s=ND&pt=9&Product=citrus+aurantium&btnSearch.x=13&btnSearch.y=5. Accessed September 14, 2010.
77. Natural Medicines Comprehensive Database. Chromium picolinate. Available at: http://0-naturaldatabase.therapeuticresearch.com.libcat.ferris.edu/nd/Search.aspx?cs=MHSLA~CP&s=ND&pt=9&Product=chromium+picolinate&btnSearch.x=12&btnSearch.y=9. Accessed September 14, 2010.
78. Natural Medicines Comprehensive Database. Garcinia cambogia. Available at: http://0-naturaldatabase.therapeuticresearch.com.libcat.ferris.edu/nd/Search.aspx?

cs=MHSLA~CP&s=ND&pt=9&Product=garcinia+cambogia&btnSearch.x=
15&btnSearch.y=8. Accessed September 14, 2010.

79. Natural Medicines Comprehensive Database. Chitosan. Available at: http://
0-naturaldatabase.therapeuticresearch.com.libcat.ferris.edu/nd/Search.aspx?
cs=MHSLA~CP&s=ND&pt=9&Product=chitosan&btnSearch.x=9&btnSearch.
y=7. Accessed September 14, 2010.

80. Natural Medicines Comprehensive Database. Pyruvate. Available at: http://
0-naturaldatabase.therapeuticresearch.com.libcat.ferris.edu/nd/Search.aspx?
cs=MHSLA~CP&s=ND&pt=9&Product=Pyruvate&btnSearch.x=8&btnSearch.
y=14. Accessed September 14, 2010.

81. Natural Medicines Comprehensive Database. Gingko biloba. Available at: http://
0-naturaldatabase.therapeuticresearch.com.libcat.ferris.edu/nd/Search.aspx?
cs=MHSLA~CP&s=ND&pt=9&Product=ginkgo+biloba&btnSearch.x=13&btn
Search.y=11. Accessed September 14, 2010.

Pharmacotherapy for Anxiety Disorders in Children and Adolescents

Ian Kodish, MD, PhD[a],*, Carol Rockhill, MD, PhD, MPH[a],
Sheryl Ryan, MD[b], Chris Varley, MD[a]

KEYWORDS

- Anxiety disorders • Pharmacotherapy
- Selective serotonin reuptake inhibitor • Children

Anxiety is an adaptive response to danger that helps promote safety by facilitating avoidance of perceived threats. Children and adolescents have common fears and worries, which are often normal and typically follow predictable developmental periods (eg, fear of storms in toddlerhood, urges to avoid leaving home when starting school). However, anxiety can be functionally impairing when it becomes excessive and enduring or occurs outside the expected developmental timeline, in which case a clinical diagnosis and treatment are warranted. In youth with anxiety, exposure to a trigger (such as a feared object or separation from an attachment figure) results in anxious reactivity, often with thoughts of catastrophic consequences. This distress typically elicits escape urges that, when followed, bring about immediate relief of anxiety (such as leaving class, washing hands). The relief is often so rewarding that the escape behavior rapidly becomes habitual, and subsequent stressors may lead to similar escape behavior, resulting in increasingly impaired functioning. Treatment requires breaking the cycle of avoidance behaviors by reducing the reinforcement associated with avoidance and gradually empowering children and youth to tolerate anxiety in the face of potentially stressful challenges. Pharmacologic interventions are believed to confer clinical benefit by reducing the degree of anxious reactivity and thereby increase the range of opportunities for children to relearn more adaptive responses to stressful stimuli. Emerging evidence also points to subtle neurotrophic

---

Disclosure: Dr Varley has been on the Speakers' Bureau for Novartis.
[a] Department of Psychiatry and Behavioral Sciences, University of Washington School of Medicine, Seattle Children's Hospital, 4800 Sandpoint Way NE, Seattle, WA 98105, USA
[b] Department of Pediatrics, Yale University School of Medicine, PO Box 208064, New Haven, CT 06520-8064, USA
* Corresponding author.
E-mail address: ian.kodish@seattlechildrens.org

Pediatr Clin N Am 58 (2011) 55–72
doi:10.1016/j.pcl.2010.10.002
0031-3955/11/$ – see front matter © 2011 Elsevier Inc. All rights reserved.

changes induced by selective serotonin reuptake inhibitors (SSRIs) that may contribute to clinical effectiveness through enhanced neuroplasticity.[1]

Anxiety disorders are highly prevalent, and cross-sectional screens of pediatric outpatients find 20% score more than the identified clinical cutoffs for one or more anxiety disorders.[2] Even among community samples of preschool children, almost 10% are found to have an anxiety disorder using *Diagnostic and statistical manual of mental disorders fourth edition* criteria.[3] Anxiety disorders occur at similar rates among young boys and girls, but gradually become more common in females, with a 2:1 to 3:1 female preponderance by adolescence.[4,5] Longitudinal studies of community samples have also shown that once a child is diagnosed with an anxiety disorder, that child is at increased future risk for recurrence of the same disorder, as well as for the subsequent development of depressive disorders and additional anxiety disorders.[6,7]

Functional neuroimaging studies of anxiety disorders in children and adolescents reveal functional impairments in brain regions that modulate emotion and fear. The basic components of this circuitry are believed to be preserved across species, and include regions in the amygdala involved in fear conditioning and responses, in the hippocampus for contextual processing, and in prefrontal cortical regions in modulation of fear and extinction of fear responses.[8] In general, the amygdala is believed to be responsible for rapid interpretation of danger, and stress-induced hormones and other neurotransmitters operate on the amygdala to strengthen memories associated with fearful stimuli, thus improving adaptive responses to threats in our environment.[9] Although prefrontal regions typically serve to modulate this amygdala responsivity, children and adults with anxiety disorders show a deficiency in this dampening of fear responses by prefrontal cortical circuits.[10]

ASSESSMENT AND DIAGNOSIS OF ANXIETY

Assessment for anxiety disorders typically starts with pediatricians or other primary care providers, often by initially addressing behavioral concerns or physical complaints such as headaches or stomachaches, which are particularly common at younger ages.[11] In addition to anxiety, associated symptoms include fatigue, muscle tension, malaise, dry mouth, or a poorly defined sense of discomfort, palpitations, syncope, chest pain, shortness of breath, dizziness, paresthesias, numbness, trembling, memory loss, difficulty concentrating, vague gastrointestinal symptoms, and urinary frequency.[12] Obtaining a timeline of physical, psychological, and behavioral symptoms of concern, preferably elicited from both the child and parents, is also recommended. A broad review focused on psychosocial stress and developmental course is also recommended, and for older children, a review of substance use, including energy drinks, caffeine, inhalants, methamphetamines, and stimulant diet pills. Evaluation for anxiety disorders should also include a review of past medical history, including previous trauma that may have precipitated posttraumatic stress disorder (PTSD), family history of psychiatric illnesses, and substance abuse.

General screening measures are available for providers to help identify children at risk for psychosocial difficulties and to add important clinical information beyond what may be obtained through a medical history. Youth self-reports may be an important tool because of the internalizing nature of anxiety disorders and because affected children may not be forthcoming with their symptoms during direct questioning.[13] Screening tools tailored to developmental level are available, and clinical judgment is required in interpreting the results.[14]

MEDICAL EVALUATION

Consideration of common medical issues that can present similarly to anxiety disorders is essential.[12,15] Physical examination and targeted laboratory testing directed at evaluation of medical disorders that are suspected based on history should be performed. In general, children do not need exhaustive diagnostic workups for their somatic symptoms. Instead, judicious use of laboratory tests can generally comprise the medical workup; these tests are indicated from a consideration of both the history and the physical examination.[16] Thus, it may be necessary to obtain screens for endocrine abnormalities such as hyperthyroidism, hypoglycemia, and hyperglycemia, as well as screens for drugs of abuse. Other considerations include pulmonary function tests to evaluate for underlying respiratory abnormalities, sleep studies to evaluate for sleep disorders, electrocardiograms to evaluate arrhythmias or when considering tricyclic agents, and electroencephalograms to rule out seizure.

TREATMENT OF ANXIETY DISORDERS

A multimodal approach to clinical treatment of youth with anxiety disorders is optimal, because studies not only show benefit of both therapeutic and pharmacologic interventions but also suggest they work in tandem to confer greater improvement in symptoms. In terms of psychotherapy, cognitive-behavioral therapy (CBT) has shown efficacy in individual, group, and family formats.[17] Randomized controlled trials (RCTs) of CBT have shown benefit in generalized anxiety disorder (GAD),[18–22] social anxiety disorder,[18–22] panic disorder,[21] obsessive-compulsive disorder (OCD),[23–25] and PTSD.[26] A recent review has further found these benefits are maintained or improved over time.[27] When youth meet criteria for an anxiety disorder, the American Academy of Child and Adolescent Psychiatry recommends the use of psychoeducation for patients and family, and when functional impairments are mild, initial intervention with CBT is preferred over starting a medication.[28]

However, an increased intensity of treatment is often needed for youth with moderate to severe symptoms of anxiety disorder, in which case a combination of medication and CBT is recommended.[29] Consistent evidence, including multiple RCTs, supports the benefit of SSRIs, both alone and in combination with therapy, for the treatment of anxiety disorders in children and adolescents. Medication intervention may be started concurrently with psychotherapy, may be needed to reduce the impairing nature of severe symptoms before psychotherapy can proceed in an effective manner, or may be used as an augmentation strategy if initial psychotherapy does not provide relief of symptoms. This review focuses on SSRIs, but also discusses other medications that have shown some degree of efficacy for treating anxiety disorders.

EVIDENCE FOR EFFECTIVENESS OF SSRIS AND SELECTIVE NOREPINEPHRINE REUPTAKE INHIBITORS

RCTs provide the highest degree of evidence for efficacy and drive evidence-based treatment algorithms. A limited, but increasing, number of RCTs have evaluated anti-anxiety agents in children and adolescents. Regarding specific anxiety subtypes, pediatric OCD has the largest number of positive RCTs, including effective benefits of sertraline,[23,30] fluoxetine,[31,32] fluvoxamine,[33] and paroxetine.[34,35] Evidence for citalopram is limited to open-label studies[36–38] and comparison with fluoxetine without placebo.[39] No RCTs have yet examined escitalopram. A recent meta-analysis of RCTs examining the tolerability and efficacy of pharmacotherapy for anxiety disorders found that the studies of SSRIs and selective norepinephrine reuptake inhibitors (SNRIs) showed a clear benefit, with an overall response rate almost double that of placebo treatment.[40] Three of the 4 medications approved by the US Food And Drug Administration (FDA) specifically for treatment of OCD in children and adolescents are SSRIs: sertraline (6 years and older), fluoxetine (7 years and older), and fluvoxamine (8 years and older).[41] No medications have yet been approved by the FDA for treatment of non-OCD anxiety in youth.

Medication and placebo response rates range across studies, and protocols may differ in definitions of clinical response. For youth with OCD, response is often defined by reductions in the children's Yale-Brown obsessive-compulsive scale[14] or improvement in clinician ratings of severity.

The effectiveness of sertraline in treating pediatric OCD was examined in 2 12-week RCTs,[23,30] including the Pediatric OCD Treatment Study (POTS), the most extensive RCT of pediatric OCD, which serves as a model for clinical trials examining the effect of both manualized psychotherapy and medications. The 4 treatment groups included sertraline, CBT, their combination, and placebo. Each active treatment arm proved superior to placebo, and combined treatment was superior to either CBT or sertraline alone. Remission rates were 53.6% for the combined group, 39% in the CBT-only group, 21% in the sertraline-only group, and 4% for placebo, yet the CBT and sertraline-only groups did not statistically differ.[23] The other RCT examining sertraline for OCD found 42% of subjects very much improved after active treatment, compared with 26% on placebo, with lasting effects in 70% of patients who were examined 12 months later.[42]

Fluvoxamine was also shown to be effective in a 10-week RCT of pediatric outpatients with OCD, with an overall 42% response rate from active treatment. Clinical symptoms improved beyond placebo response by the first week and continued to show gains through the course of treatment.[33]

Multiple placebo-controlled RCTs for paroxetine[34,35] and fluoxetine[31,32] have also shown the effectiveness of these medications for OCD in youth. Paroxetine showed significantly lower response rates among youth with comorbid illness such as ADHD, tic disorder, or oppositional defiant disorder (ODD),[35] and whereas the lower dose of fluoxetine showed effectiveness after 8 weeks, the higher-dose fluoxetine study did not differ from placebo until the 16-week evaluation. These studies suggest an overall moderate treatment effect for OCD that is similar across multiple SSRIs.[40]

Despite the greater prevalence of non-OCD anxiety disorders in children and adolescents, fewer studies have examined these other anxiety subtypes. RCTs of SSRIs have shown efficacy in the treatment of GAD, separation anxiety disorder (SAD), and social anxiety disorder, often in mixed populations that include children and adolescents with any one of or a combination of these (**Table 1**). To date, no such studies have specifically examined childhood panic disorder or PTSD. When pharmacologic treatments in RCTs are segregated by anxiety subtype (OCD vs non-OCD), treatment responses for non-OCD disorders seem slightly greater than for OCD.[40]

The largest RCT of non-OCD anxiety disorders to date is the Childhood Anxiety Multimodal Study (CAMS), a 12-week study including 488 youth with one or more of the diagnoses of SAD, GAD, and social phobia.[43] Treatment arms were sertraline only, CBT only,[44] sertraline and CBT combined, or placebo. All 3 active treatment arms showed superior responses than placebo, with 81% in the combined condition, 60% in the CBT group, and 55% in the sertraline-only group, compared with 24% in the placebo group. Similar to POTS, these findings suggest that although monotherapy with either medication or psychotherapy can be effective for treating anxiety

Table 1
Randomized controlled trails of SSRIs and SNRIs in pediatric non-OCD anxiety disorders

RCT Author	Medication	Length (Weeks)	Dosing (Mean)	Total N	Ages (Years) and Diagnoses	Effect Size of Treatment	Number Needed to Treat	Clinical Outcome/ Response Rate	Notable Side Effects
RUPP Anxiety Study Group, 2001[47]	Fluvoxamine (FLV)	8	Fixed-flexible (4.0 mg/kg/d)	128	6–17 GAD, SoP, SAD	1.1	2	CGI-I ≤ 2 FLV 76% PBO 29%	Abdominal discomfort, ↑ activity
Rynn et al, 2001[50]	Sertraline (SER)	9	Fixed (50 mg)	22	5–17 GAD	1.9	1	CGI-I ≤ 2 SER 90% PBO 10%	—
Birmaher et al,[49] 2003	Fluoxetine (FLX)	12	Fixed (20 mg)	74	7–17 GAD, SoP, SAD	0.4	4	CGI-I ≤ 2 FLX 61% PBO 35%	Abdominal pain, agitation
Wagner et al,[42] 2004	Paroxetine (PAR)	16	Flexible 10–50 mg/d (24.8 mg)	322	8–17 SoP	N/A	3	CGI-I ≤ 2 PAR 78% PBO 38%	Insomnia, ↓ appetite, vomiting, agitation
Black & Uhde,[108] 1994	Fluoxetine (FLX)	12	Fixed (0.6 mg/kg/d)	15	6–11 Elective mutism	0.67	N/A	CGI-I ≤ 3 FLX 80%, PBO 40%	—
Walkup et al,[43] 2008	Sertraline (SERT)	12	Fixed-flexible COMB (133.7 mg) SERT (146.0 mg)	488	7–17 GAD, SoP, SAD	COMB = 0.86 SERT = 0.45 CBT = 0.31	COMB = 1.7 SERT = 3.2 CBT = 2.8	CGI-I ≤ 2 COMB = 80.7% SERT = 54.9% CBT = 59.7% PBO = 23.7%	Insomnia, fatigue, restlessness
March et al,[52] 2007	Venlafaxine ER (VFX)	16	Weight-based flexible (141.5 mg)	293	8–17 SoP	0.46	5	CGI-I ≤ 2 VFX = 56% PBO = 37%	Anorexia, asthenia, nausea
Rynn et al,[51] 2007 (pooled studies)	Venlafaxine ER (VFX)	8	Weight-based, flexible	320	6–17 GAD	0.42	N/A	CGI-I ≤ 2 VFX = 69% PBO = 48%	Headache, abdominal pain, anorexia

Abbreviations: CGI-I, Clinical Global Impressions-Improvement Scale; COMB, combined; N/A, not applicable; PBO, placebo; SoP, social phobia.

disorders, a multimodal approach is more likely to be successful. The recommendation of a combination of medication and therapy for anxiety disorders also mirrors recommendations for pediatric depression[45] and complex forms of ADHD.[46]

Fluvoxamine has also been shown to be superior to placebo in an 8-week RCT of 82 youth with non-OCD anxiety disorders, which showed a strong 76% response rate for the fluvoxamine group compared with 29% in a placebo group, a difference that became significant by week 2.[47] This study design had a lead-in period of 3 weeks with supportive psychotherapy, and several subjects were excluded after responding to this brief intervention, likely reducing placebo response rates. An open-label follow-up study of the same population with continued fluvoxamine treatment showed that 94% of the responders experienced a sustained benefit when evaluated again 6 months after study completion.[48] Also, when nonresponders were subsequently switched to an open-label trial of fluoxetine, 71% did eventually show a response. Another RCT of 74 youth with mixed non-OCD anxiety disorders found that 12 weeks of fluoxetine, 20 mg, resulted in 61% as much improved or very much improved, compared with 35% of placebo subjects.[49] Subgroup analyses indicated that severe symptoms and family history of anxiety predicted poorer response, whereas youth with diagnoses of generalized anxiety or social phobia showed a better response to the medication than those with separation anxiety.

Only a few studies have examined cohorts with specific non-OCD anxiety disorders. An RCT examining 319 youth with diagnosis of social phobia showed efficacy for paroxetine, with 78% response rate for medicine versus 38% for placebo.[42] A small 9-week RCT examining just 22 children and adolescents with GAD showed efficacy for sertraline, up to doses of 50 mg, with 90% response rate for medicine versus 10% for placebo.[50]

Only one agent with dual inhibiting actions on serotonin and norepinephrine, termed SNRIs, has been tested in youth with anxiety disorders. Venlafaxine XR was examined in 2 8-week RCTs in a combined total of 320 children specifically with GAD.[51] Despite high placebo rates and lack of significant improvement on primary measures in one of the trials, pooled results show significantly greater response in the active medication group (69%) compared with placebo (48%). Another study of venlafaxine XR in 293 children with social anxiety found that 16 weeks of treatment showed a significant medication response of 56% compared with 37% in the placebo group.[52] However, studies of venlafaxine in children have raised concerns for an association with increased blood pressure, decreased growth rate, and increased suicidal ideation, so these risks should be discussed with families before initiating treatment. A recent meta-analysis of RCTs examining the tolerability and efficacy of pharmacotherapy for anxiety disorders found that the studies of SSRIs and SNRIs showed a clear benefit, with an overall response rate almost double that of placebo treatment, with SSRIs providing slightly more benefit than venlafaxine XR.[40]

There have not been head-to-head RCTs comparing effectiveness and side effects of SSRI or SNRI medications. Choice of agent is therefore often based on common side effect profiles, drug interactions, and family history of medication response. Furthermore, only short-term benefits have been evaluated in RCTs, and research findings may not generalize to clinic populations because of exclusion of youth with medical or psychiatric comorbidities.

Despite age-related differences in metabolism, and observations that SSRIs may be more effective in the treatment of adolescent depression compared with children, findings from RCTs in anxious youth do not show any differential effects on outcome based on age group.[40,53] However, data are limited regarding prescribing medication in children less than the age of 6 years. In a review of the peer-reviewed journals,

Fanton and Gleason[54] found only 16 children younger than 6 years whose response to pharmacologic treatment is described. Two case reports of fluoxetine showed effectiveness in decreasing anxiety in a preschooler with multiple anxiety disorders and in one with selective mutism, believed to be a form of social anxiety.[55,56] Data are currently too limited to provide evidence-based pharmacologic treatment recommendations for preschool children with anxiety disorders. Psychotherapy tailored to young children is instead considered to be the first-line treatment. In cases of a high severity of symptoms that are unresponsive to CBT, a trial of medication may be considered.

SAFETY CONCERNS WITH SSRIS AND SNRIS

When recommending and initially prescribing SSRIs or SNRIs, it is important to provide informed consent to the parents, and when appropriate, to the child or adolescent. States may vary on the requirements of consent and the ability of the youth to receive care without the knowledge of parents. Issues that must be discussed before prescribing include the FDA black-box warning, potential for activation side effects or less commonly sedation, and potential for nausea and headaches with dose initiation and changes.

Common side effects include nausea and stomachaches, headaches, insomnia, and restlessness. These side effects may intermittently emerge in the context of dosage adjustments and may resolve spontaneously. However, a meta-analysis of RCTs showed that dropouts because of drug-related adverse events from SSRIs and SNRIs were almost twice as common among patients taking active medication compared with placebo.[40] Clinical practice suggests that children with anxiety tend to be more sensitive to the potential side effects of these medications, and lower starting doses may be considered to mitigate these effects. Adolescents should also be cautioned regarding potential sexual side effects. Furthermore, SSRIs and SNRIs have been given a black-box warning from the FDA as a result of concern that they may potentiate suicidal thinking, a low-frequency event that nevertheless warrants informed consent[57,58] and the development of a monitoring strategy. Suicidal thoughts may be related to the potential activating effects of SSRIs, resulting in heightened somatic experiences of anxiety, increased emotional lability, and features of impulsivity. A recent RCT examining activation as a side effect of fluvoxamine in anxious youth recommended monitoring for signs of activation throughout the course of titration.[59]

Patients and families should also be cautioned that medications may need to be taken for 4 to 8 weeks to provide clinical benefit, particularly when starting with low doses. This strategy may also prevent families from abandoning trials prematurely and allow for a more systematic approach to treatment. Despite their relative safety and tolerance, abrupt discontinuation of shorter-acting agents often results in flulike symptoms.

TRICYCLIC ANTIDEPRESSANTS

Tricyclic antidepressants, including imipramine[60–62] and clomipramine,[63] have shown efficacy in several older RCTs of social anxiety or school refusal. Clomiprimine has an FDA indication for treatment of OCD based on results from 3 RCTs. The largest of these was a crossover trial in which clomipramine treatment for 20 weeks showed a 22% to 47% reduction in symptoms compared with 0% to 27% for placebo.[64] Although these agents may be considered for patients who have experienced activation problems on SSRIs, or as augmentation to SSRIs for partial response in youth with OCD,[65] tricyclic agents are less preferred because of the potential for problematic side effects, including cardiac abnormalities, constipation, sedation, and risk of fatality in overdose.

OTHER AGENTS

Buspirone (BuSpar) is a partial agonist of serotonin receptors with some evidence for treatment of generalized anxiety in adults but there are no data regarding youth with anxiety. Similarly, buproprion (Wellbutrin), an inhibitor of dopamine and norepinephrine, has not been studied in children or adolescents with anxiety.

Clonidine, an α-2 agonist, was shown to decrease arousal, aggression, and anxiety in a small open trial (n = 7) of patients ages 3 to 6 years with PTSD.[66] A crossover pilot study of propranolol in 11 pediatric patients with PTSD also showed improvements in hyperarousal and intrusivity in most patients.[67]

The sedating and appetite-stimulating properties of mirtazapine make it a consideration for patients with insomnia or prominent appetite suppression, and for those taking medications with high potential for interactions. However, there are no RCTs to support the use of mirtazapine in youth with anxiety.

Controlled trials do not support the use of benzodiazepines in children,[68–70] yet there is an extensive history of clinical use for anxious children and considerable evidence of effectiveness in adults. Clinical severity may warrant consideration of their use early in treatment of severe symptoms and as an adjunct treatment to SSRIs, particularly during initial titration, to achieve more rapid reduction in symptoms. Benzodiazepines can cause paradoxic disinhibition in some children, but are often used clinically to provide effective short-term relief, particularly if acute insomnia or disabling paniclike symptoms are present. However, this relief can produce psychological dependence in adults, and carries risks of tolerance and seizure from abrupt discontinuation.[71]

TREATMENT COURSE

A treatment algorithm is summarized in **Table 2** with clinical guidelines for each agent. These recommendations are based on our interpretation of the current literature, and are expected to need refinement as new studies offer further guidance. We recommend frequent visits when initiating medications, along with regular communication with the treating therapist. Planned increases in dose may be useful when initiating subtherapeutic doses in the context of concern for sensitivity to side effects. More frequent contact is also recommended when there is a history of depression, a strong familial preference, or when compliance is a concern. After an effective dose of medication is reached, visit frequency can be reduced. We further recommend use of standardized rating scales to measure the ongoing effectiveness of treatment. Even after symptoms resolve with an effective dose, we recommend keeping medication in place for 1 year, followed by a gradual taper to allow observation of any recurrence of symptoms, and reinstatement of prior effective dose if indicated.[72]

TREATMENT CONSIDERATIONS FOR COMMON COMORBIDITIES

Youth who are diagnosed with one anxiety disorder are likely to have 2 or more anxiety disorders concurrently.[73,74] CAMS, which included children and adolescents with social phobia, GAD, or SAD, found 78.6% of the sample had 2 or more of those disorders and 35.9% met criteria for all 3 diagnoses.[43] Providers should therefore evaluate for multiple anxiety disorders, and assess the degree of impairment from each to prioritize treatment.

Table 2
Treatment algorithm for pediatric anxiety and prescribing information

Treatment algorithm:	Select SSRI. Titrate up every 2–4 weeks until symptoms respond, until side effects preclude further dose increases, or when reach max dose. If ineffective or intolerable, use alternate SSRI for second trial					→ After 2 failed SSRI trials, reassess → or consult, consider → clomipramine for OCD; VFX → for non-OCD		→ If still no response, or familial preference, consider buspirone → or mirtazapine, alone or as → augmentation		Consider benzodiazepines for acute relief of severe symptoms or after no response to multiple trials	
Class	SSRI					Tricyclic	SNRI	5-HTa PA	Tetracyclic	Benzodiazepine	
Medication	Sertraline	Fluoxetine	Fluvoxamine	Citalopram	Paroxetine[a]	Clomipramine	Venlafaxine XR (VFX)	Buspirone	Mirtazapine	Clonazepam	Lorazepam
Starting dose	12.5–25 mg	5–10 mg	12.5–25 mg	5–10 mg	5–10 mg	25 mg	37.5 mg	5 mg 3 times a day	7.5–15 mg	0.25–0.5 mg	0.5–1 mg
Total therapeutic dose range	50–200 mg	10–60 mg	50–200 mg (Rx twice a day more than 50 mg)	10–40 mg	10–40 mg	100–150 mg	75–225 mg (Rx every night or twice a day)	15–60 mg (Rx 3 times a day)	7.5–30 mg (Rx every night)	0.25–3 mg (Rx every day 3 times a day)	0.5–6 mg (Rx every day 4 times a day)
Common side effect profile	Nausea, sedation, headache	Activation, nausea, insomnia	Hyperactivity, abdominal discomfort	Somnolence, insomnia, diaphoresis	Sedation, nausea, dry mouth	Dry mouth, constipation, diaphoresis	Nausea, sedation, dizziness	Sedation, disinhibition, headache	Hunger, sedation, dizziness	Sedation, confusion	Sedation, confusion
Special warning/ monitoring	Suicidality, activation (restlessness, impulsivity), serotonin syndrome; develop safety plan and means to assess early side effects, which may resolve in 1–2 wk; avoid abrupt discontinuation with paroxetine, sertraline, fluvoxamine, and citalopram.					HTN, rebound HTN, lethal in OD; level ≤400	HTN, tachycardia, suicidality	Safe with benzodiazepines	Weight gain	Disinhibition, tolerance, seizure from discontinuation	Disinhibition, tolerance, seizure from discontinuation
Specific indications	GAD	Long half-life		No RCTs; few interactions	Social phobia; nondepressed	OCD; EKG, BP monitoring to minimize overdose risk	GAD; nondepressed	Augmentation; sexual side effects	Appetite stimulation, insomnia; few interactions	Short-term relief of acute anxiety; longer acting	Short-term relief of acute anxiety; shorter acting; liver impaired
FDA approval	For OCD; ≥6	For OCD; ≥7	For OCD; ≥8	For adults	For adults	For OCD; ≥10	For adults	For adults	For adults	For adults	For adults

Abbreviations: 5-HTa PA, serotonin partial agonist; BP, blood pressure; EKG, electrocardiogram; HTN, hypertension; OD, overdose; Rx, prescribe.

a In June 2003, the FDA recommended against the use of paroxetine for major depressive disorder in children and adolescents.

Common comorbidities include major depressive disorder, attention-deficit/hyperactivity disorder (ADHD), ODD, and Tourette disorder.[43,73,74] In the CAM study, for example, among youth who met criteria for one or more anxiety disorders, 46% met criteria for other internalizing disorders, 11.9% for ADHD, 9.4% for ODD, and 2.7% for tic disorders. Attention to comorbidities is therefore essential.

Although there is some overlap in symptoms for anxiety and depressive disorders, only a subgroup ranging from 28% to 69% of children or adolescents who have anxiety or depression have both at the same time.[73] Risk factors for having a combination of depression and anxiety are older age and higher severity of anxiety symptoms.[73] The RCTs of youth anxiety that also included secondary measures of comorbid depression revealed little improvement in depressive features after treatment with SSRIs.[75] Although most RCTs of anxiety exclude depressive disorder diagnosis from entry, an open-label citalopram study also showed significantly lower rate of response in patients with comorbid anxiety and depression versus either alone (36.3%; vs 50% for depression, and 69.7% for anxiety).[38]

Children with behavioral dysregulation often display oppositionality, and may display symptoms of disruptive behavior disorder or ODD. Anxious children may intently refuse to comply with demands of authority figures, such as leaving the house on time. In cases when the underlying motivation for oppositionality is an attempt to avoid an anxiety trigger or to perform a compulsive ritual, an anxiety disorder is the more appropriate diagnosis. Once anxiety is treated, features of externalizing disorders should be reevaluated.

Anxiety disorders and ADHD often co-occur, with 15% to 24% of children with anxiety disorders meeting criteria for ADHD, and 25% of children with ADHD meeting criteria for an anxiety disorder.[76] Anxious children often have difficulty paying attention and concentrating on schoolwork because of hypervigilance or preoccupation with worries about peers. Carefully assessing anxiety symptoms during an ADHD evaluation is therefore essential to address the core impairments, and also to monitor for potential anxiogenic effects of medications during stimulant trials. However, addressing both impairments pharmacologically may not be indicated, because children with comorbid ADHD and anxiety who continued to exhibit anxious features following stimulant treatment were found not to show any further anxiety benefit from the addition of fluvoxamine to their stimulant regimen when compared with adding a placebo.[76] Co-occurrence of Tourette disorder with OCD is common, and evidence shows that a common set of genetic factors likely contribute to both disorders, yet treatment of one disorder neither protects from nor exacerbates the symptoms of the other.[77,78]

Limited evidence shows a strong association between substance-use disorders and anxiety disorders.[79] Most adolescents with substance-abuse disorders have comorbid psychiatric diagnoses, with anxiety disorders being a common co-occurrence.[80] When anxiety disorders begin in childhood, there is increased risk for the development of substance abuse during adolescence and adulthood.[81] Active substance use further confers risk for traumatic events and often interferes with appropriate detection of anxiety disorders.[82,83] Anxiety often escalates during periods of sobriety, particularly early in the course of recovery, warranting a greater degree of support. Epidemiologic findings suggest that severe trauma and PTSD are 5 times more prevalent in substance-abusing populations than nonsubstance-using populations, with 30% of adolescents who actively use substances meeting criteria for current PTSD and 50% meeting criteria for having had PTSD during their lifetime.[84–86] Although some studies in adults with PTSD show benefit from SSRIs,[87] no controlled studies have examined SSRIs in youth with PTSD. Trauma-focused

CBTs have shown more consistent effectiveness,[88] yet more studies are needed in this important area.

Anxiety disorders have also been associated with greater risk for developing eating disorders,[89] including anorexia nervosa in adolescent girls,[90,91] and binge eating in children.[92] Children and adolescents may vigilantly attend to severe food restriction as a means of addressing their anxiety, with nutritional deficits further impairing brain function. Patients may further exhibit extreme avoidance to psychotherapy, and there is minimal evidence supporting the use of SSRIs to aid weight restoration.[93] Pharmacologic management may nevertheless be helpful to address premorbid features of anxiety and facilitate multimodal treatment approaches.

Anxiety symptoms are also often prominent in children with autism spectrum disorders (ASDs). Bartack and Rutter,[94] in their classic study of autistic children, found that most of the autistic sample showed ritualistic and obsessive behaviors. Simonoff and colleagues[95] found that the most common comorbid diagnosis of youth with ASDs was social anxiety disorder (29%). A meta-analysis of the limited data on treatment of children with ASDs found that the use of SSRIs was associated with reduced anxiety, decreased repetitive behaviors, and improved global function.[96] However, a large study using citalopram in children with autism did not show improvement in symptomatic behaviors when compared with placebo, and another recent meta-analysis raised concerns for lack of efficacy and risk of side effects.[97,98] Nevertheless, clinical recommendations include consideration of the use of SSRIs with symptoms of anxiety, because they may still offer benefit in some children and adolescents with comorbid ASD.[99]

Although trichotillomania, or impulsive repetitive hair-pulling, is listed as an impulse control disorder, the triggers for repetitive hair-pulling are often anxious thoughts,[100,101] and urges to pull are typically accompanied by increased anxiety symptoms.[101–103] However, treatment studies using SSRIs have shown low rates of response.[104–106] Limited adult trials have revealed efficacy for clomipramine, risperidone, and olanzapine, yet the lack of child and adolescent evidence and the problematic side effects of these medications suggest pharmacotherapy should be reserved for individuals with high functional impairment or comorbid disorders.[107] CBT with habit reversal therapy has been found to be effective in reducing hair-pulling in a small open trial of adolescent patients with trichotillomania, and is the recommended first-line treatment.[104]

In children with features of social anxiety and avoidance of talking to strangers, it is important to inquire about selective mutism, which may generalize to significantly impair functioning. An RCT including 15 children aged 6 years to 12 years diagnosed with selective mutism showed significant symptomatic improvements and improved ratings by parents of anxiety and mutism when compared with placebo following fluoxetine treatment, yet continued to be symptomatic at the end of the study and did not show improvements on clinical scales.[108] An open trial of fluoxetine in 50 children with selective mutism revealed decreased anxiety and an increase in speech in social settings in 76% of the children.[109] Despite limited evidence, the treatment of choice includes SSRIs and CBT.[110]

Complementary and Alternative Medicines

Parents often seek complementary and alternative remedies before pharmacologic agents. Anxiety and stress was the third most common reason for the use of complementary and alternative medicines in children and adolescents.[111,112] Although rigorous evidence is lacking to support the use of naturopathic medications, kava, a plant found in the North Pacific, has evidence of effectiveness in 7 treatment trials.[113]

SUMMARY

Anxiety disorders are the most common mental health disorders in children and adolescents, and increasing evidence suggests pharmacotherapy can provide effective treatment. Pediatricians are increasingly faced with the challenges of assessment and pharmacologic treatment of anxious youth, many of whom have comorbid impairments, including somatic complaints, disruptive behaviors, or other clinical disorders. Psychotherapeutic options should also be considered before, and in conjunction with, medication. SSRIs have been used in the greatest number of positive pediatric anxiety trials, showing benefits in clinical response and reduction of symptoms. Tricyclic agents have also revealed benefit, particularly in OCD, but carry concerns for arrhythmia and overdose. Benzodiazepines have not been supported by efficacy studies and raise concerns for physiologic tolerance, yet may provide acute relief of impairing symptoms. Primary providers who do not feel comfortable managing the mental health needs of anxious youth should routinely seek consultation to ensure comprehensive treatment. These efforts serve to reduce the future risk of future mental health impairments, and empower anxious youth to increasingly master symptoms on their own, supported by an available and collaborative network.

REFERENCES

1. Krystal JH, Tolin DF, Sanacora G, et al. Neuroplasticity as a target for the pharmacotherapy of anxiety disorders, mood disorders, and schizophrenia. Drug Discov Today 2009;14(13/14):690–7.
2. Chavira D, Stein M, Bailey K, et al. Comorbidity of generalized social anxiety disorder and depression in a pediatric primary care sample. J Affect Disord 2004;80(2-3):163–71.
3. Egger H, Angold A. Common emotional and behavioral disorders in preschool children: presentation, nosology, and epidemiology. J Child Psychol Psychiatry 2006;47(3/4):313–7.
4. Craske M. Origin of phobias and anxiety disorders: why more women than men? Oxford (UK): Elsevier; 2003.
5. Costello EJ, Mustillo S, Erkanli A, et al. Prevalence and development of psychiatric disorders in childhood and adolescence. Arch Gen Psychiatry 2003;60(8): 837–44.
6. Last C, Perrin S, Hersen M, et al. A prospective study of childhood anxiety disorders. J Am Acad Child Adolesc Psychiatry 1996;35(11):1502–10.
7. Beesdo K, Bittner A, Pine D, et al. Incidence of social anxiety disorder and the consistent risk for secondary depression in the first three decades of life. Arch Gen Psychiatry 2007;64(8):903–12.
8. Shin LM, Liberzon I. The neurocircuitry of fear, stress, and anxiety disorders. Neuropsychopharmacology 2010;35:169–91.
9. Roozendaal B, McEwen BS, Chattarji S. Stress, memory and the amygdala. Nat Rev Neurosci 2009;10(6):423–33.
10. Pine DS, Guyer AE, Leibenluft E. Functional magnetic resonance imaging and pediatric anxiety. J Am Acad Child Adolesc Psychiatry 2008;47(11): 1217–21.
11. Centers for Disease Control and Prevention, NCHS Health eStat. U.S. children 4–17 years of age who received treatment for emotional or behavioral

difficulties: preliminary data from the 2005 National Health Interview Survey. Available at: http://www.cdc.gov/nchs/data/hestat/children2005/children2005. htm. Accessed August 28, 2010.

12. Irwin C. The adolescent visit. In: Rudolph C, Rudolph A, Hostetter M, et al, editors. Rudolph's pediatrics. 21st edition. New York: McGraw-Hill; 2002. p. 234–8.

13. Jellinek M, Murphy J, Robinson J, et al. Pediatric symptom checklist (PSC): screening school-age children for psychosocial dysfunction. J Pediatr 1988; 112(2):201–9.

14. Rockhill CM, Kodish I, DiBattisto C, et al. Anxiety disorders in children and adolescents. Curr Probl Pediatr Adolesc Health Care 2010;40:67–99.

15. Chiang O. Anxiety disorders. In: Garfunkel L, Kaczorowski J, Christy C, editors. Mosby's pediatric clinical advisor; instant diagnosis and treatment. 2nd edition. St Louis (MO): Mosby; 2007. p. 41–3.

16. Varley C, Varley J, Smith C. Anxiety disorders in children and adolescents. In: Greydanus D, Patel D, Pratt H, editors. Behavioral pediatrics. 2nd edition. New York: iUniverse; 2006. p. 618–50.

17. McClellan JM, Werry JS. Evidence-based treatments in child and adolescent psychiatry: an inventory. J Am Acad Child Adolesc Psychiatry 2003;42(12): 1388–400.

18. Barrett PM. Evaluation of cognitive behavioral group treatments for childhood anxiety disorders. J Clin Child Psychol 1998;27(4):459–68.

19. Kendall PC. Treating anxiety disorders in children: results of a randomized clinical trial. J Consult Clin Psychol 1994;62(1):100–10.

20. Kendall PC, Flannery-Schroeder E, et al. Therapy for youths with anxiety disorders: a second randomized clinical trial. J Consult Clin Psychol 1997;65(3): 366–80.

21. Manassis K, Mendlowitz SL, Scapillato D, et al. Group and individual cognitive-behavioral therapy for childhood anxiety disorders: a randomized trial. J Am Acad Child Adolesc Psychiatry 2002;41(12):1423–30.

22. Wood JJ, Piacentini JC, Southam-Gerow M, et al. Family cognitive behavioral therapy for child anxiety disorders. J Am Acad Child Adolesc Psychiatry 2006;45(3):314–21.

23. The Pediatric OCD Treatment Study (POTS) Team. Cognitive-behavior therapy, sertraline, and their combination for children and adolescents with obsessive-compulsive disorder: the Pediatric OCD Treatment Study (POTS) randomized controlled trial. JAMA 2004;292(16):1969–76.

24. Barrett P, Healy-Farrell L, March JS. Cognitive-behavioral family treatment of childhood obsessive-compulsive disorder: a controlled trial. J Am Acad Child Adolesc Psychiatry 2004;43(1):46–62.

25. Storch EA, Geffken GR, Merlo LJ, et al. Family-based cognitive-behavioral therapy for pediatric obsessive-compulsive disorder: comparison of intensive and weekly approaches. J Am Acad Child Adolesc Psychiatry 2007;46(4): 469–78.

26. King NJ, Tonge BJ, Mullen P, et al. Treating sexually abused children with post-traumatic stress symptoms: a randomized clinical trial. J Am Acad Child Adolesc Psychiatry 2000;39(11):1347–55.

27. Nevo GA, Manassis K. Outcomes for treated anxious children: a critical review of long-term-follow-up studies. Depress Anxiety 2009;26(7):650–60.

28. Connolly SD, Bernstein GA. Work group on quality issues. practice parameter for the assessment and treatment of children and adolescents with anxiety disorders. J Am Acad Child Adolesc Psychiatry 2007;46(2):267–83.

29. Southam-Gerow M, Kendall P, et al. Examining outcome variability: correlates of treatment response in a child and adolescent anxiety clinic. J Clin Child Psychol 2001;30(3):422–36.
30. March JS, Biederman J, Wolkow R, et al. Sertraline in children and adolescents with obsessive-compulsive disorder: a multicenter randomized controlled trial. JAMA 1998;280(20):1752–6.
31. Liebowitz MR, Turner SM, Piacentini J, et al. Fluoxetine in children and adolescents with OCD: a placebo-controlled trial. J Am Acad Child Adolesc Psychiatry 2002;41(12):1431–8.
32. Riddle MA, Scahill L, King RA, et al. Double-blind, crossover trial of fluoxetine and placebo in children and adolescents with obsessive-compulsive disorder. J Am Acad Child Adolesc Psychiatry 1992;31(6):1062–9.
33. Riddle MA, Reeve EA, Yaryura-Tobias JA, et al. Fluvoxamine for children and adolescents with obsessive-compulsive disorder: a randomized, controlled, multicenter trial. J Am Acad Child Adolesc Psychiatry 2001;40(2):222–9.
34. Geller DA, Wagner KD, Emslie G, et al. Paroxetine treatment in children and adolescents with obsessive-compulsive disorder: a randomized, multicenter, double-blind, placebo-controlled trial. J Am Acad Child Adolesc Psychiatry 2004;43(11):1387–96.
35. Geller DA, Biederman J, Stewart SE, et al. Impact of comorbidity on treatment response to paroxetine in pediatric obsessive-compulsive disorder: is the use of exclusion criteria empirically supported in randomized clinical trials? J Child Adolesc Psychopharmacol 2003;13(Suppl 1):s19–29.
36. Mukaddes NM, Abali O, Kaynak N. Citalopram treatment of children and adolescents with obsessive-compulsive disorder: a preliminary report. Psychiatry Clin Neurosci 2003;57(4):405–8.
37. Thomsen PH. Child and adolescent obsessive-compulsive disorder treated with citalopram: findings from an open trial of 23 cases. J Child Adolesc Psychopharmacol 1997;7(3):157–66.
38. Schirman S, Kronenberg S, Apter A, et al. Effectiveness and tolerability of citalopram for the treatment of depression and anxiety disorders in children and adolescents: an open-label study. J Neural Transm 2010;117:139–45.
39. Alaghband-Rad J, Hakimshooshtary M. A randomized controlled clinical trial of citalopram versus fluoxetine in children and adolescents with obsessive-compulsive disorder (OCD). Eur Child Adolesc Psychiatry 2009;18(3):131–5.
40. Ipser JC, Stein DJ, Hawkridge S, et al. Pharmacotherapy for anxiety disorders in children and adolescents. Cochrane Database Syst Rev 2009;3:CD005170.
41. US Department of Health and Human Services. Food and Drug Administration: drugs. Available at: http://www.fda.gov/Drugs/DrugSafety/UCM085729. Accessed August 20, 2010.
42. Wagner KD, Berard R, Stein MB, et al. A multicenter, randomized, double-blind, placebo-controlled trial of paroxetine in children and adolescents with social anxiety disorder. Arch Gen Psychiatry 2004;61(11):1153–62.
43. Walkup JT, Piacentini J, Birmaher B, et al. Cognitive behavioral therapy, sertraline, or a combination in childhood anxiety. N Engl J Med 2008;359(26):2753–66.
44. Kendall P, Hedtke K. Cognitive-behavioral therapy for anxious children: therapist manual. 3rd edition. Ardmore (PA): Workbook Publishing; 2006.
45. March J, Silva S, Petrycki S, et al. Fluoxetine, cognitive-behavioral therapy, and their combination for adolescents with depression: treatment for Adolescents With Depression Study (TADS) randomized controlled trial. JAMA 2004;292(7):807–20.

46. The MTA Cooperative Group. A 14-month randomized clinical trial of treatment strategies for attention-deficit/hyperactivity disorder. Arch Gen Psychiatry 1999; 56(12):1073–86.

47. The Research Units on Pediatric Psychopharmacology Anxiety Study Group (RUPP). Fluvoxamine for the treatment of anxiety disorders in children and adolescents. N Engl J Med 2001;344(17):1279–85.

48. Walkup J, Labellarte M, Riddle MA, et al. Treatment of pediatric anxiety disorders: an open-label extension of the research units on pediatric psychopharmacology anxiety study. J Child Adolesc Psychopharmacol 2002;12(3):175–88.

49. Birmaher B, Axelson DA, Monk K, et al. Fluoxetine for the treatment of childhood anxiety disorders. J Am Acad Child Adolesc Psychiatry 2003;42(4):415–23.

50. Rynn MA, Siqueland L, Rickels K. Placebo-controlled trial of sertraline in the treatment of children with generalized anxiety disorder. Am J Psychiatry 2001; 158(12):2008–14.

51. Rynn MA, Riddle MA, Yeung PP, et al. Efficacy and safety of extended-release venlafaxine in the treatment of generalized anxiety disorder in children and adolescents: two placebo-controlled trials. Am J Psychiatry 2007;164(2):290–300.

52. March JS, Entusah AR, Rynn M, et al. A randomized controlled trial of venlafaxine ER versus placebo in pediatric social anxiety disorder. Biol Psychiatry 2007; 62(10):1149–54.

53. Safer DA. Should selective serotonin reuptake inhibitors be prescribed for children with major depressive and anxiety disorders? Pediatrics 2006;118(3): 1248–51.

54. Fanton J, Gleason M. Psychopharmacology and preschoolers: a critical review of current conditions. Child Adolesc Psychiatr Clin N Am 2009;18(3):753–71.

55. Wright H, Cuccaro M, Leonhardt T, et al. Case study: fluoxetine in the multimodal treatment of a preschool child with selective mutism. J Am Acad Child Adolesc Psychiatry 1995;34(7):857–62.

56. Avci A, Diler R, Tamam L. Fluoxetine treatment in a 2.5 year old girl. J Am Acad Child Adolesc Psychiatry 1998;37(9):901–2.

57. Food and Drug Administration. New warnings proposed for antidepressants. Available at: http://www.fda.gov/ForConsumers/ConsumerUpdates/ucm048950. htm. Accessed December 12, 2010.

58. Singh T, Prakash A, Rais T, et al. Decreased use of antidepressants in youth after US Food and Drug Administration black box warning. Psychiatry (Edgemont) 2009;6(10):30–4.

59. Reinblatt SP, DosReis S, Walkup JT, et al. Activation adverse events induced by the selective serotonin reuptake inhibitor fluvoxamine in children and adolescents. J Child Adolesc Psychopharmacol 2009;19(2):119–26.

60. Gittelman-Klein R, Klein DF. School phobia: controlled imipramine treatment. Calif Med 1971;115(3):42.

61. Klein RG, Koplewicz HS, Kanner A. Imipramine treatment of children with separation anxiety disorder. J Am Acad Child Adolesc Psychiatry 1992; 31(1):21–8.

62. Bernstein GA, Borchardt CM, Perwien AR, et al. Imipramine plus cognitive-behavioral therapy in the treatment of school refusal. J Am Acad Child Adolesc Psychiatry 2000;39(3):276–83.

63. Berney T, Kolvin I, Bhate SR, et al. School phobia: a therapeutic trial with clomipramine and short-term outcome. Br J Psychiatry 1981;138:110–8.

64. Flament MF, Rapoport JL, Kilts C. A controlled trial of clomipramine in childhood obsessive compulsive disorder. Psychopharmacol Bull 1985;21(1):150–2.

65. Figueroa Y, Rosenberg DR, Birmaher B, et al. Combination treatment with clomipramine and selective serotonin reuptake inhibitors for obsessive-compulsive disorder in children and adolescents. J Child Adolesc Psychopharmacol 1998; 8(1):61–7.
66. Harmon R, Riggs P. Clonidine for posttraumatic stress disorder in preschool children. J Natl Med Assoc 1999;91(8):475–7.
67. Famularo R, Kinscherff R, Fenton T. Propranolol treatment for childhood posttraumatic stress disorder, acute type. A pilot study. Am J Dis Child 1988; 142(11):1244–7.
68. Bernstein GA, Garfinkel BD, Borchardt CM. Comparative studies of pharmacotherapy for school refusal. J Am Acad Child Adolesc Psychiatry 1990;29(5): 773–81.
69. Graae F, Milner J, Rizzotto L, et al. Clonazepam in childhood anxiety disorders. J Am Acad Child Adolesc Psychiatry 1994;33(3):372–6.
70. Simeon JG, Ferguson HB, Knott V, et al. Clinical, cognitive, and neurophysiological effects of alprazolam in children and adolescents with overanxious and avoidant disorders. J Am Acad Child Adolesc Psychiatry 1992;31(1):29–33.
71. Longo L, Johnson B. Addiction: part I. Benzodiazepines–side effects, abuse risk and alternatives. Am Fam Physician 2000;61:2121–8.
72. Pine DS. Treating children and adolescents with selective serotonin reuptake inhibitors: how long is appropriate? J Am Acad Child Adolesc Psychiatry 2002;2002(12):189–203.
73. Kovacs M, Devlin B. Internalizing disorders in childhood. J Child Psychol Psychiatry 1998;39(1):47–63.
74. Costello EJ, Farmer EM, Angold A, et al. Psychiatric disorders among American Indian and white youth in Appalachia: the Great Smoky Mountains Study. Am J Public Health 1997;87(5):827–32.
75. Anderson J. Epidemiological issues. In: Ollendick T, King N, Yule W, editors. International handbook of phobia and anxiety disorders in children and adolescents. New York: Plenum Press; 1994. p. 43–66.
76. Abikoff H, McGough J, Vitiello B, et al. Sequential pharmacotherapy for children with comorbid attention-deficit/hyperactivity and anxiety disorders. J Am Acad Child Adolesc Psychiatry 2005;44(5):418–27.
77. Pauls D, Alsobrook JP, Goodman W, et al. A family study of obsessive compulsive disorder. Am J Psychiatry 1995;152:76–84.
78. Pauls D, Alsobrook J. The inheritance of obsessive-compulsive disorder. Child Adolesc Psychiatr Clin N Am 1999;8(3):481–96.
79. Kendall P, Hedtke K, Aschenbrand S. Behavioral and emotional disorders in adolescents. Nature, assessment and treatment. In: Wolfe DA, Mash EJ, editors. Anxiety disorders. New York: Guilford Press; 2006. p. 259–99.
80. Jaffe S. Adolescent substance abuse and dual disorders. Child Adolesc Psychiatr Clin N Am 1996;5(1):1–261.
81. Weissman M, Wolk S, Wickramaratne P, et al. Children with prepubertal-onset major depressive disorder and anxiety grown up. Arch Gen Psychiatry 1999; 56:794–801.
82. Clark DB, Bukstein OG. Psychopathology in adolescent alcohol abuse and dependence. Alcohol Health Res World 1998;22(2):117–21.
83. Bukstein O, Brent D, Kaminer Y. Comorbidity of substance abuse and other psychiatric disorders in adolescents. Am J Psychiatry 1989;146:1131–41.
84. Deykin E, Buka S. Prevalence and risk factors for posttraumatic stress disorder among chemically dependent adolescents. Am J Psychiatry 1997;154:752–7.

85. Clark D, Bukstein O, Smith M, et al. Identifying anxiety disorders in adolescents hospitalized for alcohol abuse or dependence. Psychiatr Serv 1995;46: 618–20.

86. Clark D, Lesnick L, Hegedus A, et al. Traumas and other adverse life events in adolescents with alcohol abuse and dependence. J Am Acad Child Adolesc Psychiatry 1997;36(12):1744–51.

87. Stein DJ, Ipser JC, McAnda N. Pharmacotherapy of posttraumatic stress disorder: a review of meta-analyses and treatment guidelines. CNS Spectr 2009;14(1 Suppl 1):25–31.

88. Cohen JA, Bukstein O, Walter H, et al. Practice parameter for the assessment and treatment of children and adolescents with posttraumatic stress disorder. J Am Acad Child Adolesc Psychiatry 2010;49(4):414–30.

89. Babio N, Canals J, Pietrobelli A, et al. A two-phase population study: relationships between overweight, body composition, and risk of eating disorders. Nutr Hosp 2009;24(4):485–91.

90. Halmi KA. Anorexia nervosa: an increasing problem in children and adolescents. Dialogues Clin Neurosci 2009;11:100–3.

91. Salbach-Andrae H, Lenz K, Simmendinger N, et al. Psychiatric comorbidities among female adolescents with anorexia nervosa. Child Psychiatry Hum Dev 2008;39(3):261–72.

92. Czaja J, Rief W, Hilbert A. Emotion regulation and binge eating in children. Int J Eat Disord 2009;42(4):356–62.

93. Powers PS, Bruty H. Pharmacotherapy for eating disorders and obesity. Child Adolesc Psychiatr Clin N Am 2009;18(1):175–87.

94. Bartak L, Rutter M. Differences between mentally retarded and normally intelligent autistic children. J Autism Dev Disord 1976;6(2):109–20.

95. Simonoff E, Pickles A, Charman T, et al. Psychiatric disorders in children with autism spectrum disorders: prevalence, comorbidity, and associated factors in a population-derived sample. J Am Acad Child Adolesc Psychiatry 2008; 47(8):921–9.

96. Kolevzon A, Mathewson K, Hollander E, et al. Selective serotonin reuptake inhibitors in autism: a review of efficacy and tolerability. J Clin Psychiatry 2006;67(3): 407–14.

97. King BH, Hollander E, Sikich L, et al. Lack of efficacy of citalopram in children with autism spectrum disorders and high levels of repetitive behavior: citalopram ineffective in children with autism. Arch Gen Psychiatry 2009;66(6): 583–90.

98. Williams K, Wheeler DM, Silove N, et al. Selective serotonin reuptake inhibitors for autism spectrum disorders. Cochrane Database Syst Rev 2010;8:CD004677.

99. Volkmar F, Cook EH, Palmeroy R, et al. Practice parameters for the assessment and treatment of children, adolescents, and adults with autism and other pervasive developmental disorders. J Am Acad Child Adolesc Psychiatry 1999;38- (Suppl 12):325–45.

100. Flessner C, Woods D, Franlkin M, et al. Cross-sectional study of women with trichotillomania: a preliminary examination of pulling styles, severity, phenomenology, and functional impact. Child Psychiatry Hum Dev 2009;40(1):153–67.

101. Duke D, Bodzin D, Tavares P, et al. The phenomenology of hairpulling in a community sample. J Anxiety Disord 2009;23(8):1118–25.

102. Lewin A, Piacentini J, Flessner C, et al. Depression, anxiety, and functional impairment in children with trichotillomania. Depress Anxiety 2009;26(6): 521–7.

103. Franklin M, Flessner C, Woods D, et al. The child and adolescent trichotillomania impact project: descriptive psychopathology, comorbidity, functional impairment, and treatment utilization. J Dev Behav Pediatr 2008;29(6):493–500.

104. Tolin D, Franklin M, Diefenbach G, et al. Pediatric trichotillomania: descriptive psychopathology and an open trial of cognitive behavioral therapy. Cogn Behav Ther 2007;36(3):129–44.

105. Stein D, Bouwer C, Maud C. Use of the selective serotonin reuptake inhibitor citalopram in treatment of trichotillomania. Eur Arch Psychiatry Clin Neurosci 1997; 247(4):234–6.

106. Christenson G, MacKenzie T, Mitchell J, et al. A placebo-controlled, double-blind crossover study of fluoxetine in trichotillomania. Am J Psychiatry 1991; 148:1566–71.

107. Welsh K, McDougle C. Pharmacological strategies for trichotillomania. Expert Opin Pharmacother 2005;6(6):975–84.

108. Black B, Uhde TW. Treatment of elective mutism with fluoxetine: a double-blind, placebo-controlled study. J Am Acad Child Adolesc Psychiatry 1994;33(7): 1000–6.

109. Dummit ES, Klein RG, Trancer NK, et al. Systematic assessment of 50 children with selective mutism. J Am Acad Child Adolesc Psychiatry 1997;36(5):653–60.

110. Viana AG, Beidel DC, Rabian B. Selective mutism: a review and integration of the last 15 years. Clin Psychol Rev 2009;29(1):57–67.

111. ADAA. Anxiety Disorder Association of America, complimentary and alternative therapies. Available at: http://www.adaa.org/finding-help/treatment/complementary-alternative-treatment. Accessed May 29, 2010.

112. National Institutes of Health. National Center for Complimentary and Alternative Medicine, complimentary and alternative medicine and children. Available at: http://nccam.nih.gov/health/children/. Accessed August 28, 2010.

113. Ernst E. The risk-benefit profile of commonly used herbal therapies: Ginko, St. John's Wort, Ginseng, Echinacea, Saw Palmetto, and Kava. Ann Intern Med 2002;136(1):42–53.

Psychopharmacologic Control of Aggression and Violence in Children and Adolescents

Joseph L. Calles Jr, MD[a,b],*

KEYWORDS

- Adolescents • Aggression • Children
- Psychopharmacologic agents

It is an unfortunate fact that aggressive, violent, dangerous, and potentially lethal behaviors are rather common in the lives of American youth. The Centers for Disease Control and Prevention, of the US Department of Health and Human Services, conducts the national Youth Risk Behavior Surveillance every 2 years; the most recent complete data have been published for 2009.[1] In that survey, representative samples of public high school students (grades 9–12) were carefully questioned about various risk behaviors. Regarding those behaviors that have relevance to aggression, the following statistics were reported for the year preceding the survey: of all students, 31.5% had been in at least 1 fight, 3.8% had been in at least 1 fight that led to an injury that required medical intervention, 11.1% had been in at least 1 fight on school property, and 9.8% had experienced dating violence. In the preceding 30 days, of all students, on at least 1 occasion 17.5% had carried a weapon (eg, gun, knife, or club), 5.9% had carried a gun, 5.6% had carried a weapon on school property, and 7.7% of students had been threatened or injured with a weapon on school property.

Aggressive behaviors are the final step in a sequence that begins with some type of provoking stimulus (**Fig. 1**).[2] The initiating event can be objective and obvious, such as a person being pushed or hit, or it can be subjective and subtle (and not necessarily

---

[a] Department of Psychiatry, College of Human Medicine, Michigan State University, A236 East Fee Hall, East Lansing, MI 48824, USA
[b] Child and Adolescent Psychiatry, Psychiatry Residency Training Program, Michigan State University/Kalamazoo Center for Medical Studies, 1722 Shaffer Road, Suite 3, Kalamazoo, MI 49048, USA
* Child and Adolescent Psychiatry, Psychiatry Residency Training Program, Michigan State University/Kalamazoo Center for Medical Studies, 1722 Shaffer Road, Suite 3, Kalamazoo, MI 49048.
E-mail address: calles@kcms.msu.edu

Pediatr Clin N Am 58 (2011) 73–84
doi:10.1016/j.pcl.2010.11.002
0031-3955/11/$ – see front matter © 2011 Elsevier Inc. All rights reserved.

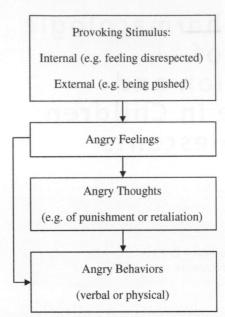

Fig. 1. The affective-cognitive-behavioral sequence of aggression. (*From* Calles JL. Aggressive behaviors. In: Greydanus DE, Patel DR, Pratt HD, et al, editors. Behavioral pediatrics. 3rd edition. Hauppauge (NY): Nova Science Publishers; 2009. p. 185–203; with permission.)

obvious to an observer), such as a person being disrespected or ignored. In individuals who display reactive aggression, disruptive behaviors are fueled by an immediate, intense emotional reaction to a real or perceived threat. Rational thinking is briefly and strongly influenced by their feelings, or is bypassed altogether. Another type of aggression, proactive aggression, may initially be triggered by negative emotions (eg, anger, envy, or greed), but that is overridden by a relatively dispassionate thought process that allows for a delayed and calculated response (ie, the person can wait to get their revenge). This article focuses on the reactive type of aggression, the more common type that is seen in clinical settings.

Anger is the most common emotion that leads to aggression. Aggressive behaviors can be diverse and are highly variable between individuals (**Fig. 2**).[2] Patterns of aggression tend to be more predictable in any given individual. For example, some people only display verbal forms of aggression, such as yelling, using profanities, or making threats to harm others. Aggression that is outwardly directed is more frightening for those who witness it, and is associated with more serious consequences. By the time that aggression causes damage to property, and especially to people (also called violent behavior), there is a high likelihood that the aggressive person will come into contact with either the medical or legal systems.

To eliminate current, or prevent future, aggression, it is important to keep in mind that there are many developmental, substance-related, and psychiatric disorders that can increase the risk for the emergence of aggressive behaviors. What follows is a review of the most common mental disorders associated with aggression and their treatments, focusing on psychopharmacologic agents. (The treatment of anger and aggression associated with developmental disorders is addressed in the article by Joseph L. Calles Jr elsewhere in this issue.)

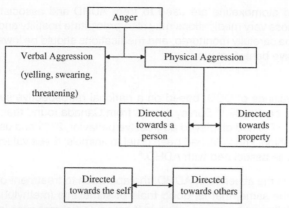

Fig. 2. The hierarchy of aggression. (*From* Calles JL. Aggressive behaviors. In: Greydanus DE, Patel DR, Pratt HD, et al, editors. Behavioral pediatrics. 3rd edition. Hauppauge (NY): Nova Science Publishers; 2009. p. 185–203; with permission.)

PSYCHIATRIC DISORDERS ASSOCIATED WITH AGGRESSION
Attention-deficit and Disruptive Behavior Disorders

In the *Diagnostic and statistical manual of mental disorders (4th edition, text revision)* (DSM-IV-TR)[3] this category is made up of attention-deficit/hyperactivity disorder (ADHD), oppositional defiant disorder (ODD), and conduct disorder (CD). As the term implies, disruptive behaviors, including aggression and violence, are a core feature of all 3 disorders. In a Canadian study of 129 consecutive children and adolescents who were referred for aggressive behavior, 93.02% were diagnosed with ODD, 88.37% with ADHD, and 38.75% with CD.[4]

ADHD

ADHD is fairly common in the general population. A national survey of 3042 youths (8–15 years of age) found the 12-month prevalence rate for ADHD to be 8.6%.[5] The previously cited Canadian study found that, in those diagnosed with ADHD, 80% had displayed aggressive behavior, 27% had used weapons in an aggressive fashion, and 28% had been cruel to animals.[4]

Treatment The recommended first choice for medication treatment of ADHD-related aggressive behaviors is usually a psychostimulant or atomoxetine. A meta-analysis of the effects of stimulants on aggression-related behaviors in ADHD[6] found the overall, average, weighted effect size to be a strong 0.84 for overt aggression. For the 7 studies (of the 28 total studies) that identified ADHD as the primary diagnosis, without comorbid ODD and/or CD, the average effect size of stimulants on overt aggressive behaviors is 0.745, which is still fairly strong.

The evidence for the efficacy of atomoxetine (a selective norepinephrine reuptake inhibitor) in the treatment of aggressive behaviors associated with ADHD is indirect, in that studies have looked at reductions in ODD behaviors, but not specifically at reductions in aggressive behaviors.[7,8] However, given that ODD is a further risk factor for aggression (see later discussion) and that 40% to 60% of children with ADHD also have ODD,[9] the use of atomoxetine should be considered, especially if patients are refractory to, intolerant of, or worsened by stimulant medications. To achieve a good clinical response, atomoxetine dosing may have to be higher (1.8 mg/kg/d) than is usually used (1.2 mg/kg/d).[7]

Stimulants and atomoxetine are used to treat ADHD and associated aggressive behaviors, but those very medications may also precipitate hostility and aggression.[10] Patients should be carefully monitored, and medications should be lowered or discontinued if aggressive behaviors worsen.

ODD

The lifetime prevalence of ODD, based on a national retrospective survey of adults, was estimated to be 10.2%.[11] Survey results from Canada found that, in those diagnosed with ODD, 77% had displayed aggressive behavior, 27% had used weapons in an aggressive fashion, and 28% had been cruel to animals; these values are not much different than those associated with ADHD.[4]

Treatment Even in the absence of ADHD, the approach to treatment of aggression in ODD starts out the same, that is, good trials of stimulants (methylphenidate and/or amphetamines) followed by atomoxetine.[12] If only a partial response is achieved with maximum doses of those medications, augmentation can be tried with divalproex,[13] risperidone,[14] or clonidine.[15]

CD

CD is fortunately not very common in the general population; only 2.1% of those aged 8–15 years meet the diagnostic criteria.[5] The Canadian study on disruptive behavior disorders found that, in those diagnosed with CD, 90% had displayed aggressive behavior, 52% had used weapons in an aggressive fashion, and 54% had been cruel to animals.[4] Although the rate of aggressive behavior in CD is somewhat higher than the rates seen in ADHD and ODD, the rates for weapon use and animal cruelty are almost twice those seen in the other 2 disorders.

Treatment It is readily apparent that CD is the most disturbing disorder in this category, the successful treatment of which should be a high clinical and societal priority. Many different psychotropic medications have been used to treat CD, especially to try and reduce aggression. The most common therapeutic agent has been lithium carbonate, used alone or in combination with other agents. A 4-week study of very aggressive, hospitalized youth (median age 12.5 years) found lithium to be clinically and statistically superior to placebo in reducing the ratings of aggressive behaviors.[16] A more recent study of children and adolescents (8–17 years; mean 14.2 years) with CD who were treated with lithium carbonate, with or without an atypical antipsychotic (AA; either risperidone or olanzapine), were retrospectively followed up 6 to 12 months after initiating treatment.[17] Almost one-half showed a significant reduction in overt aggression scores; however, the lithium-plus AA/lithium-alone ratio was about 2:1.

Various trials of AA monotherapy have been conducted in the treatment of CD-related aggression, including with aripiprazole (open-label study),[18] quetiapine (randomized, double-blind, placebo-controlled pilot study),[19] olanzapine (retrospective chart review),[20] and risperidone (randomized, double-blind, placebo-controlled pilot study).[21] With the exception of quetiapine, the AAs significantly reduced aggressive behaviors compared with placebo.

As had been previously mentioned, divalproex can be used as an augmentation agent in ODD; it can also be used as monotherapy to treat CD. A study of youth with CD, most (66%) incarcerated for violent offenses, compared 2 different levels of divalproex dosing: high-dose (500–1,500 mg daily) and low-dose (≤250 mg daily).[22] There were no significant reductions in suppression of anger scores between the 2 groups; however, the high-dose group did have a significant improvement in impulse control. Given that overt affective aggression is impulsive by nature, the use of divalproex in patients with CD may help to reduce impulsivity and, by extension, associated aggressive behaviors.[23]

Mood Disorders

Major depressive disorder

Depression is another psychiatric disorder that is relatively common in youth. In a meta-analysis of studies over 30 years, overall prevalence estimates were 2.8% for those less than 13 years of age and 5.6% for those aged 13 to 18 years.[24] Depression is also associated with aggression, beginning at a very young age. A survey of caregivers of 3- to 6-year-old children, who were placed into 1 of 4 diagnostic groups, found that the group rates of physical aggression were in the following descending order: comorbid depressed/disruptive; pure disruptive; pure depressed; and, healthy.[25] Although not as common as in the presence of disruptive behaviors, the risk for aggression in depressed children is increased compared with nondepressed children. In a study of adolescents (aged 13–17 years) with diagnosed major depressive disorder (MDD), rates of aggression were high, with 70% reporting frequent verbal aggression, 24% with frequent physical aggression, and 14% being arrested for aggressive behaviors.[26]

Treatment The agents of choice for pediatric depression, with or without aggression, have been the selective serotonin reuptake inhibitors (SSRIs). Their ameliorative effects on aggression derive from decreases in negative affect and impulsivity, and an increase in social assertiveness.[27] Given that the US Food and Drug Administration (FDA) has approved fluoxetine and escitalopram for the treatment of pediatric MDD, those should be the initial agents of choice for the treatment of depression comorbid with aggression, although theoretically any antidepressant with serotonergic activity may work. Any antidepressant may also cause or exacerbate aggression, but, in the case of fluoxetine, a meta-analysis did not support an association between its use and aggression and/or hostility-related events compared with placebo.[28]

Bipolar disorder

The prevalence of bipolar disorder is much less common than depression in the general pediatric population, estimated at 1.0% to 1.5%, but is much higher (17%–30%) in pediatric psychiatric clinics.[29] It is generally agreed that aggressive behaviors are very common in pediatric bipolar disorder. This seems to be a combination of the mood disturbance (mostly irritability) and the high rates of comorbid ADHD (60%–90%) and CD (40%–70%).[30]

Treatment It is fortunate that many of the medications that have demonstrated efficacy in the treatment of aggression (lithium carbonate, divalproex, AAs) are also the medications used to treat bipolar disorder. Treatment guidelines should be followed regarding the initial and sequenced selections of psychopharmacologic agents.[31]

Severe mood dysregulation

The term severe mood dysregulation (SMD), or a variant thereof, is being considered for inclusion as a diagnosis in the next (fifth) edition of the DSM. The concept of SMD evolved from clinical observations of children who were being diagnosed with bipolar disorder, but who had continuous (not cyclic) irritability and the absence of mania, hyperarousal (eg, insomnia vs decreased need for sleep in bipolar disorder), and increased reactivity to negative stimuli.[32] Lifetime prevalence is estimated at 3.3% in mostly white, mostly male 9- to 19-year-olds. The most common disorders comorbid with SMD are ADHD, CD, and ODD. What is relevant to the topic of this article is that the reactivity of SMD presents as frequent (≥3 times weekly) temper tantrums, verbal rages, and/or aggression toward people or property.

Treatment A 6-week randomized, double-blind, placebo-controlled trial of lithium was conducted with 7- to 17-year-olds diagnosed with SMD.[33] There were 2 surprising results: a 45% improvement during the 2-week placebo run-in; and, no significant differences between the lithium and placebo groups on outcome measures. This is consistent with the findings from a retrospective, community-based study of patients with ADHD (6–18 years), with comorbid bipolar disorder or mood disorder not otherwise specified (NOS; under which SMD was subsumed).[34] Despite similar treatments, including pharmacotherapy (mostly aripiprazole), the patients with mood disorder NOS/SMD improved significantly less than the patients with bipolar disorder.

A different approach to treatment can be tried in patients with comorbid ADHD and SMD. A study of 5- to 12-year-old children with both diagnoses used a combination of methylphenidate and behavior modification.[35] Results showed a 45% improvement in irritability and aggression in the active treatment group, double that seen in the placebo group. Based on their findings, the investigators make the statement that "the use of mood-stabilizing medications as a first-line treatment may not be necessary to achieve improvement in children with ADHD and SMD."

Anxiety Disorders

Anxiety disorders are some of the most common psychiatric disorders in children and adolescents, with prevalence rates in the 6% to 20% range.[36] Based on a review of the literature, there seems to be an association between anxiety disorders and disruptive behavior disorders, and between anxiety symptoms and reactive aggression.[37] However, the explanation for the observed comorbidity is unclear, and could include coincidence, mutual predispositions, or shared risk factors.

Posttraumatic stress disorder

In 1 urban sample, the lifetime prevalence of posttraumatic stress disorder (PTSD) in the general youth population was found to be 9.2%, whereas in a national sample of 12- to 17-year-olds 3.7% of boys and 6.3% of girls met the diagnostic criteria for PTSD.[38] Of the 3 symptom clusters in PTSD (reexperiencing, avoidance, and hyperarousal) it is the hyperarousal that is most likely to contribute to aggressive behaviors. In young children new-onset aggressive and oppositional behaviors could be manifestations of an experienced traumatic event.

Treatment There are very few studies of pharmacologic agents in child and adolescent PTSD, and there are no FDA-approved medications for PTSD in the pediatric population. As such, medication interventions are usually extrapolated from adult studies. A reasonable first choice of medication would be an SSRI, especially sertraline or paroxetine (as they are approved for PTSD in adults).[39] Dosing should start low to prevent an exacerbation of irritability and aggressiveness, a known side effect of serotonergic agents. If the SSRIs are partially effective, or noneffective, they may be augmented with or replaced by an AA, a mood stabilizer, or an alpha2-agonist (especially clonidine).

Panic disorder

It is currently appreciated that children and adolescents can experience panic attacks, and suffer with actual panic disorder at the rate of 0.5% to 5.0% in the general population and 0.2% to 10.0% in psychiatric settings.[40] That knowledge was not always available, however, as research on panic disorder in younger people lagged for many years, because of ongoing debates about whether or not it existed in that age group. An adult study evaluated anger in patients with panic disorder, obsessive-compulsive disorder, social phobia (also known as social anxiety disorder), and specific phobia, and compared it to nonclinical controls.[41] With the exception of the specific phobia group, the other anxiety groups experienced higher levels of anger than did controls. However, when comorbid depression was accounted for, the anger differential disappeared, except in those with panic disorder, who were prone to "lose their temper and express their anger aggressively."[41]

Treatment There are currently no FDA-approved medications for the treatment of panic disorder in children and adolescents. The antidepressants that are approved for panic disorder in adults (fluoxetine, sertraline, paroxetine, and venlafaxine) are often used off label in younger patients. The same caution about worsening aggression that was mentioned regarding the SSRIs in PTSD also applies to panic disorder. The benzodiazepines are also used to treat panic disorder in adults, but their use in younger patients with aggressive tendencies runs the great risk of behavioral disinhibition and worsening of symptoms.[42]

Schizophrenia and Other Psychotic Disorders

The development of schizophrenia before adulthood is so uncommon, and before age 13 years so rare, that the designations early-onset schizophrenia (EOS), with onset before age 18 years, and very-early-onset schizophrenia (VEOS), with onset before age 13 years, have been adopted for research and clinical use.[43] An Australian study examined 85 patients (aged 13–25 years; two-thirds male) with new-onset psychosis and varied diagnoses, including 44.7% with schizophrenia and 10.6% with schizophreniform disorder.[44] Results found physically aggressive behaviors in 43.5% of patients, and 27.1% of the sample had assaulted another person or used a weapon. The most serious offenses were associated with regular cannabis use and behavioral disinhibition, both common in younger ages, which was also a risk factor.

Treatment

Compared with the adult schizophrenia literature, there is a paucity of information on the treatment of aggression associated with EOS or VEOS. Some information can, therefore, be derived from adult studies to try and inform the treatment of younger, aggressive patients with schizophrenia. A 2-year follow-up study of community-living adults with schizophrenia demonstrated a significant reduction in the risk of violent behavior with the use of AAs (clozapine, risperidone, or olanzapine) compared with typical antipsychotics, such as haloperidol.[45] In another study involving adults with treatment-resistant schizophrenia, clozapine demonstrated superiority (over olanzapine and risperidone) in the reduction of aggressive behaviors.[46] In one of the few studies involving children and adolescents with schizophrenia, a small number of aggressive patients with childhood-onset schizophrenia, who were previously nonresponsive to either olanzapine or risperidone, showed reductions in violent episodes and thoughts when treated with clozapine.[47] Given the potentially serious side effects associated with clozapine, olanzapine and risperidone are safer agents to use initially.

Tourette and Other Tic Disorders

Tourette disorder (also called Tourette syndrome) is a chronic motor and vocal tic disorder, with strong familial aggregation and high comorbidity, especially with

Table 1
Disorders associated with aggressive behaviors and recommended pharmacotherapeutic strategies

Disorder	Medications[a]		
	First-line	Second-line	Third-line
ADHD	MPH or MAS	Stimulant not tried as first-line treatment	Atomoxetine
ODD	MPH or MAS	Atomoxetine	VPA, RIS, or clonidine
CD	Li ± AA	ARI, OLZ, or RIS	VPA
MDD	Fluoxetine	Escitalopram	A third SSRI or an SNRI
Bipolar disorder	Li, VPA, CBZ, OLZ, QUE or RIS	Drug class not tried as first-line treatment	Drug class not tried as first-line or second-line treatment
SMD	First-line treatment depends on the presence of comorbid conditions, eg, ADHD		
PTSD	Sertraline	Paroxetine or another SSRI	AA, AED, or clonidine
Panic disorder	SSRI	A second SSRI	A third SSRI or an SNRI
Schizophrenia	RIS or OLZ	AA not tried as first-line treatment	Clozapine
Tourette disorder	RIS	A second AA	A third AA
IED	Lithium or AED	Drug class not tried as first-line treatment	A second AED or an AA

Abbreviations: AA, atypical antipsychotic; ADHD, attention-deficit/hyperactivity disorder; AED, antiepileptic drug; ARI, aripiprazole; CBZ, carbamazepine; IED, intermittent explosive disorder; Li, lithium; MAS, mixed amphetamine salts; MDD, major depressive disorder; MPH, methylphenidate; ODD, oppositional defiant disorder; OLZ, olanzapine; PTSD, posttraumatic stress disorder; QUE, quetiapine; RIS, risperidone; SMD, severe mood dysregulation; SNRI, serotonin-norepinephrine reuptake inhibitor; SSRI, selective serotonin reuptake inhibitor; VPA, valproic acid.
[a] If the first-line agent is ineffective, or exacerbates the behavior, the second- or third-line agents may be selected.

obsessive-compulsive disorder and, to a lesser degree, ADHD.[48] Prevalence figures vary widely from 1:100 to 1:10,000, depending on the diagnostic criteria used. In addition to comorbid psychiatric disorders, approximately 25% to 70% of children with Tourette disorder display recurrent episodes of explosive anger or aggression (rage attacks), which are often described as the most impairing symptoms.[49]

Treatment
Considering the high degree of comorbidity with other psychiatric disorders, the initial treatment of Tourette disorder with medications will depend on identifying and prioritizing the other diagnoses.[50] However, a reasonable first choice to address both tics and aggression would be one of the AAs,[50,51] with many clinicians electing to start with risperidone.

Intermittent Explosive Disorder

As the name implies, intermittent explosive disorder (IED) is defined as episodic aggressive outbursts that are excessive in response to environmental stressors, and are not caused by medical, substance-use, or other psychiatric disorders.[3] IED is actually more common than was once believed, with a current diagnostic lifetime rate of 2.37% and 6.32% in a community sample.[52] The histories of adults with IED are notable for the onset of the disorder, on average, sometime in early adolescence.[53]

Table 2
Medications used to treat aggressive behaviors in children and adolescents with psychiatric disorders

Class	Agent	Dose Range (mg)[a]
Psychostimulants 　Methylphenidate 　Amphetamines	Methylphenidate[b] Dextroamphetamine[b] MAS[b]	0.15–0.7 mg/kg per dose: 10–80[c] 0.08–0.3 mg/kg per dose: 5–80[c] 2.5–40[c]
Antipsychotics 　Atypical 　Partial DA agonist	Risperidone Olanzapine Quetiapine Clozapine Aripiprazole	0.02–0.06 mg/kg: 0.5–6 0.15–0.20 mg/kg: 2.5–20 25–600 6.25–25 initially; 75–500[d] 2–30
Alpha-agonists	Clonidine Guanfacine[b]	0.05–0.3 0.5–4
Mood stabilizers[c] 　Lithium salts 　Antiepileptic drugs	Lithium carbonate[e] Valproic acid[b,e] Carbamazepine[b,e] Lamotrigine Oxcarbazepine	10–30 mg/kg (<12 y) 25–35 mg/kg (≥12 y) 20 mg/kg 7 mg/kg 25 (weeks 1 and 2), 50 (weeks 3 and 4), increase by 50 mg every 1–2 wk; 225–375 maximum 20–29 kg: 900 30–39 kg: 1200 >39 kg: 1800
Antidepressants 　SSRIs 　SNRIs 　Other (for ADHD)	Fluoxetine Sertraline Fluvoxamine[b] Paroxetine[b] Citalopram Escitalopram Venlafaxine[b] Atomoxetine	10–60 25–200 25–300 10–50 10–40 5–20 37.5–225 0.5–1.2 mg/kg[c] 1.4 mg/kg or 100 mg maximum

Abbreviation: MAS, mixed amphetamine salts.
[a] Total daily dose, unless otherwise specified.
[b] Also available in extended-release form for once-daily dosing.
[c] Given in divided doses.
[d] Dose increases dependent on white blood cell counts.
[e] Monitoring of blood levels required.

Treatment

Given the likely under-recognition, underdiagnosis, or misdiagnosis of IED (as, eg, bipolar disorder) in clinical settings, it is not surprising that there are no good quality psychopharmacologic studies to help guide treatment. What is available suggests trials of essentially all of the medications that have been mentioned for the other disorders in this article.[54] My preference is to start with one of the mood stabilizers, either lithium carbonate or an anticonvulsant, which are usually well tolerated by younger patients.

SUMMARY

Aggression has always been a part of the human condition, and children and adolescents are not immune to its effects. When younger people become aggressive, they can negatively affect those around them, and can also adversely affect their own psychological, social, emotional, academic, and occupational development. Therefore health care providers must identify the causes of the aggressive behaviors and intervene in a therapeutic manner. The purpose of this article is to review common psychiatric disorders associated with aggression and provide recommendations for their treatment using psychotropic medications (**Tables 1** and **2**).

REFERENCES

1. Centers for Disease Control and Prevention. Youth risk behavior surveillance-United States, 2009. MMWR Surveill Summ 2010;59(No SS-5):1–142.
2. Calles JL. Aggressive behaviors. In: Greydanus DE, Patel DR, Pratt HD, et al, editors. Behavioral pediatrics. 3rd edition. Hauppauge (NY): Nova Science Publishers; 2009. p. 185–203.
3. American Psychiatric Association. Diagnostic and statistical manual of mental disorders (4th edition, text revision). Washington, DC: American Psychiatric Association; 2000.
4. Turgay A. Aggression and disruptive behavior disorders in children and adolescents. Expert Rev Neurother 2004;4(4):623–32.
5. Merikangas KR, He JP, Brody D, et al. Prevalence and treatment of mental disorders among US children in the 2001–2004 NHANES. Pediatrics 2010;125(1):75–81.
6. Connor DF, Glatt SJ, Lopez ID, et al. Psychopharmacology and aggression. I: a meta-analysis of stimulant effects on overt/covert aggression-related behaviors in ADHD. J Am Acad Child Adolesc Psychiatry 2002;41(3):253–61.
7. Newcorn JH, Spencer TJ, Biederman J, et al. Atomoxetine treatment in children and adolescents with attention-deficit/hyperactivity disorder and comorbid oppositional defiant disorder. J Am Acad Child Adolesc Psychiatry 2005;44(3):240–8.
8. Bangs ME, Hazell P, Danckaerts M, et al, Atomoxetine ADHD/ODD Study Group. Atomoxetine for the treatment of attention-deficit/hyperactivity disorder and oppositional defiant disorder. Pediatrics 2008;121(2):e314–20.
9. August GJ, Realmuto GM, MacDonald AW 3rd, et al. Prevalence of ADHD and comorbid disorders among elementary school children screened for disruptive behavior. J Abnorm Child Psychol 1996;24(5):571–95.
10. Polzer J, Bangs ME, Zhang S, et al. Meta-analysis of aggression or hostility events in randomized, controlled clinical trials of atomoxetine for ADHD. Biol Psychiatry 2007;61(5):713–9.
11. Nock MK, Kazdin AE, Hiripi E, et al. Lifetime prevalence, correlates, and persistence of oppositional defiant disorder: results from the National Comorbidity Survey Replication. J Child Psychol Psychiatry 2007;48(7):703–13.
12. Turgay A. Psychopharmacological treatment of oppositional defiant disorder. CNS Drugs 2009;23(1):1–17.
13. Blader JC, Schooler NR, Jensen PS, et al. Adjunctive divalproex versus placebo for children with ADHD and aggression refractory to stimulant monotherapy. Am J Psychiatry 2009;166(12):1392–401.
14. Armenteros JL, Lewis JE, Davalos M. Risperidone augmentation for treatment-resistant aggression in attention-deficit/hyperactivity disorder: a placebo-controlled pilot study. J Am Acad Child Adolesc Psychiatry 2007;46(5):558–65.
15. Connor DF, Barkley RA, Davis HT. A pilot study of methylphenidate, clonidine, or the combination in ADHD comorbid with aggressive oppositional defiant or conduct disorder. Clin Pediatr (Phila) 2000;39(1):15–25.
16. Malone RP, Delaney MA, Luebbert JF, et al. A double-blind placebo-controlled study of lithium in hospitalized aggressive children and adolescents with conduct disorder. Arch Gen Psychiatry 2000;57(7):649–54.

17. Masi G, Milone A, Manfredi A, et al. Effectiveness of lithium in children and adolescents with conduct disorder: a retrospective naturalistic study. CNS Drugs 2009;23(1):59–69.
18. Findling RL, Kauffman R, Sallee FR, et al. An open-label study of aripiprazole: pharmacokinetics, tolerability, and effectiveness in children and adolescents with conduct disorder. J Child Adolesc Psychopharmacol 2009;19(4):431–9.
19. Connor DF, McLaughlin TJ, Jeffers-Terry M. Randomized controlled pilot study of quetiapine in the treatment of adolescent conduct disorder. J Child Adolesc Psychopharmacol 2008;18(2):140–56.
20. Masi G, Milone A, Canepa G, et al. Olanzapine treatment in adolescents with severe conduct disorder. Eur Psychiatry 2006;21(1):51–7.
21. Findling RL, McNamara NK, Branicky LA, et al. A double-blind pilot study of risperidone in the treatment of conduct disorder. J Am Acad Child Adolesc Psychiatry 2000;39(4):509–16.
22. Steiner H, Petersen ML, Saxena K, et al. Divalproex sodium for the treatment of conduct disorder: a randomized controlled clinical trial. J Clin Psychiatry 2003; 64(10):1183–91.
23. Khanzode LA, Saxena K, Kraemer H, et al. Efficacy profiles of psychopharmacology: divalproex sodium in conduct disorder. Child Psychiatry Hum Dev 2006;37(1):55–64.
24. Costello EJ, Erkanli A, Angold A. Is there an epidemic of child or adolescent depression? J Child Psychol Psychiatry 2006;47(12):1263–71.
25. Belden AC, Thomson NR, Luby JL. Temper tantrums in healthy versus depressed and disruptive preschoolers: defining tantrum behaviors associated with clinical problems. J Pediatr 2008;152(1):117–22.
26. Knox M, King C, Hanna GL, et al. Aggressive behavior in clinically depressed adolescents. J Am Acad Child Adolesc Psychiatry 2000;39(5):611–8.
27. Bond AJ. Antidepressant treatments and human aggression. Eur J Pharmacol 2005;526(1–3):218–25.
28. Tauscher-Wisniewski S, Nilsson M, Caldwell C, et al. Meta-analysis of aggression and/or hostility-related events in children and adolescents treated with fluoxetine compared with placebo. J Child Adolesc Psychopharmacol 2007;17(5):713–8.
29. Youngstrom E, Duax J. Evidence-based assessment of pediatric bipolar disorder, Part I: base rate and family history. J Am Acad Child Adolesc Psychiatry 2005;44(7):712–7.
30. Biederman J, Mick E, Faraone SV, et al. Pediatric bipolar disorder or disruptive behavior disorder? Prim Psychiatry 2004;11(9):36–41.
31. Kowatch RA, Fristad M, Birmaher B, et al, The Child Psychiatric Workgroup on Bipolar Disorder. Treatment guidelines for children and adolescents with bipolar disorder. J Am Acad Child Adolesc Psychiatry 2005;44(3):213–35.
32. Brotman MA, Schmajuk M, Rich BA, et al. Prevalence, clinical correlates, and longitudinal course of severe mood dysregulation in children. Biol Psychiatry 2006;60(9):991–7.
33. Dickstein DP, Towbin KE, Van Der Veen JW, et al. Randomized double-blind placebo-controlled trial of lithium in youths with severe mood dysregulation. J Child Adolesc Psychopharmacol 2009;19(1):61–73.
34. Bastiaens L, Bastiaens J. Severely mood-disordered youth respond less well to treatment in a community clinic than youth with bipolar disorder. Psychiatry (Edgmont) 2008;5(10):37–41.
35. Waxmonsky J, Pelham WE, Gnagy E, et al. The efficacy and tolerability of methylphenidate and behavior modification in children with attention-deficit/hyperactivity disorder and severe mood dysregulation. J Child Adolesc Psychopharmacol 2008;18(6):573–88.

36. Connolly SD, Bernstein GA, Work Group on Quality Issues. Practice parameter for the assessment and treatment of children and adolescents with anxiety disorders. J Am Acad Child Adolesc Psychiatry 2007;46(2):267–83.
37. Bubier JL, Drabick DA. Co-occurring anxiety and disruptive behavior disorders: the roles of anxious symptoms, reactive aggression, and shared risk processes. Clin Psychol Rev 2009;29(7):658–69.
38. Cohen JA, Work Group on Quality Issues. Practice parameter for the assessment and treatment of children and adolescents with posttraumatic stress disorder. J Am Acad Child Adolesc Psychiatry 2010;49(4):414–30.
39. Donnelly CL. Pharmacologic treatment approaches for children and adolescents with posttraumatic stress disorder. Child Adolesc Psychiatr Clin N Am 2003;12(2):251–69.
40. Diler RS. Panic disorder in children and adolescents. Yonsei Med J 2003;44(1): 174–9.
41. Moscovitch DA, McCabe RE, Antony MM, et al. Anger experience and expression across the anxiety disorders. Depress Anxiety 2008;25(2):107–13.
42. Paton C. Benzodiazepines and disinhibition: a review. Psychiatr Bull R Coll Psychiatr 2002;26(12):460–2.
43. McClellan J, Werry J, Work Group on Quality Issues. Practice parameter for the assessment and treatment of children and adolescents with schizophrenia. J Am Acad Child Adolesc Psychiatry 2001;40(7 Suppl):4S–23S.
44. Harris AW, Large MM, Redoblado-Hodge A, et al. Clinical and cognitive associations with aggression in the first episode of psychosis. Aust N Z J Psychiatry 2010;44(1):85–93.
45. Swanson JW, Swartz MS, Elbogen EB. Effectiveness of atypical antipsychotic medications in reducing violent behavior among persons with schizophrenia in community-based treatment. Schizophr Bull 2004;30(l):3–20.
46. Volavka J, Czobor P, Nolan K, et al. Overt aggression and psychotic symptoms in patients with schizophrenia treated with clozapine, olanzapine, risperidone, or haloperidol. J Clin Psychopharmacol 2004;24(2):225–8.
47. Chalasani L, Kant R, Chengappa KN. Clozapine impact on clinical outcomes and aggression in severely ill adolescents with childhood-onset schizophrenia. Can J Psychiatry 2001;46(10):965–8.
48. Keen-Kim D, Freimer NB. Genetics and epidemiology of Tourette syndrome. J Child Neurol 2006;21(8):665–71.
49. Budman CL, Rockmore L, Stokes J, et al. Clinical phenomenology of episodic rage in children with Tourette syndrome. J Psychosom Res 2003;55:59–65.
50. Budman CL. Treatment of aggression in Tourette syndrome. Adv Neurol 2006;99: 222–6.
51. Budman C, Coffey BJ, Shechter R, et al. Aripiprazole in children and adolescents with Tourette disorder with and without explosive outbursts. J Child Adolesc Psychopharmacol 2008;18(5):509–15.
52. Coccaro EF, Schmidt CA, Samuels JF, et al. Lifetime and 1-month prevalence rates of intermittent explosive disorder in a community sample. J Clin Psychiatry 2004;65(6):820–4.
53. McElroy SL, Soutullo CA, Beckman DA, et al. DSM-IV intermittent explosive disorder: a report of 27 cases. J Clin Psychiatry 1998;59(4):203–10.
54. Olvera RL. Intermittent explosive disorder: epidemiology, diagnosis and management. CNS Drugs 2002;16(8):517–26.

Psychopharmacology of Autistic Spectrum Disorders in Children and Adolescents

Ahsan Nazeer, MD

KEYWORDS

- Autism • Psychopharmacology • Stereotypes • Aggression
- Compulsion • Ritualistic behavior • Anxiety

Autism is a neurodevelopmental disorder with core symptom domains of impairment in social interactions and communication, and restricted, repetitive behaviors and interests. The disorder was initially described by Kanner[1] in 1943. In his seminal paper he described these children to be born without the ability to make social relationships and identified some characteristic features including limited ability to develop relationships, language delays, aloofness, lack of imagination, and persistence on sameness. Bleuler[2] had already used the term "autism" in 1912 to describe "self-absorption" or "withdrawal from reality" as one of the pathognomonic features of schizophrenia. Rutter[3,4] later identified four core symptom clusters in autistic disorder: (1) social impairment, (2) language disturbances, (3) insistence on sameness, and (4) onset before 30 months of age. These criteria, with modifications and changes, were later incorporated into the *Diagnostic and Statistical Manual of Mental Disorders* (DSM)-III systems of classification.[5]

DSM-IV text-revision (TR) identifies five disorders under the category of autism spectrum disorder (ASD): (1) autistic disorder, (2) Asperger syndrome, (3) childhood disintegrative disorder, (4) Rett syndrome, and (5) pervasive developmental disorder not otherwise specified. DSM-V, scheduled for publication in 2013, has proposed the following changes to this category.[6] Rett syndrome will be excluded from DSM-V; childhood disintegrative disorder, Asperger syndrome, and pervasive developmental disorder not otherwise specified will be merged into a single diagnosis of autistic disorder; and diagnostic criteria for autistic disorder will be changed as follows: the domains of "social interaction" and "communication" will be merged into "social/communication deficits," and "restricted interests" will be renamed "fixed

---

The author has nothing to disclose.

Child and Adolescent Psychiatry, Department of Psychiatry, College of Human Medicine, Michigan State University, Kalamazoo Center for Medical Studies, 1722 Shaffer Street, Suite 3, Kalamazoo, MI 49048–1633, USA

E-mail address: nazeer@kcms.msu.edu

interests/repetitive behaviors." In the social/communication domain, DSM-V will require all of the following criteria to be met: deficits in nonverbal and verbal communication, lack of social reciprocity, and lack of peer relationships. In the fixed interests/repetitive behaviors domain, DSM-V will require any two of the following three criteria to be met: (1) stereotypic behaviors or unusual sensory symptoms, (2) adherence to routines, and (3) restricted interests.

There continues to be a possibility of further changes in the proposed DSM-V criteria until its publication in 2013. Until that time, it is advisable for clinicians to continue using the DSM-IV-TR criteria to diagnose and document ASD.

ASDs are associated with numerous comorbidities and disabling symptoms including aggression and self-injurious behaviors (SIB). Behavioral and pharmacologic interventions are the mainstay of treatment. This article summarizes the current state of knowledge on the pharmacotherapy of ASDs.

Medications are usually not the first-line treatment to target the core symptoms of autism, which respond to intensive behavioral interventions. Instead, pharmacotherapy in these individuals is limited to the management of the comorbid symptoms of aggression, hyperactivity, impulsivity, inattention, obsessions, anxiety, depression, and repetitive behaviors. Studies[7] have reported a 9% to 10% prevalence rate of comorbid psychiatric disorders in this population. One recent study[8] has found 70% of their ASD sample to have at least one comorbid psychiatric disorder and 41% with two or more comorbid disorders. The same study also reported social anxiety disorder, attention-deficit/hyperactivity disorder (ADHD), and oppositional defiant disorder to be the three most common comorbid disorders. Treatment of these associated symptoms is necessary when they cause psychosocial dysfunction and impairment in the individual's life. What follows is a review of the symptom-specific treatments of these disorders.

AGGRESSION

Aggressive symptoms in autism are common, and if severe, they can be an indicator of poor long-term prognosis. Aggression, as a term, is commonly used to define a broad range of behaviors including intentional or unintentional violence toward others, SIB, sexual offenses, fire setting, and defiance toward caretakers. Identifying the triggers and nature of the behavior aids in the treatment because behavioral interventions can be effectively implemented to target these symptoms.[9] Recent studies have identified the effectiveness of combined use of medications with intensive behavioral treatments. In one recent study, the authors sought to identify the cumulative benefit of these treatments.[10] After implementation of intensive behavioral interventions while keeping medication use stable, the authors noticed substantial reduction in the number of average aggressive behaviors. The addition of neuroleptic medications enhanced the success of behavioral interventions in managing aggression. Some of the causes of aggression that need to be identified before the initiation of pharmacotherapy **Box 1**.

Evaluating the intensity of aggression is an important initial step of management. An understanding of the target behavior including the predictors of aggression helps in selecting appropriate treatment settings. Less serious events warrant further evaluation in an outpatient setting for implementation of behavioral plans and psychopharmacology. More serious events, however, warrant an immediate assessment in an urgent care or emergency room setting with goals to maintain safety and to prevent further deterioration in functioning. Once the medical and psychosocial factors are considered in the differential diagnosis, and believed not to be the contributing factor, consideration can be given to psychopharmacologic agents to target the aggressive behaviors.

Box 1
Common causes of aggression in autistic children
Impaired understanding of actions and consequences
Impaired ability to communicate and express wants and needs
Impaired coping skills
Conflict with peers and authority figures
Psychosocial dysfunction
Undiagnosed pain, constipation, underlying seizures, hypoglycemia
Psychiatric factors: Psychosis, depression, mania, suicidal or homicidal ideation

There are limited evidence-based psychopharmacologic options to treat the aggressive symptoms in autistic individuals, because few studies have used aggression and SIB as primary outcome measures. Given the limitations in the medical literature on this matter, medications usually are directed at the underlying neurobiologic deficits that are believed to trigger those symptoms. Briefly, dopaminergic, adrenergic, serotonergic, and opioid systems are thought to be associated with aggression. One review of 21 trials covering 12 medications[11] found only methylphenidate and risperidone to be effective; however, this review was published before the 2009 Food and Drug Administration (FDA) approval of aripiprazole for the treatment of irritability associated with autism.

Antipsychotics

Both first- and second-generation antipsychotic (neuroleptic) medications can be used to manage aggressive symptoms in autism and have shown efficacy across different studies. Among this group, haloperidol and risperidone have extensive literature support for their use in this population,[12–14] and in 2006 risperidone received FDA approval for the treatment of irritability and aggression in children with autism aged 5 to 16 years.[15] Haloperidol has been shown to reduce social isolation and stereotypes while improving learning, anger-related behaviors, hyperactivity, and tasks of language acquisition.[12,16] Chlorpromazine and fluphenazine also have shown efficacy, although sedation, dystonic reactions, and withdrawal dyskinesias have limited their effectiveness. Because of the different mechanisms of action, atypical antipsychotics have slightly lower propensity of causing extrapyramidal symptoms and are considered to be the first choice for the management of aggression and SIB. Nevertheless, when prescribed at high dose, these medications are as prone to cause extrapyramidal symptoms as the conventional antipsychotics.[17]

Three randomized controlled trials (RCTs) of the use of risperidone in autistic disorders have shown its efficacy in controlling irritability and aggression and these results are consistent across other studies. Initial studies on the short- and long-term effects of risperidone were published by the Research Units on Pediatric Psychopharmacology Autism Network (RUPPAN).[14,18] During their 8-week trial, 101 individuals were evaluated for irritability, aggression, and SIB using the Aberrant Behavior Checklist (ABC) and then randomized for risperidone or placebo. At a mean dose of 1.8 mg/day, the risperidone group was found to have 57% reduction in their ABC scores compared with 14% in the placebo group. Reduction in the stereotype and hyperactivity subscales of ABC was more pronounced, but no statistically significant improvement in core symptoms of social withdrawal and inappropriate speech subscales was noticed. During the long arm of the trial, subjects who initially responded to risperidone were enrolled in an open-label continuation phase for an additional 16 weeks followed by 8 weeks of randomized double-blind placebo-controlled discontinuation phase. During the open-label continuation phase, most of the initial responders (51 of 63) continued to remain stable without any worsening of symptoms. The mean irritability score (ABC-I) showed 59% reduction from the rating at the initiation of trial. In the second phase of this trial, 36 individuals were initially enrolled, whereas 32 completed this phase. Among 32 that were randomized to continued risperidone treatment (N = 16) and to placebo (N = 16), 62.5% (N = 10) from the placebo group relapsed compared with 12.5% (N = 2) from the risperidone group whose symptoms worsened. The median time to relapse was 34 days for placebo group compared with 57 days for the risperidone group. The results of this study underscore the need for long-term medication management in individuals with autism.

Fewer studies have evaluated the efficacy of risperidone among preschool children with ASD. A 3-year-long open-label naturalistic study reviewed the clinical outcomes of risperidone monotherapy among 53 children with ASD, ages ranging from 3.6 to 6.6 years, at a mean dose of 0.55 mg/day.[19] Improvement in behavior and affect regulation was noticed in 47.2% of the children who continued to take risperidone throughout the study period. For the remaining 52.8% of subjects who discontinued the medication, side effects including increased appetite, elevated prolactin levels without clinical symptoms, and lack of efficacy were major concerns. In a double-blind, placebo-controlled trial,[20] researchers evaluated the safety and effectiveness of risperidone among 24 preschool children aged 2.5 to 6 years who were also undergoing applied behavioral analysis. The Childhood Autism Rating Scale and the Gilliam Autism Rating Scale were the primary outcome measures. The group was randomized to risperidone (0.5–1.5 mg/day) or placebo for 6 months. The risperidone group tolerated the medication well except for sedation, hypersalivation, and increased appetite, which were noted to be the most common adverse effects. Findings suggest superior improvements in global measurements of autism symptoms in the risperidone group compared with the placebo group but no specific change in the core autistic symptoms of language, stereotypes, social deficits, and restricted interests was found in the study sample.

Efficacy of olanzapine is suggested by a few open-label trials and case reports. One double-blind placebo-controlled trial of olanzapine among 11 children aged 6 to 14 years has shown promise at a mean dose of 10 mg/day.[21] On the Clinical Global Impression-Improvement Rating (CGI-I) scale, 50% of the olanzapine group showed improvement compared with 20% of the placebo group. Sedation and weight gain were the main side effects among the study sample.

Aripiprazole has recently received FDA approval for its use in the treatment of irritability in autistic children aged 6 to 17 years. Two double-blind, placebo-controlled trials have shown aripiprazole to be efficacious in the treatment of aggression associated with ASD. In the first 8-week trial, 98 subjects aged 6 to 17 years were randomly assigned to flexible-dose aripiprazole (5–15 mg/day) or placebo treatment.[22] The ABC and the CGI-I irritability subscale were the primary outcome measure. Among the sample, 76.5% of subjects completed the trial, and the aripiprazole group showed greater improvement in the ABC and the CGI irritability subscale across weeks 1 through 8. The remaining 10.6% of the aripiprazole group discontinued the medication because of side effects including extrapyramidal symptoms. Aripiprazole treatment was associated with a greater than 7% increase in weight compared with the placebo. At the end of the study, fasting blood glucose and lipid values were comparable across both groups without any statistically significant increase in the aripiprazole group. Suicide-related adverse events were common in the placebo group compared with the aripiprazole group. In the second 8-week parallel group trial, 218 children and adolescents with aggressive behaviors were randomized to flexible-dose aripiprazole or placebo.[23] This study found all aripiprazole doses to be effective in reducing the mean ABC irritability subscales. Sedation and weight gain were the most common side effects and on average, the aripiprazole group gained 1.3 kg through the 8-week trial.

No RCTs are available for ziprasidone and quetiapine, but open-label trials have shown efficacy in individuals with autism. In the most recent open-label trial, 12 adolescents were treated with ziprasidone with doses ranging from 20 to 160 mg/day.[24] Authors noted 75% of their sample to be treatment responders according to the parameters on CGI-I. On ABC, irritability and hyperactivity subscales showed improvement. Ziprasidone was found to be weight neutral, but the mean QTc increase was 14.7 milliseconds among the sample.

Movement disorders including tardive dyskinesia are an important limiting factor in the use of the older first-generation antipsychotic medications. Recent studies have documented a lower risk of tardive dyskinesia with second-generation antipsychotics compared with first-generation medications. A recent review[25] has noted a 0.35% incidence rate of tardive dyskinesia among children with atypical antipsychotics compared with 7.7% in adults using conventional antipsychotics. All of the antipsychotics pose the risk of metabolic syndrome that is characterized by elevations in weight, blood pressure, and lipids and glucose.[26] Because of the complex array of side effects, it is recommended to periodically check the patient's weight, waist circumference, blood pressure, and fasting blood glucose and lipid levels. Counseling about nutrition and activity levels needs to be included in the treatment sessions.

Selective Serotonin Reuptake Inhibitors

The serotonergic system has been implicated in the pathogenesis of aggression since 1961 when researchers noticed elevated blood 5-HT levels in six children among a cohort of 23 individuals with autism.[27] Depletion of dietary tryptophan, a precursor of 5-HT, has been found to worsen autistic symptomatology. Considering these findings, theoretically selective serotonin reuptake inhibitor (SSRI) medications seem to be the best possible choice to treat either the core or comorbid symptoms of autism. Unfortunately, at this time there is no clear evidence suggesting the efficacy of these medications for aggressive behaviors in autism. Altogether there are seven RCT involving fluoxetine, citalopram, and fluvoxamine with various outcome measures suggesting no specific evidence of the benefits of SSRI use for aggression in children with autism.[28]

α_2-Agonists

Adrenergic stimulation has been postulated in the pathophysiology of tics, ADHD, and aggression in children. Individuals with autism have difficulty in filtering out unwanted stimuli and are easily hyperaroused suggesting underlying adrenergic stimulation. Clonidine and guanfacine are two available α-agonists that have different side effect profiles and are efficacious in the treatment of aggression. In clinical practice, these agents have been used effectively in the management of irritability and mild aggression particularly in the children with associated impulsive and hyperactive behaviors. One small, double-blind, placebo-controlled crossover study, involving eight children and adolescents with ADHD-like symptoms has showed improvement in the measures of aggression and SIB.[29] Sedation and hypotension seemed to be the most common adverse effects. Guanfacine, a longer acting α_2-agonist with less sedative potential, was effective in only 23.8% of the patients in a retrospective analysis of 80 children aged 3 to 18 years old.[30]

Psychostimulants

Psychostimulants are effective in the treatment of individuals in whom the aggression is associated with impulsivity and hyperactivity. In others, when aggression is not comorbid with hyperactive and impulsive behaviors, these medications show modest results and seem to cause worsening in irritability, insomnia, and paradoxic aggression. Methylphenidate is among the most studied psychostimulant in children and adolescents with autism; two RCTs show aggression as an outcome measure.[31,32] In the first controlled trial, 10 children aged 7 to 10 years were administered methylphenidate, 10 mg twice a day for 1 week, and 20 mg twice a day for the next week. Methylphenidate was significantly more effective in improving the primary outcome measures of aggression and SIB measured with ABC-I. The other controlled trial of 13 children with ADHD and autism studied the efficacy of flexible-dose methylphenidate (0.3–0.6 mg/kg in twice a day and three times a day dosing). Subjects showed improvement on aggression subscales of the IOWA Conners'. Higher methylphenidate dose was associated with more side effects of irritability and social withdrawal.

Mood Stabilizers

The adult and pediatric literature has supported the role of mood stabilizers in aggressive symptoms associated with mania and conduct disorders.[33–35] Because of these effects on overt aggression it was thought that mood stabilizers play an efficacious role in the management of aggression associated with autism. This possibility, however, is based only on anecdotal reports. Except for one positive trial in an autistic sample, published RCTs of divalproex sodium, lamotrigine, and levetiracetam have not supported this notion.

In a trial of divalproex sodium 30 individuals with autism, aged 6 to 20 years, with aggression and SIB were randomized to 20 mg/kg daily dose of divalproex versus placebo.[36] After 8 weeks, no significant differences were found among the groups on the aggression subscale of ABC-I and on the Overt Aggression Scale. Increased appetite was the major side effect in the divalproex group. In the most recent RCT, 27 subjects with ASD at a mean age of 9.46 years were randomized to divalproex sodium versus placebo for 12 weeks.[37] Primary outcome measures were ABC-I and CGI-I. Medication was titrated on the basis of weight to achieve a minimum plasma level of 50 µg/ml. The authors found an overall improvement of 62.5% in the divalproex group as compared with 9% in the placebo group. Worsening aggression in two subjects from the active group was the only major side effect noticed.

Open-label trials of lamotrigine also have shown efficacy in improving behavioral problems in individuals with autism. The only RCT of lamotrigine was conducted in 27 subjects with autism aged 3 to 11 years who were randomized to lamotrigine, 5 mg/kg/d, versus placebo over 8 weeks.[38] After initial titration, the optimal dose of lamotrigine was maintained for 4 weeks. This phase was followed by 2 weeks tapering down and 4 weeks medication-free period. No significant differences were found among groups on the primary outcome measure of ABC-I.

Levetiracetam is another mood stabilizer that has shown promise in open-label trials but the only RCT[39] has not supported its use for aggression.

Risperidone, methylphenidate, and clonidine had the most published support for efficacy in the treatment of irritability, aggression, and SIB in individuals with ASD.[11]

Mood stabilizers also have good clinical support for use in this population, but further studies are needed to replicate these effects.

HYPERACTIVITY AND IMPULSIVITY IN ASD

Hyperactive, impulsive, and inattentive behaviors in individuals with autism usually represent a comorbid diagnosis of ADHD, despite the DSM-IV qualifier that autism and ADHD should not be diagnosed concurrently. These symptoms are increasingly prevalent in individuals with autism and in one study, authors noted the incidence of ADHD in ASDs to be as high as 74%.[40] Genetic factors play an important role in the transmission of this disorder and D_2 and D_4 dopamine receptor and dopamine transporter genes have been implicated in the pathophysiology.

The diagnosis of comorbid ADHD is easier to establish in individuals with high-functioning rather than low-functioning autism. The usual initial presentation is of a child who fidgets, needs constant reminders, is disruptive and impulsive in the classroom, displays poor frustration tolerance, and gets irritable and aggressive. It is important to rule out any medical causes of hyperactivity including hyperthyroidism that can mimic these behaviors. Depression, anxiety, and cognitive deficits with resultant limited coping skills also can mimic these behaviors and need to be considered in the differential diagnosis.

There is evidence[41] of shared genetic influence in the pathophysiology of these disorders. It is a common clinical perception that these disorders are relatively difficult to treat if they coexist. Children tend to have more side effects from the medications used, and the treatment response is usually suboptimal. Standard medications that improve symptoms in children with either diagnosis alone tend to cause numerous side effects including irritability, dysphoria, and behavioral disinhibition. The dopaminergic system has been implicated in the pathophysiology and so is a natural target for pharmacologic management. Perhaps because of the mutually exclusionary criterion in the DSM-IV-TR that the diagnosis of ADHD and ASD should not be made concurrently, fewer studies have looked into the management of these patients in which both disorders coexist.[42] **Table 1** summarizes the evidence for the use of psychostimulants and α-agonists based on a recent review.[43]

Among psychostimulants, methylphenidate seems to have most support in the literature for its use in this population.[31,32,44,45] Atomoxetine has shown promise in one RCT,[46] whereas clonidine[29,47] and guanfacine[48] have shown mixed results. Guanfacine was effective in one open-label trial.[48]

Numerous other medications including atypical antipsychotics, antidepressants, anxiolytics, and mood stabilizers have been proposed for the potential treatment of hyperactivity in children with ASD. The data to support these treatments are scant and mostly consist of case reports, open-label trials, and chart reviews. Among these medications, typical and atypical antipsychotics have held more promise in comparison with others. Haloperidol is among the most studied typical antipsychotic with 11 clinical trials showing efficacy in the management of hyperactivity associated with ASD. Dystonic reactions, withdrawal, and tardive dyskinesias are the major side effects associated with this medication. Among atypical antipsychotics, risperidone has the most literature support for its use; numerous controlled trials, including one from RUPPAN, have supported its role in ASD children with hyperactivity. The RUPPAN trial included 101 children age 5 to 17 years with pervasive developmental disorder.[18] Risperidone was begun at 0.5 mg/day and was titrated up and maintained at a mean dose of 1.8 mg/day. Sixty-nine percent were considered responders with improvement in hyperactivity and irritability scores. Increased appetite, drowsiness,

Table 1
Medications used to treat hyperactivity and impulsive behaviors with ASD

Medications	Efficacy	Literature Support	Common Side Effects
Psychostimulants			
Methylphenidate	Effective	Many double-blind placebo-controlled trials and open-label studies Research Units of Pediatric Psychopharmacology (RUPP): effective at doses of 0.25–0.5 mg/kg; 49% subjects were labeled as responders; 18% withdrew from the study because of side effects.[44] Posey et al[45]: methylphenidate at doses of 0.125–0.50 mg/kg; subjects from the original RUPP study. Hyperactivity and impulsivity improved more than inattention.	Irritability, dysphoria, worsening aggression
Nonstimulants			
Atomoxetine	Effective	Many open-label trials. Only double-blind placebo-controlled crossover trial in 16 children with pervasive developmental disorder and ADHD. Atomoxetine group, 56% responders; placebo group, 25% responders.[46]	Sedation, irritability, constipation, nausea
α-Agonists			
Clonidine	Mixed results	Two double-blind placebo-controlled cross-over studies. Mixed results with both showing improvement in parent-rated end points.[29,47]	Sedation the most common side effect
Guanfacine	Effective	Open-label trial and one retrospective chart review.[48]	Irritability and agitation

and fatigue were the major side effects in that trial. Literature on the use of SSRIs, mood stabilizers, and anxiolytics has not been encouraging with numerous trials showing lack of efficacy.

Methylphenidate, atomoxetine, and risperidone have most of the literature support for their use in the treatment of ADHD-related symptoms among individuals with ASD. Despite the perception of increased side effects with psychostimulants, recent studies[49] have reported that these medications are usually well-tolerated in this comorbid population. If present, dysphoric mood and irritability can be managed by a trial of another stimulant or a nonstimulant medication or atomoxetine. Because these individuals often have complicated presentations of multiple symptoms, trials of atypical antipsychotics to target the comorbid aggression and stimulant-resistant hyperactivity of SSRIs for stimulant-induced anxiety and stereotypical behaviors may be helpful. In case of partial response to stimulants, the addition of α-agonists is sometimes warranted.

REPETITIVE BEHAVIORS

Repetitive and stereotypic behaviors constitute the core domain of ASD but are also present in numerous other conditions. These behaviors are fixed, repetitive, rhythmic, and nonfunctional, and worsen with stress and anxiety. Some studies have noticed higher rates of repetitive behaviors in individuals with increased severity of autism.[50] When present with ASD, these behaviors at times are ego-syntonic and provide a self calming purpose for the individual. It is when these behaviors include repetitive self-injury or obsessions that behavioral or pharmacologic interventions are considered. On occasion, differentiating between autism-based repetitive behaviors and ego-dystonic rituals of obsessive-compulsive disorder becomes challenging. Characteristics of the repetitive behaviors can help with this differential diagnosis. One study found fewer obsessions of symmetry and contamination and more of tapping, touching, and rubbing in ASD individuals compared with individuals with obsessive-compulsive disorder.[51]

Table 2			
Medications used to treat repetitive behaviors based on RCTs in children and adolescents			
Medications	**Efficacy**	**Literature Support**	**Common Side Effects**
SSRIs			
Fluoxetine	Effective	Double-blind, placebo-controlled trial; 45 children and adolescents aged 5–16 years. Three-phased 20-week, trial separated by a 4-week washout phase. Mean dose of 0.4 mg/kg/d. Improvement in repetitive behaviors measured by C-YBOCS. Low-dose fluoxetine was superior to placebo to manage the repetitive behaviors.[55]	Headache, diarrhea, weight gain
Citalopram	Ineffective	National Institute of Health sponsored randomized, multicenter 12-week study; 149 subjects with ASDs age 5–17 years. Randomized to citalopram versus placebo with mean citalopram dose of 16.5 mg/day. No difference was noted on C-YBOCS or on CGI-improvement subscale between groups.[52]	Increased energy, impulsiveness, diarrhea
Atypical antipsychotics			
Risperidone	Effective	Double-blind placebo-controlled trial (RUPP). Follow-up study based on the original data from RUPP trial and 16-week open-label continuation phase. Effects on secondary outcome measures were noted. Significant improvement in restrictive repetitive behaviors on C-YBOCS.[56]	Weight gain
Mood stabilizers			
Valproate	Effective	Double-blind, placebo-controlled 8-week trial; 13 individuals (12 children and 1 adult) with ASD. Mean dose of 500–1500 mg/day and levels were maintained at 50–100 µg/ml. Improvement in repetitive behaviors was noted on C-YBOCS.[57]	Weight gain, irritability

Anxiety is a subjective feeling of inner tension and distress. Because of the relatively preserved communication skills, higher-functioning individuals with autism tend to better describe this subjective sense of distress compared with lower-functioning individuals. Worsening in repetitive behaviors and regression in daily functioning can be an indication of underlying anxiety disorder. In individuals with autism anxiety can be an expression of the genetic transmission of the disorder or of environmental stressors, including a change in routines, school changes, conflicts with teachers or caretakers, or physical illnesses. Collateral information from caregivers about the nature of core repetitive behaviors, their recent worsening, and change in character is very valuable in the differential diagnosis.

Although, the data regarding the efficacy of pharmacologic agents to manage these behaviors are limited, some controlled trials have shown effectiveness of certain medications including SSRIs and antipsychotics. Serotonin dysfunction has been postulated in the pathophysiology of ASD and repetitive behaviors. Despite some controversies,[52] the current state of knowledge supports the use of SSRIs as the first-line of management of these disabling symptoms. Medications that have shown promise[53–57] are listed in **Table 2**.

In one review,[54] the authors suggest eliciting family history of bipolar disorder and using it as a guiding factor in the choice of medications to target repetitive behaviors. They recommend using atypical antipsychotics as the initial medication of choice with later augmentation by SSRIs in individuals with a positive family history of bipolar disorder. In the absence of such a history, they recommend using SSRIs as the first-line of treatment with later augmentation with atypical antipsychotics if warranted. Other authors have recommended using SSRIs as the initial medication of choice with later substitution of mirtazapine in case of no response. In my clinical experience, using an SSRI while evaluating for worsening suicidal ideations and behavioral activation is usually the safest initial choice.

SUMMARY

Psychiatric comorbidities are the norm rather than the exception in ASDs. Aggressive behaviors and ADHD constitute the bulk of psychiatric comorbid disorders in this patient population. Early recognition and proper treatment of these comorbidities is an important step in the long-term psychosocial management of ASDs.

ACKNOWLEDGMENTS

The author gratefully acknowledges the editorial contributions of Dr Michael R. Liepman in the preparation of this manuscript.

REFERENCES

1. Kanner L. Autistic disturbances of affective contact. Nerv Child 1943;2:217–50.
2. Bleuler E. The theory of schizophrenic negativism. Nervous and mental disease monograph series no. 11. Translated by William A. White (MD). New York: The Journal of Nervous and Mental Disease Publishing Company; 1912.
3. Rutter M. Concepts of autism: a review of research. J Child Psychol Psychiatry 1968;9(1):1–25.
4. Rutter M. Diagnosis and definition. In: Rutter M, Schopler E, editors. Autism: a reappraisal of concepts and treatment. New York: Plenum Press; 1978.
5. American Psychiatric Association. Diagnostic and statistical manual of mental disorders. 3rd edition. Washington: American Psychiatric Publishing; 1987.

6. American Psychiatric Association. DSM-V development. Washington: APA;; 2010.
7. Ghaziuddin M, Tsai L, Ghaziuddin N. Comorbidity of autistic disorder in children and adolescents. Eur Child Adolesc Psychiatry 1992;1(4):209–13.
8. Simonoff E, Pickles A, Charman T. Psychiatric disorders in children with autism spectrum disorders: prevalence, comorbidity, and associated factors in a population-derived sample. J Am Acad Child Adolesc Psychiatry 2008;47(8):921–9.
9. Schreibman L. Intensive behavioral/psychoeducational treatments for autism: research needs and future directions. J Autism Dev Disord 2000;30:373–8.
10. Frazier TW, Youngstrom EA, Haycook T, et al. Effectiveness of medication combined with intensive behavioral intervention for reducing aggression in youth with autism spectrum disorder. J Child Adolesc Psychopharmacol 2010;20(3): 167–77.
11. Parikh MS, Kolevzon A, Hollander E. Psychopharmacology of aggression in children and adolescents with autism: a critical review of efficacy and tolerability. J Child Adolesc Psychopharmacol 2008;18:157–78.
12. Anderson LT, Campbell M, Grega DM, et al. Haloperidol in the treatment of infantile autism: effects on learning and behavioral symptoms. Am J Psychiatry 1984; 141:1195–202.
13. Malone RP, Gratz SS, Delaney MA, et al. Advances in drug treatments for children and adolescents with autism and other pervasive developmental disorders. CNS Drugs 2005;19:923–34.
14. Research Units on Pediatric Psychopharmacology Autism Network. Risperidone treatment of autistic disorder: longer-term benefits and blinded discontinuation after 6 months. Am J Psychiatry 2005;162:1361–9.
15. Food and Drug Administration. FDA approves the first drug to treat irritability associated with autism, risperdal. FDA News; 2006. Available at: http://www.fda.gov/NewsEvents/Newsroom/PressAnnouncements/2006/ucm108759.htm. Accessed June 14, 2010.
16. Campbell M, Anderson LT, Meier M, et al. A comparison of haloperidol and behavior therapy and their interaction in autistic children. J Am Acad Child Adolesc Psychiatry 1978;17(4):640–55.
17. Pierre JM. Extrapyramidal symptoms with atypical antipsychotics: incidence, prevention and management. Drug Saf 2005;28:191–208.
18. Research Units on Pediatric Psychopharmacology Autism Network (RUPPAN). Risperidone in children with autism for serious behavioral problems. N Engl J Med 2002;347:314–21.
19. Masi G, Cosenza A, Mucci M, et al. A 3-year naturalistic study of 53 preschool children with pervasive developmental disorders treated with risperidone. J Clin Psychiatry 2003;64:1039–47.
20. Luby J, Mrakotsky C, Stalets MM, et al. Risperidone in preschool children with autistic spectrum disorders: an investigation of safety and efficacy. J Child Adolesc Psychopharmacol 2006;16:575–87.
21. Hollander E, Wasserman S, Swanson EN, et al. A double blind placebo-controlled pilot study of olanzapine in childhood/adolescent pervasive developmental disorder. J Child Adolesc Psychopharmacol 2006;16(5):541–8.
22. Owen R, Sikich L, Marcus R, et al. Aripiprazole in the treatment of irritability in children and adolescents with autistic disorder. Pediatrics 2009;124(6): 1533–40.
23. Marcus RN, Owen R, Kamen L, et al. A placebo-controlled, fixed dose study of aripiprazole in children and adolescents with irritability associated with autistic disorder. J Am Acad Child Adolesc Psychiatry 2009;48(11):1110–9.

24. Malone RP, Delaney MA, Hyman SB, et al. Ziprasidone in adolescents with autism: an open-label pilot study. J Child Adolesc Psychopharmacol 2007;17(6):779–90.
25. Correll CU, Schenk EM. Tardive dyskinesia and new antipsychotics. Curr Opin Psychiatry 2008;21:151–6.
26. Mackin P, Watkinson HM, Young AH. Prevalence of obesity, glucose homeostasis disorders and metabolic syndrome in psychiatric patients taking typical or atypical antipsychotic drugs: a cross-sectional study. Diabetologia 2005;48:215–21.
27. Schain RJ, Freedman D. Studies on 5-hydroxyindole metabolism in autistic disorder and other mentally retarded children. J Pediatr 1961;58:315–20.
28. Williams K, Wheeler DM, Silove N, et al. Selective serotonin reuptake inhibitors (SSRIs) for autism spectrum disorders (ASD). Cochrane Database Syst Rev 2010;8:CD004677.
29. Jaselskis CA, Cook EH, Fletcher KE, et al. Clonidine treatment of hyperactive and impulsive children with autistic disorder. J Clin Psychopharmacol 1992;12:322–7.
30. Posey DJ, Puntney JI, Sasher TM, et al. Guanfacine treatment of hyperactivity and inattention in pervasive developmental disorders: a retrospective analysis of 80 cases. J Child Adolesc Psychopharmacol 2004;14(2):233–41.
31. Quintana H, Birmaher B, Stedge D, et al. Use of methylphenidate in the treatment of children with autistic disorder. J Autism Dev Disord 1995;25:283–94.
32. Handen BL, Johnson CR, Lubetsky M. Efficacy of methylphenidate among children with autism and symptoms of attention-deficit hyperactivity disorder. J Autism Dev Disord 2000;30:245–55.
33. Kafantaris V, Campbell M, Padron-Gayol MV, et al. Carbamazepine in hospitalized aggressive conduct disorder children: an open pilot study. Psychopharmacol Bull 1992;28(2):193–9.
34. Malone RP, Delaney MA, Luebbert JF, et al. A double-blind placebo-controlled study of lithium in hospitalized aggressive children and adolescents with conduct disorder. Arch Gen Psychiatry 2000;57(7):649–54.
35. Carlson GA, Rapport MD, Pataki CS, et al. Lithium in hospitalized children at 4 and 8 weeks: mood, behavior and cognitive effects. J Child Psychol Psychiatry 1992;33(2):411–25.
36. Hellings JA, Weckbaugh M, Nickel EJ, et al. A double-blind, placebo-controlled study of valproate for aggression in youth with pervasive developmental disorders. J Child Adolesc Psychopharmacol 2005;15:682–92.
37. Hollander E, Chaplin W, Soorya L, et al. Divalproex sodium *vs.* placebo for the treatment of irritability in children and adolescents with autism spectrum disorders. Neuropsychopharmacology 2010;35(4):990–8.
38. Belsito KM, Law PA, Kirk KS, et al. Lamotrigine therapy for autistic disorder: a randomized, double-blind, placebo-controlled trial. J Autism Dev Disord 2001;31:175–81.
39. Wasserman S, Iyengar R, Chaplin WF, et al. Levetiracetam versus placebo in childhood and adolescent autism: a double-blind placebo-controlled study. Int Clin Psychopharmacol 2006;21(6):363–7.
40. Goldstein S, Schebach AJ. The comorbidity of pervasive developmental disorder and attention disorder: results of a retrospective chart review. J Autism Dev Disord 2004;34(3):329–39.
41. Reiersen AM, Constantino JN, Grimmer M, et al. Evidence for shared genetic influences on self-reported ADHD and autistic symptoms in young adult Australian twins. Twin Res Hum Genet 2008;11:579–85.
42. Reiersen AM, Todd RD. Co-occurrence of ADHD and autism spectrum disorders: phenomenology and treatment. Expert Rev Neurother 2008;8(4):657–69.

43. Hazell P. Drug therapy for attention-deficit hyperactivity disorder-like symptoms in autistic disorder. J Paediatr Child Health 2007;43(1–2):19–24.

44. Research Units on Pediatric Psychopharmacology Autism Network. A randomized, double-blind, placebo controlled, crossover trial of methylphenidate in children with hyperactivity associated with pervasive developmental disorders. Arch Gen Psychiatry 2005;62:1266–74.

45. Posey DJ, Aman MG, McCracken JT, et al. Positive effects of methylphenidate on inattention and hyperactivity in pervasive developmental disorders: an analysis of secondary measures. Biol Psychiatry 2007;61(4):538–44.

46. Arnold LE, Aman MG, Cook AM, et al. Atomoxetine for hyperactivity in autism spectrum disorders: placebo-controlled crossover pilot trial. J Am Acad Child Adolesc Psychiatry 2006;45(10):1196–205.

47. Fankhauser MP, Karumanchi VC, German ML, et al. Double-blind, placebo-controlled study of the efficacy of transdermal clonidine in autism. J Clin Psychiatry 1992;53(3):77–82.

48. Scahill L, Aman MG, McDougle CJ, et al. A prospective open trial of guanfacine in children with pervasive developmental disorders. J Child Adolesc Psychopharmacol 2006;16(5):589–98.

49. Santosh PJ, Baird G, Pityaratstian N, et al. Impact of comorbid autism spectrum disorders on stimulant response in children with attention deficit hyperactivity disorder: a retrospective and prospective effectiveness study. Child Care Health Dev 2006;32(5):575–83.

50. Militerni R, Bravaccio C, Falco C, et al. Repetitive behaviors in autistic disorder. Eur Child Adolesc Psychiatry 2002;11(5):210–8.

51. McDougle CJ, Kresch LE, Goodman WK, et al. A case-controlled study of repetitive thoughts and behavior in adults with autistic disorder and obsessive-compulsive disorder. Am J Psychiatry 1995;152(5):772–7.

52. King BH, Hollander E, Sikich L, et al. Lack of efficacy of citalopram in children with autism spectrum disorders and high levels of repetitive behavior: citalopram ineffective in children with autism. Arch Gen Psychiatry 2009;66(6):583–90.

53. Soorya L, Kiarashi J, Hollander E. Psychopharmacologic interventions for repetitive behaviors in autism spectrum disorders. Child Adolesc Psychiatr Clin N Am 2008;17(4):753–71.

54. Anagnostou E, Hollander E. Treatment of repetitive behaviors in autism. Curr Psychiatr 2006;5:55–64.

55. Hollander E, Phillips A, Chaplin W, et al. A placebo controlled crossover trial of liquid fluoxetine on repetitive behaviors in childhood and adolescent autism. Neuropsychopharmacology 2005;30:582–9.

56. McDougle CJ, Scahill L, Aman MG, et al. Risperidone for the core symptom domains of autism: results from the study by autism network of the Research Units on Pediatric Psychopharmacology. Am J Psychiatry 2005;162:1142–8.

57. Hollander E, Soorya L, Wasserman S, et al. Divalproex sodium vs. placebo in the treatment of repetitive behaviours in autism spectrum disorder. Int J Neuropsychopharmacol 2006;9(2):209–13.

Pharmacotherapy for Child and Adolescent Attention-deficit Hyperactivity Disorder

Gabriel Kaplan, MD[a,b,*], Jeffrey H. Newcorn, MD[c]

KEYWORDS

• ADHD • Stimulants • Atomoxetine • Guanfacine
• Pharmacotherapy

Research in the past 2 decades has demonstrated that attention-deficit/hyperactivity disorder (ADHD) is a frequently occurring psychiatric disorder that causes considerable suffering to patients and their families. ADHD begins in early childhood, and persists through adolescence and into adulthood in 70% of patients.[1] Two large epidemiologic studies in the United States have placed the prevalence of ADHD at 8.7% in children[2] and 4.4% in adults.[3] ADHD affects boys more than girls, although percentages vary across studies. Moreover, the gender ratio among youth presenting for treatment decidedly favors males. However, data from a recent 11-year follow-up study found that girls also have significant morbidity and disability associated with the disorder.[4] Pathognomonic biologic tests are not yet available so a comprehensive clinical assessment, buttressed by use of validated and normed rating scales, and structured diagnostic interviews, remains the gold standard diagnostic approach. The search for biologic markers has recently produced interesting findings, suggesting that such tests could be available in the near future. For instance, data show that ADHD is a highly heritable condition for which potentially responsible candidate genes have been identified and characteristic neuroanatomic as well as neurophysiologic findings have been confirmed.[5] Furthermore, current diagnostic criteria[6] yield similar prevalence rates across the United States and Europe, and the condition is found in most other parts of the world.[7] These data suggest there is a strong neurobiologic contribution to ADHD and support the use of medication treatments. The present paper outlines current pharmacologic ADHD treatment options and focuses on their

[a] Department of Psychiatry, Hoboken University Medical Center, 308 Willow Avenue, Hoboken, NJ 07030, USA
[b] Department of Psychiatry, University of Medicine and Dentistry of New Jersey, 65 Bergen Street, Newark, NJ 07107-3001, USA
[c] Department of Psychiatry, Mount Sinai Medical School, 1 Gustave L Levy Place, New York, NY 10029, USA
* Corresponding author. 535 Morris Avenue, Springfield, NJ 07081.
E-mail address: drgkaplan@gmail.com

Pediatr Clin N Am 58 (2011) 99–120
doi:10.1016/j.pcl.2010.10.009
0031-3955/11/$ – see front matter © 2011 Elsevier Inc. All rights reserved.
pediatric.theclinics.com

safety profile and efficacy. In addition, treatment selection, guidelines for monitoring treatment, and recent controversies in the field are addressed.

ASSESSMENT AND TREATMENT PRINCIPLES

A thorough differential diagnostic evaluation is essential, as children can present with hyperactivity, inattention, and behavioral dysregulation (ie, core symptoms of ADHD) as a result of a variety of other reasons, such as environmental stressors and other psychiatric or medical problems. Exposing children who do not have ADHD to treatment would not be expected to alleviate their condition, and could potentially worsen their symptoms. Although a comprehensive outline of assessment procedures and nonpharmacologic treatments can be consulted elsewhere,[8] a few basic principles are noted here.

Diagnosis

Diagnostic and statistical manual of mental disorders fourth edition (text revision) (DSM-IV)[6] provides diagnostic criteria that are used worldwide (although DSM-IV is not recognized in many countries). For patients to meet ADHD criteria, they must have either (1) 6 or more from a list of 9 symptoms of inattention for at least 6 months, to a degree that is maladaptive or (2) 6 or more of a list of 9 symptoms of hyperactivity/impulsivity for at least 6 months, to a degree that produces impairment in social, school, or occupational functioning. Furthermore, some symptoms that cause impairment should have been present before 7 years of age and some impairment from the symptoms must be present in 2 or more settings (eg, at school/work and at home). In addition, symptoms cannot be better accounted for by another mental disorder (although they may coexist with those of another mental disorder; ie, comorbidity).

Diagnostic Workup

ADHD is diagnosed from comprehensive psychiatric/medical histories and relevant physical and mental status examinations. All other assessments and/or tests that may be used support these primary methods. If a patient has a current or past medical problem, a thorough medical history is mandatory and consultation with specialists may be recommended. In addition to meeting with the patient, evaluators should also conduct an in-person interview of the caretakers and seek information from teachers either in person, by phone, or via completion of rating scales. Psychological testing is not essential but can be helpful, especially if learning disorders are also present. Because patients with ADHD often have co-occurring psychiatric disorders, the presence of comorbidity should be investigated as treatment necessitates taking this into account.[9,10]

Discussing Treatment Options, Medications, and Monitoring with Patients and Caretakers

Successful treatment of ADHD disorders demands significant caretaker commitment, and is best approached using a chronic care model. Few parents have had the experience of giving medication to their child on a daily basis, as is required when youth with ADHD are treated pharmacologically. For most children, prior medication use would have been limited to antibiotics or other type of acute somatic treatment. In addition to dealing with concerns regarding medication use, it is important for the clinician to instruct the family that ADHD treatment requires frequent monitoring, and to engage in a frank and realistic discussion regarding what medication can and cannot accomplish. Medical screening must be undertaken, and families should be advised regarding potential adverse effects. Medication is often highly effective in treating current symptoms of ADHD. Although the long-term effect on future functioning has not been adequately determined,[11] most patients who are treated with medication for a long period of time continue to demonstrate positive effects of treatment. However, although medications can help to improve family or peer relations acutely and potentially in the future, they cannot necessarily repair relationships or circumstances that may have been damaged or adversely affected as a result of past symptoms. A strong therapeutic alliance should be developed with both the patient and caretakers to foster a clear understanding of the condition, its potential impairments, and the reasons for pursuing medication treatment. Better understanding these issues is presumed to improve adherence to treatment. Adherence to treatment is of considerable importance, because although medication for ADHD is highly effective, many patients discontinue treatment very early on. As a general rule (recognizing that all rules have exceptions), although medication often offers the best option for acute treatment of core ADHD symptoms, a variety of evidence-based psychosocial modalities, such as summer treatment programs, teacher training, and behavioral parent training can be also be used effectively.[12] These can be offered alone or in conjunction with medications, and in some circumstances, combined medication and behavior therapy has been demonstrated to offer advantages.[13] Occasionally, patients are maintained in psychosocial treatment alone because of family preference, suboptimal response to pharmacotherapy, or unacceptable side effects. For these reasons, it is important that all available pharmacologic, nonpharmacologic, and educational options be discussed with the family at the outset of treatment.

Monitoring Tools

Several rating scales have been developed to aid in assessing the effectiveness of ADHD treatment. Some of these can also be used to improve the accuracy of the diagnostic process but should not be considered diagnostic instruments when used alone. Rating scales are available in multiple informant formats (ie, for parents, teachers, and adolescents), and in various lengths (eg, long or abbreviated formats). For instance, there are ultra brief paper and pencil scales that take less than 3 minutes to complete and have been amply validated, as well as a variety of computer-based formats. **Box 1** shows the most commonly used assessment tools. These instruments offer the opportunity to quantify data that are otherwise subjective, primarily by comparing ratings for the index patient against data derived from a large group of individuals of the same age and gender (ie, normative database). Ratings should be obtained from multiple sources before treatment is initiated and periodically thereafter to assess outcomes. Resulting scores assist the clinician in establishing when maximum symptom reduction is reached via a systematic and data-driven input process. There has been considerable recent interest in the development of scales to assess the effect of treatment on functional status, and not just symptoms. However, there is not yet an accepted gold standard method available. A comprehensive review of assessment tools is available elsewhere.[14]

PSYCHOPHARMACOLOGY OF ADHD

A brief review of the pathophysiology of ADHD is helpful in understanding the potential remedial role that pharmacologic agents can play. The behavioral and cognitive impairments that ADHD patients experience can be viewed from a unifying neuropsychological perspective as originating in deficits in executive functions.[15] These functions encompass high-level tasks such as organizing, prioritizing, focusing,

Box 1	
Most commonly used ADHD rating scales	
Name	**Main Features and Web Site**
Conners Scales	Available in parent, teacher, adolescent versions Long, short, and abbreviated (10 item) forms www.mhs.com
ADHD Rating Scale-IV	Based on the DSM-IV 18 symptoms, school and home versions available www.guilford.com
Brown ADD Scale	Available in parent, teacher, and adolescent self-report versions. Assesses executive functions www.psychcorp.pearsonassessments.com
SKAMP	Brief 10-item version for teacher or observer www.adhd.net
SNAP-IV	Public domain scales www.adhd.net/snap-iv-form.pdf
CBCL	Not ADHD specific but one of the oldest and most studied scales. Multiple informant versions www.aseba.org

sustaining effort, managing frustration, using working memory, and monitoring and selfregulating.[16] The neuronal substrates for these functions are located in the prefrontal cortex (PFC) and its various diverse connections,[17] including the striatum, thalamus, cerebellum and many other regions. Dopamine (DA) and noradrenaline (NA) are 2 neurotransmitters that are essential to PFC function, and small changes in these neurotransmitters can have marked effects. Too much or too little catecholaminergic presence can result in PFC dysfunction. DA and NA seem to exert actions at the cortical level that are both synergistic and unique. NA is often believed to strengthen attention to stimuli via enhanced network connections, sometimes referred to as increasing signal; DA is also involved in attention to stimuli but also seems to weaken unnecessary connections or decrease noise. All US Food and Drug Administration (FDA)-approved agents are believed to potentiate catecholamine transmission in the PFC, which helps to explain why they are effective in improving ADHD symptoms. The American Academy of Child and Adolescent Psychiatry (AACAP) recommends that the initial psychopharmacologic treatment of ADHD be with an FDA-approved agent.[8] These belong either to the stimulant or nonstimulant categories, as described later. Agents that have not been approved by the FDA are briefly discussed here as well because some have a fairly developed evidence base and can provide alternative options for patients who either do not benefit from or do not tolerate FDA-approved treatments.

FDA-APPROVED STIMULANT AGENTS

These include 2 types of agents: amphetamine (AMP) and methylphenidate (MPH). In 1937, Charles Bradley published a classic paper[18] describing a "spectacular" improvement in the school performance of behaviorally disordered children who were treated with dl-amphetamine (Benzedrine). This marked the beginning of modern child psychopharmacology and documented that AMP was a potentially effective treatment for the condition that subsequently became known as ADHD. MPH (Ritalin) followed in the 1950s, with reports by Knobel and colleagues,[19] and others. Stimulants are amongst the most well-researched psychotropics. Their high degree of efficacy has been demonstrated in multiple randomized controlled studies[20] in which they improved the core ADHD symptoms of hyperactivity, impulsivity, and inattention. In addition, stimulants also improve academic productivity or task completion, family interactions, aggression, school disruption, peer interactions, antisocial behaviors, and may even decrease the risk for subsequent comorbid psychiatric disorders and academic failure.[20,21] Despite the significant and desirable improvements in behavioral and cognitive symptoms, evidence for long-term improvement in academic achievement has been elusive.[22] If patients with ADHD experience acute medication improvements in several skills that are necessary for learning, why has this not resulted in verifiable enhancement of academic long-term outcomes? This apparent contradiction can be partially explained by recognizing a variety of methodological shortcomings.[23] For instance, studies have varied greatly in the types of pharmaceutical formulations used, dose ranges (some perhaps suboptimal), and times of medication administration. Perhaps duration of treatment was not sufficient enough to demonstrate change or patients did not adhere to treatment as prescribed. These issues may have interfered with the power to demonstrate effectiveness in long-term academic function, an outcome measure that is very complex and multidetermined. It is also possible that for such improvement to occur, medication alone may be insufficient, and more comprehensive wraparound modalities may be necessary. A final feasible explanation is that the nature of ADHD symptoms and impairments change with time, and it is possible that stimulant treatment is less well suited to some of the long-term deficits in organization and selfregulation that are seen in older individuals with ADHD.

Several preparations of AMP and MPH are available in the United States, in both generic and branded formulations. The different formulations of each of the 2 drug classes are similar in therapeutic and safety profiles but differ in route of administration and/or mechanism of delivery, which determine the specific formulation's kinetic profile and the resultant short or long duration of action. In the past few years, the understanding of ADHD changed from a condition that manifests only during school hours to one that can potentially impair the patient's functioning in all settings throughout the day. For this reason, short-acting immediate-release formulations (IR), despite their high degree of efficacy, present certain challenges because of the need for repeated administration over the course of the day. Longer-acting extended release preparations (ie, ER, LA, SR, XR) may improve compliance by reducing the number of times the patient must take the medication and protect confidentiality by obviating the need for administration during the school day. As reviewed later, a variety of technologies have been used to prolong duration of action.

AMP and MPH are equally efficacious at the group level when dosed comparably, with a response rate of 65% to 75%. However, individual patients can show a preferential response to either AMP or MPH. Thus, the overall stimulant response rate increases to as much as 85% if the 2 classes of medications are tried.[8] Unfortunately, there is no current method to determine which patient will respond better to which type of stimulant. A child's response to an appropriate dose of stimulant can usually be observed within 30 to 90 minutes of administration. Side effects, if any, tend to be mild, short-lived, and amenable to dose or timing adjustments. The most frequently occurring adverse effects are decreased appetite and insomnia, but other changes in affective function and mood regulation can be observed, particularly when the drug effects wear off. Occasionally, more severe adverse effects can occur, the most worrisome of which is the potential risk for catastrophic cardiovascular events, which is discussed in detail later. Other serious side effects of stimulants, such as psychosis, obsessive ruminations, and movement disorders, are infrequent and usually abate if the medication dose is lowered or stopped.[24] **Box 2** shows stimulant side effects and contraindications. **Box 3** enumerates black-boxed warnings.

Despite recent concerns addressed later in this review, when used according to clinical guidelines, stimulants have enjoyed an unparalleled track record of more

---

Box 2
Stimulant side effects and contraindications (similar for all preparations but the wording in the package insert may vary from product to product)

Side effects
  Common
    Insomnia
    Anorexia
    Headache
    Weight loss
    New onset tics
    Irritability
  Less frequent
    Nausea
    Abdominal pain
    Palpitations
    Dizziness
    Drowsiness
    Changes in pulse
  Rare
    Allergic reactions
    Fever
    Arthralgia
    Psychosis
    Depression
    Sudden death (specifically in preexisting cardiac conditions)

Contraindications
  Advanced arteriosclerosis
  Symptomatic cardiovascular disease
  Moderate to severe hypertension
  Hyperthyroidism
  Known hypersensitivity or idiosyncrasy to sympathomimetic amines
  Tics/Tourette syndrome
  Glaucoma
  Agitated states
  History of drug abuse
  During or within 14 days after the administration of monoamine oxidase inhibitors (MAOI)

Box 3
Stimulant black-boxed warnings (similar for all preparations but the wording in the package insert may vary from product to product)

MPH

Drug dependence. Should be given cautiously to patients with a history of drug dependence or alcoholism. Frank psychotic episodes can occur. Careful supervision is required during withdrawal.

AMP

Misuse may cause sudden death/serious cardiovascular adverse events. High potential for abuse. Administration for prolonged periods of time may lead to drug dependence.

---

than 7 decades of demonstrated efficacy and a relatively low incidence of side effects. Because these agents work quickly, safely, and effectively, there is probably no other mental health condition for which patients, and more frequently their parents, offer the treating clinician more laudatory comments for a job well done. And yet, for reasons not well understood, despite high response rates and level of tolerability, most patients discontinue their medication within a year.[25] The apparent disconnect between the perception of physicians that stimulants have a high degree of efficacy and tolerability and the relatively poor long-term adherence observed in patients is an important focus of research.

Amphetamine (AMP) Preparations

There are 2 kinds of AMP agents: dextroamphetamine (d-AMP) and mixed amphet-amine salts (MAS), a racemic AMP formulation bound to a mixture of salts. AMP is believed to work by enhancing DA and NA neurotransmission,[20] both by blocking reuptake and facilitating release of neurotransmitter. Existing AMP preparations are classified into short- and long-acting, and prodrug formulations. The main features are shown in **Table 1**.

Short-acting AMP formulations (about 6 hours duration)

These include generic d-AMP, branded d-AMP (Dextrostat), branded d-AMP solution (ProCentra), generic mixed amphetamine salts or MAS (50% d-AMP plus 50% dl-AMP) and branded MAS (Adderall). Different enantiomer combinations were developed because although d-AMP is more potent, some patients respond to one enantiomer but not the other.[26] AMP has been widely used for decades with excellent safety and effi-cacy. Short-acting AMP is the only FDA-approved medication for use in children as young as 3 years old. Side effects are shown in **Box 2**.

Long-acting AMP formulations (about 8 to 10 hours duration)

These comprise branded d-AMP spansules (Dexedrine), generic mixed amphetamine salts extended release (MAS XR), and branded MAS XR (Adderall XR). Dexedrine spansules are capsules that contain 2 types of beads: d-AMP IR beads that account for the initial action plus other beads covered by a polymer substance resulting in a delayed release of d-AMP. The efficacy and safety profile of the spansule is compa-rable with that of d-AMP IR. MAS XR are capsules containing Microtrol technology beads. Half of these beads contain MAS IR and the other half are coated with a substance designed to release MAS IR once the beads reach a higher pH environ-ment, usually in the intestine. The efficacy of extended release MAS has been well established in short controlled studies as well as in open label studies up to a 24-month period.[27] The side effect profile is outlined in **Box 2**.

Table 1			
AMP preparations main features			
Name/Formulation Duration	Dose Forms	Starting Dose	**Maximum Dose (May Increase as per MD Judgment)**
Short Acting (only these FDA-approved for children aged 3–5-y)			
Adderall (mixed AMP salts)	5, 7.5, 10, 12.5, 15, 20, 30 mg tablets	3–5 y: 2.5 mg every day >6y: 5 mg every day	40 mg
DextroStat (d-AMP)	5, 10 mg tablets	3–5 y: 2.5 mg every Day >6 y: 5 mg every day	40 mg
ProCentra (d-AMP)	5 mL/5 mg solution	Same as DextroStat	40 mg
Long Acting			
Dexedrine spansule (d-AMP slow release)	5, 10, 15 mg capsule	5–10 mg every day	40 mg
Adderall XR (mixed AMP salts XR)	5, 10, 15, 20, 25, 30 mg capsule	10 mg every day	30 mg; contents can be sprinkled
Prodrug			
Vyvanse (LDX)	20, 30, 40, 50, 60, 70 mg capsule	20 mg every day	70 mg; contents can be dissolved in water

Prodrug formulation

Lisdexamfetamine (LDX) or Vyvanse (brand name) is the only agent in this category. LDX is a therapeutically inactive molecule that, after ingestion, is hydrolyzed by endogenous enzymes to l-lysine, a naturally occurring essential amino acid, and active d-amphetamine, which is responsible for its therapeutic effect. Conversion of LDX to d-amphetamine and l-lysine occurs mostly in the blood.[28] Thus, its long duration of action, measured up to 13 hours in school-aged children in controlled research in a laboratory classroom,[29] is perhaps the result of a postabsorption systemic biologic conversion, in contrast to other stimulants that rely on preabsorption delayed release mechanisms.[30] The efficacy of LDX has been documented in short- and long-term studies[31] and the medication has been generally well tolerated.[32] The adverse effect profile is shown in **Box 2**. There may be an advantage for LDX with regard to abuse potential. Research showed that, at an equivalent amount of amphetamine base taken orally, LDX 100 mg had attenuated responses on measures of abuse liability compared with immediate-release d-amphetamine 40 mg.[33] LDX is highly soluble and the capsule can be opened to dissolve its contents in water.

Methylphenidate (MPH) Preparations

There are oral and transdermal formulations available in the United States. Similar to AMP, oral preparations can be subclassified according to duration of action into short- or immediate-release, intermediate, and long-acting formulations. **Table 2** shows their main features.

Oral short-acting MPH formulations (about 3 to 5 hours duration)

These include dl-MPH IR (available in generic, Methylin branded generic, including solution and chewable, and Ritalin brand) and DexMPH IR (available in generic and Focalin brand). MPH's probable mechanism of action is to block the reuptake of

Table 2
MPH preparations main features

Name/Formulation Duration	Dose Forms	Starting Dose	Maximum Dose (May Increase as per MD Judgment)
Short Acting (4 h)			
Ritalin, Methylin (MPH)	5, 10, 20 mg tablet	5 mg twice a day	40 mg
Focalin (DexMPH)	2.5, 5, 10 mg capsule	2.5 mg twice a day	30 mg
Intermediate Acting (8 h)			
Metadate ER (MPH ER)	10, 20 mg capsule	10 mg every morning	60 mg
Ritalin (MPH SR)	SR 20 mg tab	20 mg every morning	60 mg
Metadate CD (Diffucaps MPH)	10, 20, 30, 40, 50, 60 mg	20 mg every morning	60 mg; contents of the capsules can be sprinkled
Ritalin LA (SODAS MPH)	10, 20, 30, 40 mg	20 mg every morning	60 mg; contents of the capsules can be sprinkled
Long Acting (12 h)			
Concerta (OROS MPH)	18, 27, 36, 54 mg cap	18 mg every morning	72 mg; do not cut/crush
Focalin XR (SODAS DexMPH)	5, 10, 15, 20, 30 mg capsule	5 mg every morning	30 mg; contents can be sprinkled
MPH Transdermal System			
Daytrana patch	10, 15, 20, 30 mg patches	10 mg patch	30 mg; patch cannot be cut

norepinephrine and DA into the presynaptic neuron, thereby increasing the availability of these neurotransmitters to the synaptic cleft.[17] MPH IR is a racemic mixture of its d- and l-*threo* enantiomers. DexMPH IR contains only the d-*threo* enantiomer considered to be more pharmacologically active so it is administered at half the dose of the racemic compound. It was found to be significantly more effective than placebo[20] with a side effect profile similar to dl-MPH. The IR formulations are rapidly absorbed and therapeutic action can often be observed within 30 to 60 minutes. However, their half-life of 3 to 5 hours requires multiple doses during the day to achieve ongoing symptom control. The efficacy of MPH IR has been documented for the past 30 years in many short-term trials. However, only recently did 2 large randomized multisite trials study longer periods. These 2 studies, sponsored by the US National Institute of Mental Health, are the Multimodal Treatment Study of Children with ADHD (MTA) study[34] and the Preschool ADHD Treatment Study (PATS).[35]

The MTA study posed 3 questions. How do long-term medication and behavioral treatments compare with one another? Are there additional benefits when they are used together? What is the effectiveness of systematic, carefully delivered treatments versus routine community care? In this study, 579 children with ADHD Combined Type, aged 7 to 9.9 years at study entry, were randomly assigned to 14 months of treatment with: rigorous medication management; intensive behavioral treatment; the 2 combined; or standard community care (delivered by community providers who in two thirds of the cases treated patients with medications). Seventy-four percent of the MTA Study subjects in the medication management group received MPH IR 3 times per day with an average dose of approximately 31 mg/d, which was well tolerated overall. Because of ethical concerns about the duration of the trial, a placebo or sham treatment control group was not included; the community care group served as the comparator arm. Although all groups showed considerable reductions in symptoms with time, there were significant differences between the 4 groups. For core ADHD symptoms, children in the combined treatment and medication management groups showed significantly greater improvement than those given intensive behavioral treatment and community care. However, the combined treatment offered no significantly greater benefits than medication management alone for core ADHD symptoms. The MTA results validated the clinical experience that children who largely adhere to a well-titrated regimen of stimulants continue to benefit significantly for at least 14 months. After completing the controlled study, children were free to continue treatment with community providers and were followed by the MTA study group. Although the initial study was not designed to demonstrate effects beyond 14 months, researchers had hoped that such effects would be nonetheless present at follow-up. Data from an 8-year follow-up were recently published, with overall findings showing that treatment-related improvements were generally maintained but differential treatment efficacy was lost.[11] In other words, there were no differences between the 4 initially assigned treatment groups on repeated measures of psychiatric symptoms, academic function, and social functioning. The differential effects of study treatments, observed when the interventions were delivered during the controlled treatment period, softened when the rigor of treatment was relaxed. Thus, in the MTA study follow-up, the outcome of children who had received an intensive treatment protocol years earlier was no different from that of children receiving community-style treatment when assessed 8 years later. The study data did not address individual patient needs; the investigators stated that "Decisions about starting, continuing, and stopping medication may have to be made on an individualized basis, avoiding untested assumptions about continuing benefit and using periodic trial discontinuations to check for need and benefit."[11(p497)] The findings, however, generated controversy and media reports were published questioning the efficacy of stimulants, which resulted in a response from AACAP asking families to consult with a doctor before discontinuing medication abruptly.[36]

PATS is the largest and longest study of ADHD preschoolers to date. To assess the efficacy and safety of MPH IR, children aged 3 to 5.5 years were enrolled to participate in a multiphased trial including a 5-week randomized placebo controlled phase and a 40-week open label maintenance. The investigators concluded that MPH was effective in this younger population at smaller doses than were used in the MTA study and that, overall, treatment was considered safe.

Oral intermediate-acting MPH formulations (about 8 hours duration)
These include sustained or extended release formulations such as MPH SR (generic), Metadate ER and CD (branded generics), and Ritalin SR and LA (brand). To achieve longer duration, Metadate ER and Ritalin SR consist of MPH molecules that are carried within a wax matrix that liberates the active ingredient slowly as it traverses the gastrointestinal tract, thereby delaying absorption. This delivery method is known as single pulse release, in contrast to more recent double pulse release preparations described later. Although the duration of single pulse MPH is extended to approximately 6 to 8 hours, clinicians have noted that onset of action can also be delayed, so these formulations are less preferred. Side effects are the same as with the IR formulations. Metadate CD uses Diffucaps, a beaded formulation with 30% IR and 70% delayed beads.

Patients who cannot swallow the capsule may sprinkle its beads into apple sauce, pudding, and so forth, for easier ingestion. Ritalin LA uses the Spheroidal Oral Drug Absorption System (SODAS), in which the active molecule is placed in beads inside a capsule. Each bead-filled capsule contains half the dose as IR beads and half as enteric-coated, delayed-release beads. Thus, in these double pulse formulations, there is an initial immediate release of the active agent followed by a second delayed release about 4 hours later.

Long-acting MPH formulations (about 12 hours duration)

These include branded MPH (Concerta) and DexMPH (Focalin XR). Efficacy for these agents has been established in numerous clinical trials[20] and side effects are the same as for the IR formulations, although there may be individual differences (see **Box 2**). Sophisticated delivery methods are involved in prolonging duration of action. For instance, Concerta uses the Osmotic-controlled Release Oral delivery System (OROS) technology. In this case, MPH IR is found on the outer coat of the tablet to provide rapid onset of action after ingestion. Once the IR dissolves, an osmotic gradient is created that slowly releases stimulant contained inside the tablet's core. Focalin XR uses the SODAS technology.

MPH transdermal formulation

Daytrana, the only available formulation of this kind, consists of a skin patch with 3 layers: (1) a polyester/ethylene vinyl acetate laminate film backing, (2) a proprietary adhesive formulation consisting of an acrylic adhesive, a silicone adhesive, and methylphenidate (DOT Matrix transdermal technology), and (3) a protective liner that is attached to the adhesive surface to be removed before the patch can be used. In this formulation, MPH is absorbed transdermally, with the total dose delivered dependent on the patch size (which comes in 4 different strengths) and wear time. It is recommended that the patch be applied to the hip area, 2 hours before the desired onset of action. Because therapeutic effect continues after the patch is removed, it must be removed after 9 hours to achieve a 12-hour duration. Efficacy was demonstrated in laboratory classroom studies and long-term extension studies.[37] In addition to the usual potential side effects seen with orally delivered MPH, the patch may elicit skin reactions if it is worn every day, so it is generally recommended that it be applied to the opposite hip the following day. This formulation offers flexibility of therapeutic duration, which can be controlled by variations in the length of time the patch Is worn. It is also helpful for children who are unable to swallow oral preparations.

SPECIAL SAFETY CONSIDERATIONS REGARDING STIMULANTS

A significant increase in the number of patients treated with stimulants, coupled with safety concerns raised by newly available data from large original and meta-analytical studies, led to a reassessment of the risk/benefit ratio of stimulants. More specifically, interest has been focused on 4 areas: growth, substance abuse risk, tics, and cardiovascular effects.

Growth

The appetite-suppressant effects of stimulants for treating children with ADHD were described in 1937 by Bradley. Adverse consequences on growth have been understood as stemming either directly from decreased appetite or from the effects of the medication on dopaminergic neurons in the pituitary and resultant effects on growth hormone.[38] Clinicians investigating growth delay in earlier follow-up studies concluded that the loss in expected weight and height was small and drug discontinuation resulted in growth rebound. Furthermore, patients treated continuously for up to 5 years until the age of 13 years showed no difference in height when compared with untreated peers.[38] These results were generally reassuring to clinicians instituting prudent weight/height checkups. Physicians advised parents that the potentially adverse consequences of stimulants on growth were benign, although they also monitored for the appearance of any problems in selected individuals. However, new follow-up data on height differences between treated and non-treated children[39] as well as an increasingly accepted practice of continuing treatment beyond early adolescence, called for a reexamination of the issue with diverging research results. For instance, a recent comprehensive review[40] concluded, consistent with earlier findings, that treatment with stimulants in childhood can result in small reductions in expected height and weight that attenuate over time. On the other hand, the findings of a 10-year follow-up study of 124 children[41] did not support an association between deficits in growth outcomes with either ADHD or psychostimulant treatment of ADHD. Because study results aggregate group effects rather than describe individual changes, it is possible that, although immaterial to group statistics, important growth delays could be noted in specific patients, or that even very small changes could occur that are unacceptable for some patients. Thus, at the bedside, should height and weight problems develop in some patients, strategies such as drug holidays or switching to a different agent can be entertained. The context for such a treatment modification decision should be a carefully developed risk/benefit assessment, taking into account concerns regarding stature versus the potential consequences of modifying a treatment that was otherwise effective up to that point.[40]

Abuse Potential

All stimulants are classified as Controlled Class II (CII) substances and carry a warning regarding their potential for abuse. At the same time, most studies have found that the risk of abuse in patients treated for ADHD under medical supervision is very low. Some studies have even concluded that there is perhaps greater risk of developing comorbid addiction in untreated patients. However, the issue is far from resolved. The prescribing of CII agents is tightly regulated; historically, prescriptions could not exceed a 30-day supply. Possibly in recognition of the protective nature of medical supervision, the US Drug Enforcement Administration (DEA) recently eased regulations for CII agents allowing the issuing of multiple prescriptions authorizing the patient to receive a total of up to a 90-day supply. However, the various US states have different policies regarding the way this regulation may be implemented at the local level, and some states still do not allow more than 30-days of medication per prescription. The issue of diversion, in particular in the college setting, has been the focus of recent particular concern. Students increasingly seek stimulants to gain a perceived academic advantage rather than to experience a more traditional intoxicating effect. Therefore, clinicians must consider this important fact when assessing ADHD in this population. These and other addiction-related issues, such as traditional stimulant abuse and management of patients who present with comorbid substance abuse disorders, are examined elsewhere.[10]

Tics

According to current labeling, stimulants are contraindicated in patients with tic disorders. The relationship between stimulants and tics has been the subject of considerable controversy and is discussed in detail in a recent review.[42] A frequent treatment dilemma is that children with ADHD with tics are usually more impaired by symptoms of ADHD than tics, and despite the labeling, at the group level, stimulants are the most effective treatment of ADHD. Research shows that patients with comorbid tic disorder and ADHD[42] can benefit from stimulants, in particular MPH, most often without detriment. Atomoxetine and guanfacine are alternatives found to be helpful in children with comorbid tic/ADHD disorders.

Cardiovascular Effects

Although epidemiologic work has clearly demonstrated that ADHD is not a benign self-limiting childhood disorder,[3] most clinicians would agree that its treatment should not include agents with significant risk for catastrophic cardiac outcomes. The proposed mechanism of action of stimulants is to facilitate DA and NA transmission. Because the NA system also exerts a potent effect on cardiovascular functions, virtually all studies report small to moderate increases in pulse and blood pressure with treatment.[38] However, although acute stimulant toxicity and chronic nonmedical use can lead to severe and sometimes fatal cardiovascular consequences, the degree of stimulant heart risk in patients medically supervised for the treatment of ADHD, in particular the risk of sudden death, has been more difficult to quantify. For instance, the FDA reviewed 20 cases of sudden death during treatment with stimulants but the rate of death during stimulant treatment was less than the that for the general population so that a direct relationship to drug treatment could not be firmly established from the data.[38] Moreover, 2 large retrospective studies, one in the United Kingdom and the other in the United States, found no association between stimulants and sudden death.[43,44] On the other hand, a sophisticated report that used case-control and psychological autopsy methodology did find a small but significant association.[45] An editorial on the controversy concluded that although data suggesting a link between stimulants and sudden unexplained death cannot be dismissed because the sympathomimetic activity of stimulants provides biologic plausibility for cardiovascular effects, sudden unexplained death is a rare event and it is not possible to quantify the risk beyond estimating that it is very small.[46] Nonetheless, this risk, however small, is likely to be increased in children with a preexisting cardiac condition. Thus, it is recommended that before initiating stimulant therapy, physicians assess risk by reviewing findings from a physical examination and obtaining a detailed cardiac history in an effort to assess the presence of pathologic condition of the heart. Clinicians should rule out a history of congenital problems, severe heart palpitations, fainting, exercise intolerance, chest pain, previous cardiac consultations, or a family history of sudden death. In addition, blood pressure and heart rate should be monitored before and during stimulant treatment for every patient. More intensive routine pretreatment tests have not been universally accepted.[47] For instance, in April 2008, the American Heart Association (AHA) recommended that a electrocardiograph (ECG) be obtained as part of the routine assessment for children considered for treatment with stimulant medication, to identify children potentially at risk for sudden death. However, this recommendation was not sanctioned by pediatric or child psychiatric practice guidelines. In May 2008, the AHA and American Academy of Pediatrics, in a report cosponsored by AACAP, jointly issued a news release clarifying that obtaining an ECG before starting medication was reasonable but not mandatory.[48] Because cardiovascular events are fortunately a rare event in children, studies attempting to assess medication risk have been limited by sample size. A large study in progress[49] may hopefully shed more light on this issue. The investigators expect to identify nearly 500,000 ADHD medication users aged 3 to 17 years by combining data from 5 of the largest Medicaid states and a large commercial health insurance database. They will evaluate the incidence rates of serious adverse cardiovascular events in persons exposed to ADHD medications and compare them with rates in an unexposed, population-based reference group. Study results are expected by the end of 2010. Given the plausible danger of cardiac complications in children with heart problems, it has become a standard of practice to refer any patient with a history or current symptoms of heart disease for clearance by a cardiology specialist before initiating treatment.

FDA-APPROVED NONSTIMULANT AGENTS

At present, there are only 2 FDA-approved nonstimulant agents, atomoxetine and guanfacine extended release or GXR, which target noradrenergic neurotransmission preferentially. Atomoxetine is approved in children 6 years of age and older, and adults; GXR is only approved for use in children and adolescents. The main differences between these agents and the stimulants are DEA noncontrolled status, 24/7 duration, and slower onset of action. **Table 3** shows the main features of these agents.

Atomoxetine (Strattera)

This was the first nonstimulant approved by the FDA in 2002, and the first medication of any type to be approved for use in adults. Atomoxetine binds selectively to the NA transporter, thereby increasing synaptic norepinephrine diffusely and dopamine in the PFC (where dopamine reuptake is achieved via norepinephrine transporters). This agent is well absorbed after oral administration and is metabolized primarily through the cytochrome P-450 2D6 pathway, so that coadministration with some selective serotonin reuptake inhibitors (SSRIs) (eg, paroxetine and to a lesser extent fluoxetine) is not advisable because of drug/drug interactions. The efficacy of atomoxetine has been well documented in short- and long-term studies.[8] Full therapeutic effect can take up to 6 to 8 weeks, but some degree of improvement is usually evident by 4 weeks[50] and there is evidence that a later full response could be predicted by week 4.[51] The common side effect profile is benign, with symptoms such as somnolence (most often occurring early in treatment), nausea, decreased appetite, vomiting, insomnia, irritability, and mood swings. Because small reductions in height and weight can also occur with atomoxetine, it is prudent to monitor these parameters. However, effects on these are probably less substantial with atomoxetine than stimulants. Small

Table 3
FDA-approved nonstimulant agents

Name/Formulation Duration	Dose Forms	Starting Dose	Remarks
Strattera (Atomoxetine)	10, 18, 25, 40, 60, 80, 100 mg capsule	<70 kg: 0.5 mg/kg/d. Increase up to 1.2 mg/kg/d not faster than every 3 days, can be given twice a day	Max dose = 100 mg or <1.4 mg/kg. Higher doses have not shown greater efficacy
Intuniv (GXR)	1, 2, 3, 4 mg	1 mg, then increase by 1 mg/wk up to 4 wk	Max dose = 4 mg. However, if tolerated, doses up to 0.12 mg/kg may provide additional benefit. Do not crush, swallow whole

although statistically significant changes have been observed in heart rate and pulse[38] so it is important to monitor them as well. Atomoxetine was enthusiastically received because of potential advantages over stimulants, such as lower risk for abuse, long-lasting therapeutic effects, and noncontrolled status. However, an effect size lower than that of stimulants,[20] and side effect concerns contributed to a decreased rate of use. The risk of suicidal ideation, listed in a boxed warning,[52] should be discussed with patients and their families. In particular, patients should be monitored closely for suicidality during the first few months of treatment and after any dose changes. As a result of postmarketing reports, the package insert warns that atomoxetine should be discontinued if a patient develops jaundice or laboratory evidence of liver injury.[53] Despite these issues, atomoxetine is still considered a first-line treatment in children and adolescents with a history of substance abuse or dependence, in those with significant anxiety symptoms,[54] and in cases based on family preference. Investigators continue to conduct further studies with the goal of finding a more certain place for Strattera within the ADHD medication armamentarium. For instance, there is evidence that some patients may respond preferentially to atomoxetine.[55]

Guanfacine XR (Intuniv)

This is a selective alpha 2A (a2A) adrenoreceptor agonist that in its IR form was approved for the treatment of hypertension but had been used off-label for ADHD for about 15 years. GXR, a branded guanfacine extended release formulation (Intuniv), was approved by the FDA in 2009 for ADHD in children aged 6 to 17 years. Guanfacine IR had been viewed as an alternative to stimulants and a medication that could be preferentially used in patients with tics and aggression, similar to the way clonidine, another a2 agonist that is less specific for the a2A receptor, was used off-label. Although these agents were considered to have relatively lower efficacy, they had often been used for their sedating effects, either to facilitate sleep or to treat hyperactive and oppositional symptoms, and often used in conjunction with stimulants. However, clinical studies with GXR[56] and an improved understanding of the potential role of a2A receptors[57] in ADHD have offered important new information. Research in animals and humans indicates that guanfacine strengthens the regulation of attention and behavior by directly stimulating postsynaptic a2A adrenoreceptors in the PFC (mainly dorsolateral PFC). Short-term controlled studies as well as open label studies of up to 24 months duration concluded that GXR was effective and safe as monotherapy. Because studies found that GXR improves both hyperactive and inattentive symptoms, it was suggested that the extended release formulation has measurable specific effects on attention itself.[58] Other studies have shown GXR to be safe and effective when coadministered with stimulants and for oppositional behaviors.[59–61] It is recommended that dosing be titrated upwards slowly using a fixed dose approach, informed by a calculation of milligrams per kilogram. Improvement can be seen in some cases at week 2. The side effect profile is considered mild, with a preponderance of sedation that attenuates with continued use.[62] Because guanfacine is a hypotensive agent, its cardiovascular effects have been looked at in detail in both controlled and open label studies. Findings were similar across subject populations, showing mild decreases in blood pressure and heart rate that tended to normalize with continued treatment. Although there were few research instances of cardiovascular adverse effects,[58] in clinical settings, it is recommended that baseline and follow-up readings of blood pressure and pulse be obtained. Discontinuation should take place slowly because of reports that IR a2 agents can cause rebound hypertension, although this was not found with GXR. Commonly reported side effects include abdominal pain, dizziness, dry mouth, and constipation. Weight loss and delayed growth have not been observed. GXR does not carry any black-box warnings but is contraindicated in patients showing sensitivity to guanfacine.

NON–FDA-APPROVED TREATMENTS

For many years, clinicians have searched for alternatives to the traditional stimulant treatments. A few agents found effective to some degree have not been approved by the FDA. For instance, because of their effects on central neurotransmission, antidepressant agents were among the first options researched. Multiple controlled and open label studies demonstrated that imipramine and desipramine are effective for ADHD symptoms, in particular behavioral problems more than cognitive deficits.[63] Despite their efficacy, these agents are rarely used today because of concerns regarding cardiovascular toxicity and the availability of approved nonstimulant agents. Bupropion (available as generic and Wellbutrin brand), considered to be a safer antidepressant from the cardiovascular perspective, has shown efficacy in controlled studies of children and adults with ADHD, and although not approved by the FDA for this indication, can be considered a second-line agent.[20] At higher doses, bupropion is associated with an increased risk of seizure. In contrast to the tricyclics and bupropion, the SSRI antidepressants have not shown efficacy in ADHD. Modafinil (available as generic and Provigil brand), a Schedule IV atypical stimulant wake-promoting agent with actions similar to AMP and MPH, has a solid evidence base supporting efficacy in ADHD.[63] Nonetheless, the FDA rejected approval of this agent because of concerns regarding the possibility of developing Stevens-Johnson syndrome, the reason why it is less often recommended.

MEDICATION SELECTION: GENERAL GUIDELINES

As noted earlier, there are multiple agents that can be used to initiate or maintain treatment. Practice algorithms published by specialty associations are helpful in guiding clinicians, as these convey consensus recommendations. However, most algorithms are not empirically derived and should not be construed as the only path to follow. The following paragraphs offer practical advice for various issues that confront clinicians in their day-to-day practice. These recommendations are meant only to provide guidance to the clinician and serve as a template for further customization.

Pretreatment Procedures

Before beginning pharmacotherapy, it is helpful to record baseline measures such as blood pressure, heart rate, and growth rate, to determine the safety and feasibility of treatment. Also, parents and teachers often are asked to complete pretreatment symptom rating scales, the results of which can be evaluated longitudinally with treatment. The identification of target symptoms is essential to assess improvement.

Choosing a Starting Agent

The multiplicity of agents available and the variety of patient clinical presentations call for a true blending of art and science to guide the process of selecting the best medication option for individual patient circumstances. Treatment is to begin with an FDA-approved agent but should this be a stimulant or nonstimulant? Unless specific contraindications exist, stimulants are the favored first choice because of their high degree of efficacy for core ADHD symptoms, rapid onset of action, ease of use, and generally benign side effect profile. Nonstimulants may be used first because of patient/caretaker preference, patient/caretaker substance abuse (diversion or direct abuse), comorbidity, prior stimulant failure, or recent intolerance to stimulant side effects.

Short- Versus Long-acting Stimulant Formulations

Longer-acting stimulant preparations are the best first option because once-daily administration affords the patient full day symptom coverage in school, afterschool activities, homework, and evening family time. In addition, these agents may improve adherence and are potentially less likely to be abused. On the other hand, children less than 6 years of age are usually started on short-acting preparations because they are more sensitive to dose-dependent adverse effects and long-acting agents are not available in low enough strengths. However, once a safe dose of an IR formulation has been established, conversion to a longer-acting agent may be considered. In selected cases, IR formulations may also be preferable to extended release agents.

AMP Versus MPH

Several studies have compared AMP with MPH formulations and although some differences in effectiveness and side effect profiles exist, these are not clinically meaningful. Both types of stimulants have demonstrated high efficacy and when one class fails, the other can be recommended next to increase overall treatment effectiveness to as much as 85%. Individual clinicians may become comfortable with one stimulant type, which they use first in beginning treatment, and switch to the other if the first trial fails. In special circumstances, such as children who cannot swallow pills, physicians may recommend one of the various preparations that do not require ingestion of an intact pill.

Medication Titration

As with most other treatments in child psychiatry, the rule of thumb is to start with the lowest possible dose and to monitor side effects and efficacy every few days. If there is inadequate improvement and there are few significant side effects, it is reasonable to increase to the next dose level. This strategy can continue until either the desired effect is reached or severe side effects appear. In general, clinicians titrate upwards until improvements in rating scale reach scores of 40% to 50% above the baseline, and until substantial improvements in functional status are observed.

What to do When Side Effects Develop

The usual steps are either to discontinue the initial stimulant and switch to the other class or switch to a nonstimulant. Evidence-based data do not preferentially support continuation with either strategy after a first treatment fails. If intolerance to stimulant side effects develops, then switching to a nonstimulant is preferred. Combination therapy has become a relatively accepted strategy because there is evidence that adding a nonstimulant to stimulant therapy potentiates the effectiveness of the overall regimen. If no improvement after 2 ADHD treatments is noted, a reassessment is necessary. For instance, comorbidity with affective disorder, anxiety disorder, or substance abuse needs to be evaluated as well as establishing that adherence has been reasonable.

Nonimprovement with FDA-approved Treatments

If reassessment fails to identify any complicating circumstances, nonapproved treatments can be entertained. However, these treatments generally have lower effect sizes than approved agents. An additional option is to use behavior therapy, for which evidence-based efficacy data of effectiveness are available. If medication is preferred, trials of bupropion, modafinil, clonidine, or other noradrenergic agents (eg, noradrenergic tricyclic antidepressants) can be entertained, as long as appropriate informed consent is obtained.

Duration of Successful Treatment

Because some patients will no longer require pharmacotherapy with time, the need for continued therapy should be reevaluated from time to time. To minimize disruptions in school functioning, it is often recommended that treatment be maintained at least until final examinations take place, at which point it can be tapered and discontinued. Following this strategy ensures that teacher input is still available but final grades are not jeopardized as there is time to reinstitute treatment if the patient relapses off medication. While, the demand for treatment is lower when there is no school, the determination that medication is no longer necessary during summer may not hold up when school begins again. With respect to stimulant discontinuation, if a patient becomes symptomatic, routine use of off-treatment periods (ie, drug holidays) on weekends or summer is not recommended. However, as noted earlier, if there is growth delay, drug holidays are recommended as a strategy to allow for catch up. Regarding nonstimulants, it is not advisable to stop treatment during the summer as it may take several weeks to return to therapeutic levels. Weekend drug holidays are impractical for the same reason.

SUMMARY

ADHD is the most frequently occurring child and adolescent psychiatric condition for which families consult a variety of medical specialists including pediatricians, family practitioners, psychiatrists, and neurologists, as well as nonphysicians. This article has reviewed the various FDA-approved and nonapproved pharmacologic agents currently available for ADHD, and has presented information on the relative strengths of each treatment as well as their potential adverse effects. Pharmacotherapy for ADHD is generally highly effective and safe, although some patients do not respond to initial treatment efforts and other patients experience problems with tolerability. Care-optimizing strategies have been offered with these considerations in mind. It is hoped that the rapid pace of advancement in the understanding of the neurobiology and genetics will soon make available further information to tailor treatments to specific patient characteristics. In the meantime, the type of art and science medical treatment approaches described here will likely continue to offer relief for most children and adolescents with ADHD.

ACKNOWLEDGMENTS

The authors wish to thank Bennett Silver, MD, for his helpful comments during the preparation of this manuscript.

REFERENCES

1. Barkley R, Murphy K, Fischer M. ADHD in adults: what the science says. New York: Guilford Press; 2008.
2. Froehlich TE, Lanphear BP, Epstein JN, et al. Prevalence, recognition, and treatment of attention-deficit/hyperactivity disorder in a national sample of US children. Arch Pediatr Adolesc Med 2007;161(9):857–64.

3. Kessler RC, Adler L, Barkley R. The prevalence and correlates of adult ADHD in the United States: results from the National Comorbidity Survey Replication. Am J Psychiatry 2006;163(4):716–23.
4. Biederman J, Petty CR, Monuteaux MC, et al. Adult psychiatric outcomes of girls with ADHD: 11-year follow -up in a longitudinal case-control study. Am J Psychiatry 2010;167:409–17.
5. Kieling C, Goncalves R, Tannock R, et al. Neurobiology of ADHD. Child Adolesc Psychiatr Clin N Am 2008;17:285–307.
6. American Psychiatric Association. Diagnostic and statistical manual of mental disorders fourth edition (text revision) DSM-IV-TR. Washington, DC: APA; 2000.
7. Polanczyk G, de Lima MS, Horta BL, et al. The worldwide prevalence of ADHD: a systematic review. Am J Psychiatry 2007;164(6):942–8.
8. Pliszka S, AACAP Work Group on Quality Issues. Practice parameter for the assessment and treatment of children and adolescents with attention-deficit/hyperactivity disorder. J Am Acad Child Adolesc Psychiatry 2007;46(7):894–921.
9. Nazeer A, Calles JL Jr. Pediatric bipolar disorders. Int J Child Adolesc Health 2010;3(2):187–95.
10. Ivanov I, Pearson A, Kaplan G, et al. Treatment of adolescent ADHD and comorbid substance abuse. Int J Child Adolesc Health 2010;3(2):143–61.
11. Molina B, Hinshaw S, Swanson J, et al. The MTA at 8 years: prospective follow-up of children treated for combined-type ADHD in a multisite study. J Am Acad Child Adolesc Psychiatry 2009;48(5):484–500.
12. Antshel K, Barkley R. Psychosocial interventions in ADHD. Child Adolesc Psychiatr Clin N Am 2008;17:421–37.
13. Jensen PS, Hinshaw SP, Swanson JM, et al. Findings from the NIMH Multimodal Treatment Study of ADHD (MTA): implications and applications for primary care providers. J Dev Behav Pediatr 2001;22(1):60–73.
14. Collett BR, Ohan JL, Myers KM. Ten-year review of rating scales. V: Scales assessing attention-deficit/hyperactivity disorder. J Am Acad Child Adolesc Psychiatry 2003;42(9):1015–37.
15. Barkley RA. Behavioral inhibition, sustained attention, and executive functions: constructing a unifying theory of ADHD. Psychol Bull 1997;121(1):65–94.
16. Brown TE. Attention deficit disorder. New Haven (CT): Yale University Press; 2005.
17. Arnsten AF. Toward a new understanding of attention-deficit hyperactivity disorder pathophysiology: an important role for prefrontal cortex dysfunction. CNS Drugs 2009;23(Suppl 1):33–41.
18. Bradley C. The behavior of children receiving benzedrine. Am J Psychiatry 1937;94:577–85.
19. Knobel M, Wolman M, Mason A. Hyperkinesis and organicity in children. Arch Gen Psychiatry 1959;1(3):310–21.
20. Paykina N, Greenhill L. Attention deficit hyperactivity disorder. In: Findling RL, editor. Clinical manual of child and adolescent psychopharmacology. Washington, DC: American Pyschiatric Publishing; 2008. p. 33–87.
21. Biederman J, Monuteaux MC, Spencer T, et al. Do stimulants protect against psychiatric disorders in youth with ADHD? A 10-year follow-up study. Pediatrics 2009;124(1):71–8.
22. Advokat C. What exactly are the benefits of stimulants for ADHD? J Atten Disord 2009;12(6):495–8.
23. Greydanus D, Kaplan G, Antshel K. Attention deficit hyperactivity disorder: neuropsychologic and pharmacologic considerations. In: Noggle CA, Dean RS,

editors. The neuropsychology of psychopharmacology. New York: Springer; in press.

24. Greenhill LL, Pliszka S, Dulcan MK. Practice parameter for the use of stimulant medications in the treatment of children, adolescents and adults. J Am Acad Child Adolesc Psychiatry 2002;41(2):26S–49S.

25. Marcus S, Wan G, Kemner J, et al. Continuity of methylphenidate treatment for attention-deficit/hyperactivity disorder. Arch Pediatr Adolesc Med 2005;159:572–8.

26. Arnold LE, Huestis RD, Smeltzer DJ, et al. Levoamphetamine vs dextroamphetamine in minimal brain dysfunction. Arch Gen Psychiatry 1976;33(3):292–301.

27. Prince J, Wilens T. Pharmacotherpay of ADHD and comorbidities. In: Brown T, editor. ADHD comorbidities handbook. Washington, DC: American Psychiatric Publishing; 2009. p. 229–84.

28. Pennick M. Absorption of lisdexamfetamine dimesylate and hydrolysis to form the active moiety, d-amphetamine. Poster presented at: New Clinical Drug Evaluation Unit 49th Annual Meeting, Hollywood (FL), June 29 to July 2, 2009.

29. Wigal SB, Kollins SH, Childress AC, et al. The 311 Study Group. A 13-hour laboratory school study of lisdexamfetamine dimesylate in school-aged children with attention-deficit/hyperactivity disorder. Child Adolesc Psychiatry Ment Health 2009;3(1):17.

30. Haffey MB, Buckwalter M, Zhang P, et al. Effects of omeprazole on the pharmacokinetic profiles of lisdexamfetamine dimesylate and extended-release mixed amphetamine salts in adults. Postgrad Med 2009;121(5):11–9.

31. Najib J. The efficacy and safety profile of lisdexamfetamine dimesylate, a prodrug of d-amphetamine, for the treatment of attention-deficit/hyperactivity disorder in children and adults. Clin Ther 2009;31(1):142–76.

32. Findling RL, Childress AC, Krishnan S, et al. Long-term effectiveness and safety of lisdexamfetamine dimesylate in school-aged children with attention-deficit/hyperactivity disorder. CNS Spectr 2008;13(7):614–20.

33. Jasinski DR, Krishnan S. Abuse liability and safety of oral lisdexamfetamine dimesylate in individuals with a history of stimulant abuse. J Psychopharmacol 2009; 23(4):419–27.

34. The MTA Cooperative Group. A 14-month randomized clinical trial of treatment strategies for attention-deficit/hyperactivity disorder. Arch Gen Psychiatry 1999; 56:1073–86.

35. Greenhill L, Kollins S, Abikoff H, et al. Efficacy and safety of immediate-release methylphenidate treatment for preschoolers with ADHD. J Am Acad Child Adolesc Psychiatry 2006;45(11):1284–93.

36. Available at: http://www.aacap.org/cs/2009_press_releases/american_academy_of_child_and_adolescent_psychiatry_urges_parents_not_to_discontinue_adhd_treatment_abruptly. Accessed June 4, 2010.

37. Bukstein OG. Transdermal methylphenidate system: old wine in a new bottle. Expert Opin Drug Metab Toxicol 2009;5(6):661–5.

38. Vitiello B. Understanding the risk of using medications for attention deficit hyperactivity disorder with respect to physical growth and cardiovascular function. Child Adolesc Psychiatr Clin N Am 2008;17(2):459–74.

39. Swanson JM, Elliott GR, Greenhill LL, et al. Effects of stimulant medication on growth rates across 3 years in the MTA follow-up. J Am Acad Child Adolesc Psychiatry 2007;46(8):1015–27.

40. Faraone SV, Biederman J, Morley CP, et al. Effect of stimulants on height and weight: a review of the literature. J Am Acad Child Adolesc Psychiatry 2008; 47(9):994–1009.

41. Biederman J, Spencer TJ, Monuteaux MC, et al. A naturalistic 10-year prospective study of height and weight in children with attention-deficit hyperactivity disorder grown up: sex and treatment effects. J Pediatr 2010;157:635–40, 640.e1.
42. Bloch MH, Panza KE, Landeros-Weisenberger A, et al. Meta-analysis: treatment of attention-deficit/hyperactivity disorder in children with comorbid tic disorders. J Am Acad Child Adolesc Psychiatry 2009;48(9):884–93.
43. Winterstein AG, Gerhard T, Shuster J, et al. Cardiac safety of central nervous system stimulants in children and adolescents with attention-deficit/hyperactivity disorder. Pediatrics 2007;120:1494–501.
44. McCarthy S, Cranswick N, Potts L, et al. Mortality associated with attention-deficit hyperactivity disorder (ADHD) drug treatment: a retrospective cohort study of children, adolescents and young adults using the general practice research database. Drug Saf 2009;32(11):1089–96.
45. Gould MS, Walsh BT, Munfakh JL, et al. Sudden death and use of stimulant medications in youths. Am J Psychiatry 2009;166(9):992–1001.
46. Vitiello B, Towbin K. Stimulant treatment of ADHD and risk of sudden death in children. Am J Psychiatry 2009;166(9):955–7.
47. Leslie LK, Alexander ME, Trikalinos TA, et al. Reexamining the Emperor's new clothes: ambiguities in current cardiac screening recommendations for youth with ADHD. Circ Cardiovasc Qual Outcomes 2008;1:134–7.
48. Newcorn JH, Donnelly C. Cardiovascular safety of medication treatments for attention-deficit/hyperactivity disorder. Mt Sinai J Med 2009;76(2):198–203.
49. Hennessy S, Schelleman H, Daniel G, et al. Cardiovascular safety of ADHD medications: rationale for and design of an investigator-initiated observational study. Pharmacoepidemiol Drug Saf 2010;19:934–41.
50. Ledbetter M. Atomoxetine: a novel treatment for child and adult ADHD. Neuropsychiatr Dis Treat 2006;2(4):455–66.
51. Newcorn JH, Sutton VK, Weiss MD, et al. Clinical responses to atomoxetine in attention-deficit/hyperactivity disorder: the Integrated Data Exploratory Analysis (IDEA) study. J Am Acad Child Adolesc Psychiatry 2009;48(5):511–8.
52. Daughton JM, Kratochvil CJ. Review of ADHD pharmacotherapies: advantages, disadvantages, and clinical pearls. J Am Acad Child Adolesc Psychiatry 2009; 48(3):240–8.
53. US Food and Drug Administration. Atomoxetine (marketed as Strattera): serious liver injury. Postmarket Reviews 2009;2:1. Available at: http://www.fda.gov/Drugs/DrugSafety/DrugSafetyNewsletter/ucm110235.htm. Accessed October 30, 2010.
54. Geller D, Donnelly C, Lopez F, et al. Atomoxetine treatment for pediatric patients with attention-deficit/hyperactivity disorder with comorbid anxiety disorder. J Am Acad Child Adolesc Psychiatry 2007;46(9):1119–27.
55. Newcorn JH, Kratochvil CJ, Allen AJ, et al. Atomoxetine and osmotically released methylphenidate for the treatment of attention deficit hyperactivity disorder: acute comparison and differential response. Am J Psychiatry 2008;165(6):721–30.
56. Sallee FR, Lyne A, Wigal T, et al. Long-term safety and efficacy of guanfacine extended release in children and adolescents with attention-deficit/hyperactivity disorder. J Child Adolesc Psychopharmacol 2009;19(3):215–26.
57. Arnsten AF, Scahill L, Findling RL. Alpha2-adrenergic receptor agonists for the treatment of attention-deficit/hyperactivity disorder: emerging concepts from new data. J Child Adolesc Psychopharmacol 2007;17(4):393–406.
58. Biederman J, Melmed RD, Patel A, et al. Long-term, open-label extension study of guanfacine extended release in children and adolescents with ADHD. CNS Spectr 2008;13(12):1047–55.

59. Spencer TJ, Greenbaum M, Ginsberg LD, et al. Safety and effectiveness of coadministration of guanfacine extended release and psychostimulants in children and adolescents with attention-deficit/hyperactivity disorder. J Child Adolesc Psychopharmacol 2009;19(5):501–10.

60. Connor D, Spencer T, Kratochvil C, et al. Effects of guanfacine extended release on secondary measures in children with attention-deficit/hyperactivity disorder and oppositional symptoms. Paper presented at: Annual Meeting of the American Psychiatric Association. San Francisco (CA), May 16–21, 2009.

61. Stahl SM. Mechanism of action of alpha 2A-adrenergic agonists in attention-deficit/hyperactivity disorder with or without oppositional symptoms. J Clin Psychiatry 2010;71(3):223–4.

62. Faraone SV, Glatt SJ. Effects of extended-release guanfacine on ADHD symptoms and sedation-related adverse events in children with ADHD. J Atten Disord 2010;13(5):532–8.

63. Biederman J, Spencer TJ. Psychopharmacological interventions. Child Adolesc Psychiatr Clin N Am 2008;17(2):439–58.

Psychopharmacology of Eating Disorders in Children and Adolescents

Neville H. Golden, MD[a],*, Evelyn Attia, MD[b]

KEYWORDS

• Eating disorders • Pharmacology • Treatment
• Children • Adolescents

Eating disorders are prevalent in adolescents and pediatricians play an important role in their identification, diagnosis, and management. Although some pediatricians may choose to refer their patients to specialized eating disorders programs, many, especially those who practice a long distance from major medical centers, may be called on to play a central role in the management of an adolescent with an eating disorder.

One of the most challenging aspects of treating a teenager with an eating disorder is that the wishes of the adolescent, driven by the eating disorder, are often in direct conflict with those of the treatment team and the family. It would be helpful if there were a safe psychopharmacologic agent that could alleviate the preoccupation with shape and weight or distortion in body image that makes treatment so challenging. The psychopharmacologic management of adolescents with eating disorders is further complicated by the high rates of psychiatric comorbidity and the paucity of data regarding the usefulness of psychiatric medications in younger populations. Recent black-box warnings about medications frequently prescribed to treat adolescents with eating disorders further add to the confusion. This article reviews the scientific evidence for use of psychotropic medication in the treatment of children and adolescents with eating disorders and briefly reviews the major types of eating disorders and the comorbidities associated with them. The efficacy and safety of psychotropic medications for the treatment of eating disorders in general are discussed, with a focus on data that are specific to children and adolescents.

Dr Golden has nothing to disclose. Dr Attia receives research support from Eli Lilly & Co.
[a] Division of Adolescent Medicine, Stanford University School of Medicine, Palo Alto, CA, USA
[b] Columbia University Medical Center, Weill Cornell Medical College, New York, NY, USA
* Corresponding author. Division of Adolescent Medicine, Lucile Packard Children's Hospital at Stanford, 770 Welch Road, Suite 433, Palo Alto, CA 94304.
E-mail address: ngolden@stanford.edu

Pediatr Clin N Am 58 (2011) 121–138
doi:10.1016/j.pcl.2010.11.001
0031-3955/11/$ – see front matter © 2011 Elsevier Inc. All rights reserved.

pediatric.theclinics.com

MAJOR CATEGORIES OF EATING DISORDERS

The spectrum of eating disturbances varies widely, ranging from mildly abnormal eating habits to life-threatening chronic disease. The most commonly used definitions of eating disorders are provided by the American Psychiatric Association's Diagnostic and Statistical Manual of Mental Disorders, fourth edition (DSM-IV).[1] These criteria are currently being revised in the soon-to-be-published DSM-5.[2] In DSM-IV, 3 major groups of patients are identified: those who meet criteria for anorexia nervosa (AN), those who meet criteria for bulimia nervosa (BN), and those who have features of an eating disorder but who do not meet the diagnostic criteria for either AN or BN, referred to as an eating disorder not otherwise specified (EDNOS). In children and adolescents, most patients are in the EDNOS category. Changes to the diagnostic criteria being considered for DSM-5, including less-stringent frequency and severity criteria, make it likely that younger patients with weight and eating behavior disturbances will more likely meet DSM-5 criteria for the major eating disorder categories.

The core feature of AN is self-imposed weight loss, or failure to gain weight during a period of growth, leading to a weight that is less than that expected for height and age. In addition, patients have an intense fear of gaining weight, a distorted body image, and, for postmenarcheal girls, loss of at least 3 consecutive menstrual cycles. There are 2 subtypes: restricting type and binge-eating/purging type (**Box 1**). The lifetime prevalence of AN in the United States and western Europe is reported to be 0.3% to 0.5%.[3] Peak age of onset is 15 to 19 years, and 95% of sufferers develop the disorder before the age of 25 years. The female/male ratio is 9:1 with a higher ratio of boys reported in those less than 14 years old.

BN is characterized by recurrent episodes of binge eating accompanied by episodes of inappropriate compensatory behaviors, such as self-induced vomiting or misuse of laxatives, diuretics, or other medications. These behaviors are accompanied by cognitions that reflect influence of body shape and weight on self-evaluation. Diagnosis of BN requires that the behavioral disturbance not occur in the context of AN; therefore, individuals with BN are generally at normal or above normal weight. The lifetime prevalence of BN has been estimated at 1.5% to 2.0% in adult women.[4,5] The prevalence of DSM-IV BN is lower in adolescent samples because BN develops in older adolescence and young adulthood. Prevalence of BN was found to be 0.3% in a nationwide study of 12 to 23 year olds in Portugal[6] and 0.75% in a study of girls in Spain.[7] The gender ratio is slightly more balanced in BN than AN, with 20% to 30% of those affected being male.[4] DSM-IV defines BN as requiring that binge and purge episodes occur at least twice weekly for 3 months, but the criteria for BN being proposed for DSM-5 describe that once-weekly episodes for a period of 3 months is sufficient to make the diagnosis. It is likely that adolescents who had previously received the nonspecific EDNOS diagnosis for subthreshold BN will more likely meet full diagnostic criteria for BN using DSM-5.

EDNOS is a heterogeneous diagnostic category that includes patients presenting with symptoms similar to AN or BN but who do not meet all of the diagnostic criteria for those disorders. Included in this group are those who have started weight loss, but may not have reached markedly low weight for height, those who have low weight but have not lost menstrual activity, or those with binge and purge behavior but with frequency less than twice weekly or duration less than 3 months, or those who purge but do not binge, to maintain a weight they perceive to be thin and healthy. EDNOS also includes some other conditions such as binge-eating disorder (BED) and night-eating syndrome (NES).

Box 1
DSM-IV diagnostic criteria

Anorexia nervosa

Refusal to maintain body weight at or greater than a minimally normal weight for age and height (eg, weight loss leading to maintenance of body weight less than 85% of that expected; or failure to make expected weight gain during period of growth, leading to body weight less than 85% of the expected)

Intense fear of gaining weight or becoming fat, even though underweight

Disturbance in the way in which one's body weight or shape is experienced, undue influence of body weight or shape on self-evaluation, or denial of the seriousness of the current low body weight

In postmenarcheal women, amenorrhea, (ie, absence of at least 3 consecutive menstrual cycles). A woman is considered to have amenorrhea if her periods occur only following hormone (eg, estrogen) administration

Specify type

Restricting type: during the current episode of anorexia nervosa, the person has not regularly engaged in binge-eating or purging behavior (ie, self-induced vomiting or the misuse of laxatives, diuretics, or enemas)

Binge-eating/purging type: during the current episode of AN, the person has regularly engaged in binge-eating or purging behavior (ie, self-induced vomiting or the misuse of laxatives, diuretics, or enemas)

Bulimia nervosa

Recurrent episodes of binge eating. An episode of binge eating is characterized by both of the following:

Eating, in a discrete period of time (eg, within any 2-hour period), an amount of food that is definitely larger than most people would eat during a similar period of time and in similar circumstances

A sense of lack of control of eating during the episode (eg, a feeling that one cannot stop eating or control what or how much one is eating)

Recurrent inappropriate compensatory behavior to prevent weight gain, such as self-induced vomiting; misuse of laxatives, diuretics, enemas, or other medications; fasting; or excessive exercise

Binge eating and inappropriate compensatory behaviors both occur on average at least twice a week for 3 months

Self-evaluation is unduly influenced by body shape and weight

The disturbance does not occur exclusively during episodes of AN

From American Psychiatric Association. Diagnostic and Statistical Manual of Mental Disorders (fourth edition, text revision). Washington, DC: American Psychiatric Association; 2000; with permission. © 2000 American Psychiatric Association.

In BED, patients binge eat but do not engage in compensatory behaviors such as purging. In DSM-IV, BED is categorized within the EDNOS umbrella, although it is being proposed as a formal diagnostic category for DSM-5. Among adults, BED is the most common eating disorder, with lifetime prevalence estimates in the community of 3.5% among women and 2.0% among men.[4] BED is considerably more prevalent in adults than it is in children and adolescents, although it has been described in younger groups, especially because overweight and obesity are increasingly present in pediatric samples. BED is more difficult to assess in children because of the challenges inherent in self-reported dietary recall in younger samples, as well as the difficulty children may have in understanding the concept of loss of control during eating episodes. Developmentally appropriate language may be necessary to assess accurately the concept of loss-of-control eating.[8] Up to 30% of overweight children and adolescents[8–12] report episodes of loss of control during eating episodes. Binge eating equally affects boys and girls, although girls may be more willing to report disordered eating than boys.[13]

NES is characterized by morning anorexia, evening hyperphagia, and insomnia with awakenings followed by nocturnal ingestions believed to be explained by a delay in the usual circadian timing of food intake relative to the sleep-wake cycle. The female athlete triad is a syndrome occurring in female athletes consisting of 3 interrelated conditions: low energy availability, menstrual dysfunction, and low bone mineral density.[14] Although some patients with the triad have an eating disorder, many do not, but are consuming inadequate calories for their activity level. The inadequate energy consumption may be caused by body image concerns, but may also be the result of a desire to improve athletic performance. Some athletes may have a lack of knowledge regarding the true metabolic demands of their athletic training. Inadequate energy intake results in an energy imbalance, leading to suppression of the hypothalamic-pituitary-ovarian axis. The athlete develops menstrual irregularity, amenorrhea, and a low estrogen state that contributes to low bone mass and increased fracture risk.

In children and younger adolescents, there are some other distinct clinical conditions related to disturbances with eating that are sometimes grouped in the EDNOS classification. The Great Ormond Street Children's Hospital Classification includes eating disturbances in children and young adolescents in which there is no distortion in body image or preoccupation with shape or weight. Some of these conditions may be accompanied by loss of weight and growth retardation (**Box 2**).[15] DSM-5 is considering the inclusion of a new category of eating disorder called avoidant/restrictive food intake disorder (ARFID), which describes many of these eating-related disturbances (**Box 3**).[2]

COMORBIDITY

Patients with eating disorders have high rates of psychiatric comorbidity, either concurrent with the eating disorder, or manifesting earlier or later. For AN, the lifetime prevalence of affective disorders, especially depression, is 50% to 68% and the lifetime rate of anxiety disorders (especially obsessive-compulsive disorder and social phobia) is 30% to 65%. These symptoms are worsened by malnutrition, and weight restoration will contribute to improvement in mood and anxiety symptoms, in addition to improving the core eating disorder. Anxiety disorders often predate the onset of AN, and depression and anxiety may persist after recovery from the eating disorder. For BN, approximately 80% of patients report a lifetime prevalence of psychiatric comorbidity with high rates of mood disorders (50%–70%), anxiety disorders (13%–65%), substance abuse disorders (approximately 25%), and personality disorders (20%–80%). Patients with BN tend to be impulsive and may engage in high-risk activities such as sexual promiscuity, stealing, and self-injury. An anxiety disorder may predate the onset of BN, and substance abuse disorder frequently follows its onset.[16]

Box 2
The Great Ormond Street criteria for eating disorders

Food avoidance emotional disorder (FAED)

    Food avoidance or difficulty

    Weight loss

    Mood disturbance

    No cognitive distortions regarding weight or shape

    No organic brain disease, psychosis, or drug-related cause

Selective eating disorder (SED)

    Limited food choices for at least 2 years

    Unwilling to try new foods

    No cognitive distortions regarding weight or shape

    No fear of choking or vomiting

    Weight and height are usually appropriate for age

Functional dysphagia

    Food avoidance

    Fear of choking or vomiting

    Often there is a history of an episode of choking

    No cognitive distortions regarding weight or shape

    No organic brain disease or psychosis

Pervasive food refusal

    A refusal to eat, drink, walk, talk, or care for self

    Resistant to others' efforts to help

Anorexia nervosa

Bulimia nervosa

Data from Nicholls D, Chater R, Lask B. Children into DSM don't go: a comparison of classification systems for eating disorders in childhood and early adolescence. Int J Eat Disord 2000;28 (3):317–24.

PHARMACOLOGIC TREATMENT OF AN

The difficulties in conducting randomized controlled trials (RCTs) in AN have recently been reviewed.[17] Difficulties with subject recruitment, accompanied by high dropout rates, result in small sample sizes that limit statistical power and make interpretation of existing studies difficult. Medication treatments may be particularly difficult for AN patients to accept compared with psychological interventions.[17] Furthermore, although some RCTs of medication treatments have been conducted in adults with AN, there have been no published RCTs specifically conducted in children and adolescents.

Antidepressants and AN

Patients with AN often exhibit symptoms of depression and early studies examined the use of antidepressants in this disorder. There have been 4 published RCTs on the use

> **Box 3**
> **DSM-5 proposed diagnostic criteria for ARFID**
>
> *ARFID*
>
> Eating or feeding disturbance as manifested by persistent failure to meet appropriate nutritional and/or energy needs associated with 1 or more of the following:
>
> 1. Significant weight loss (or failure to achieve expected weight gain or faltering growth in children)
> 2. Significant nutritional deficiency
> 3. Dependence on enteral feeding
> 4. Marked interference with psychosocial functioning
>
> There is no evidence that lack of available food, an associated culturally sanctioned practice, or a general medical condition or other mental disorder alone is sufficient to account for the disorder
>
> The eating disturbance does not occur exclusively during the course of AN or BN
>
> If the eating disturbance occurs exclusively in the context of another mental disorder (eg, mental retardation or a pervasive developmental disorder), it is sufficiently severe to warrant independent clinical attention
>
> *Adapted from* American Psychiatric Association. Diagnostic and Statistical Manual of Mental Disorders version 5: proposed criteria. dsm5.org; with permission. © 2010 American Psychiatric Association. Available at: http://www.dsm5.org/proposedrevisions/pages/eatingdisorders.aspx. Accessed September 1, 2010.

of antidepressants in adults with AN. Lacey and Crisp[18] conducted an RCT on the use of clomipramine, a tricyclic agent with antidepressant and antiobsessional properties, in 16 adult patients with AN who were hospitalized for refeeding. Clomipramine was associated with increased hunger and appetite but a reduced rate of weight gain. Halmi and colleagues[19] conducted an RCT on the use of the tricyclic antidepressant amitriptyline, the appetite stimulant cyproheptadine, and placebo in 72 subjects with AN, and found that amitriptyline did not increase the rate of weight gain or improve depression in patients with AN. Cyproheptadine increased rate of weight gain and reduced depressive symptoms in those who were not purging, but impaired treatment efficacy for those who were purging. In a 5-week double-blind RCT conducted by Biederman and colleagues,[20] 11 subjects were treated with amitriptyline and 14 received placebo. Amitriptyline was associated with significant side effects and did not improve weight gain, eating disorder symptoms, or symptoms of depression. Tricyclic antidepressants are associated with several cardiac side effects including tachycardia, hypotension, and cardiac arrhythmias, in particular prolongation of the QT interval, and should only be used with extreme caution in malnourished patients with AN.

The selective serotonin reuptake inhibitors (SSRIs) have a better safety profile than the tricyclic antidepressants and also have proven efficacy for obsessive-compulsive disorder in children and adolescents.[21] The findings of altered levels of serotonin metabolites in the cerebrospinal fluid of low-weight and weight-restored subjects with AN suggest alterations in the serotonergic pathways in this disorder.[22,23] The SSRIs increase serotonin levels available to the postsynaptic receptor and, on a theoretic basis, might be useful as an adjunct in the treatment of AN. Attia and colleagues[24] randomized 31 adult women with AN, who were hospitalized on an inpatient clinical research unit, to receive 7 weeks of fluoxetine at a target daily dose of 60 mg, or placebo in a double-blind fashion. However, although both groups improved in weight and psychological symptoms, there was no additional benefit associated with fluoxetine compared with placebo. A retrospective study of adolescents with AN, who were assessed during their inpatient stay and at 3 and 6 months following hospitalization, compared 19 subjects treated with an SSRI during inpatient and/or outpatient periods with 13 who did not receive an SSRI, and found no difference between the 2 groups in body mass index (BMI), eating disorder symptoms, or depressive symptoms at discharge from the inpatient program or at follow-up 6 months after discharge.[25]

Two studies have examined the use of fluoxetine in relapse prevention in adults with AN. After an inpatient stay intended to restore weight, Kaye and colleagues[26] assigned 16 subjects to receive fluoxetine and 19 to receive placebo in a randomized double-blind fashion. Subjects were then followed for a year without controlling for other treatments the subjects may have received. Compared with those receiving placebo, the subjects on fluoxetine had improved weight gain and a reduction in core eating disorder symptoms and symptoms of depression and anxiety, suggesting that fluoxetine may play a role in relapse prevention in AN. Walsh and colleagues[27] were not able to replicate these findings in a large, carefully designed multisite study of 96 subjects with AN from the New York State Psychiatric Institute and Toronto General Hospital. Subjects were weight restored in inpatient or partial hospital programs and then randomly assigned to fluoxetine or placebo, together with cognitive behavioral therapy (CBT), and followed as outpatients for 1 year in a double-blind manner. Time to relapse, BMI, and clinical measures of depression at follow-up did not differ between the groups. Moreover, there was no difference in response to fluoxetine between clinical sites, suggesting that the findings of the study can be generalized.

Atypical Antipsychotic Medication and AN

Isolated case reports, retrospective studies, and some uncontrolled case series have generated considerable interest in the possible role of the atypical antipsychotic medications in the management of AN. Atypical antipsychotic medications block both the serotonergic and dopaminergic receptors and reduce anxiety, agitation, depression, and obsessional thinking in clinical populations with psychotic disorders for whom these medications are generally prescribed. An added potential advantage in the management of patients with AN is that, both in laboratory animals and in humans, the atypical antipsychotic medications are associated with weight gain. Although most of the studies on the atypical antipsychotics have been conducted in adults, both olanzapine[28,29] and quetiapine[30] have been used safely in children and adolescents with AN. The atypical antipsychotic most studied is olanzapine, but other atypicals with published reports include quetiapine and risperidone. In a series of 5 hospitalized children with AN described by Boachie and colleagues,[28] administration of olanzapine was associated with significant increases in rate of weight gain and a reduction in agitation and anxiety before and after meals.[28] In Mehler and colleagues'[29] series of 5 adolescents with AN treated with olanzapine, preoccupation with body image and anxiety related to gaining weight also improved but, in contrast to the findings of Boachie and colleagues,[28] the rate of weight gain in adolescents treated with olanzapine did not exceed the rate of weight gain before initiating treatment with olanzapine. Uncontrolled open-label trials in larger numbers of subjects with AN have documented more significant weight gain in short periods of time in adults,[31,32] as well as in adolescents.[33] In the adolescent study, 13 subjects aged 9.6 to 16.3 years (mean age 13.7 ± 2.3 years) were treated with olanzapine for 6 months. BMI increased significantly after 1 month of treatment and continued to increase until the end of the study. Eating attitudes and global functioning scores improved, and there was a reduction in anxiety, hyperactivity, and symptoms of depression.[33] However, none of these studies included a control group, and it is not clear how much of the response to treatment was secondary to the multidisciplinary and multimodal treatment that subjects were receiving.

There have been 2 published placebo-controlled RCTs examining the use of olanzapine in AN, both conducted in adults. One compared olanzapine with placebo, and both groups received CBT.[34] The other compared olanzapine with placebo in patients who were attending a specialized eating disorders day program.[35] Both studies found that treatment as usual resulted in increases in BMI as well as improvement in eating disorder symptoms, obsessionality, and depression. Both studies also found that olanzapine improved obsessionality more than standard treatment plus placebo. Brambilla and colleagues'[34] study of 30 subjects, 15 of whom were treated with olanzapine and 15 who received placebo, found no difference in the rate of change of BMI between the 2 groups. Bissada and colleagues'[35] study of 34 subjects, 16 assigned to olanzapine and 18 assigned to placebo, found that treatment with olanzapine resulted in greater and more rapid weight gain than placebo. The Bissada and colleagues[35] used a higher target dose of olanzapine (10 mg) than did Brambilla and colleagues[34] (5 mg). Although we are aware of ongoing studies examining the use of olanzapine in children and adolescents with eating disorders, to our knowledge, there have been no published RCTs on the use of olanzapine in children and adolescents with AN.

Quetiapine is an atypical antipsychotic that is less likely to cause dramatic weight gain and may be more acceptable to patents with AN who fear gaining weight. In 2 open-label studies, adults treated with quetiapine showed improvement in anxiety, depression, and eating disorders scores, but weight gain was modest.[36,37] Quetiapine has been used safely in a series of 3 treatment-resistant children and adolescents with AN.[30] The 3 subjects, aged 11, 14, and 15 years reported improvement in the delusional quality of their body image distortion when treated with quetiapine. As with olanzapine, we are not aware of any RCTs on the use of quetiapine for children and adolescents with AN.

There have been 3 published case reports on the use of risperidone in adolescents with AN.[38,39] The first described a young girl who was diagnosed with an autistic disorder at age 4 years and then at age 13 years developed AN. Treatment with risperidone was associated with a decrease in agitation and aggression, lessening of her rigidity, and loss of paranoid ideation.[38] The 2 cases described by Newman-Toker[39] were adolescents, aged 12 and 19 years, with restrictive AN but no other psychopathologic disorder. Within a week of adding risperidone to an SSRI, both patients reported improvement in anxiety and obsessions about food and both patients began to gain weight. Both patients believed that the risperidone contributed to the improvement of their cognitive distortions around eating and allowed them to feel more in control of their thinking.[39]

Common side effects of the atypical antipsychotic medications include somnolence and dry mouth, but more serious side effects include metabolic abnormalities such as insulin resistance, hyperlipidemia and diabetes, and the emergence of extrapyramidal symptoms, the most serious of which is tardive dyskinesia. Further study is needed to determine whether the side effect profile for this class of medications is the same among individuals with AN as it is in other clinical populations.

In summary, none of the RCTs conducted in adults with AN found significant benefit associated with antidepressant medication, either in promoting weight gain or in alleviating the core eating disorder symptoms. It has been postulated that, with malnutrition, depletion of tryptophan, a precursor of serotonin, may interfere with the action of antidepressants, and in particular the SSRIs.[40] However, in the malnourished state, even after supplementation with tryptophan, fluoxetine has not been shown to improve weight gain or eating disorder symptoms.[41] In addition, even after partial weight restoration and nutritional rehabilitation, the SSRIs have not proved to prevent relapse. Case reports and open-label studies suggest that olanzapine may be useful in reducing anxiety related to eating, obsessive thinking, depression, and some eating disorder symptoms, but the effect on weight again, beyond that achieved by standard treatment, is not clear. A recent systematic review concluded that, based on the results of existing studies, "there is insufficient evidence to confirm that the atypical antidepressants enhance weight gain in AN."[42] There may be a role for psychopharmacology in individual patients with AN, for example, in those with overwhelming anxiety or obsessionality, or in those with comorbid depression or obsessive-compulsive disorder, especially when the depressive and obsessional symptoms predated the onset of the eating disorder, but the sample sizes in the existing studies have been too small to identify those patients most likely to benefit from the addition of psychotropic medication. At present, the results regarding the role of the atypical antipsychotics remain inconclusive. What is clear is that psychopharmacology should not be the first line of treatment of AN.

PHARMACOLOGIC TREATMENT OF BN

In contrast to AN, several classes of medication have been found in RCTs to be helpful in reducing core symptoms in BN. However, as in AN, there is a paucity of data about children and adolescents, and further study is needed to determine whether medications that are beneficial to adults with BN are applicable to children and adolescents. Because of the limited information about medication effects in children and adolescents, safety concerns about some psychiatric medications in younger patients, and because behavioral interventions such as CBT are helpful for BN, medications are usually not used as a first-line intervention for most children and adolescents who present with BN. Medication is more commonly used as part of a multimodal treatment plan, and, when prescribed, should be offered with adequate education about, and attention to, possible side effects.

Antidepressants were the first class of agents examined for possible usefulness in BN, and essentially all RCTs of antidepressants have found that medication is more beneficial than placebo at decreasing binge and purge behavior. These effects are independent of effects on mood, and the medications are helpful irrespective of baseline mood status.[43–45] The earliest studies of antidepressants in BN used tricyclic antidepressants[46] and monoamine oxidase inhibitors (MAOIs).[43,47,48] These studies consistently found that the study medication reduced the frequency of binge and purge episodes for the duration of the trial. Side effects of these medications, including dry mouth, orthostasis, and weight gain, were described and considerably limited the acceptability of these treatments to clinical populations. These studies were additionally limited by their small sample sizes, short durations, and lack of follow-up. The dopamine antagonist bupropion has been studied in a single clinical trial in which bupropion was associated with significant improvement in bulimic symptoms but was associated with grand mal seizures in 4 of the 55 participants receiving the active medication, leading to a strong advisory against use of bupropion in BN.[49]

Fluoxetine is the only medication to have received a specific approval from the US Food and Drug Administration (FDA) for therapeutic use for BN, and is the most commonly used medication for the treatment of BN in adults. The evidence base for the use of this medication is significant, with 6 RCTs supporting its usefulness.[50–55] Five of these 6 trials support the usefulness of 60 mg of fluoxetine, a dose higher than that commonly used for the treatment of depression. This dose is well tolerated by individuals with BN and can be started at the recommended dose or titrated quickly to reach it. In the large Fluoxetine Bulimia Nervosa Collaborative Study Group's study of 387 subjects with BN who received fluoxetine or placebo, medication response at study termination was predictable at 3 weeks into medication treatment. In BN, response to medication treatment seems to occur within the first few weeks of initiating the medication.[56,57]

Although no RCT has been completed in children or adolescents, one open trial reported significant decreases in binge and purge behavior in 10 adolescents with BN receiving fluoxetine 60 mg with no significant side effects or other adverse events reported.[58] Fluoxetine is the only antidepressant medication that has received FDA approval for use in children and adolescents with depression, which makes it a likely first-choice medication for younger patients with BN in need of pharmacotherapy. However, because of concerns about reports of increased suicidality in children and adolescents who have been prescribed antidepressants, in October 2004 the FDA issued a black-box warning alerting families and providers to the increased risk of suicidal thoughts and the need for closer monitoring of children and adolescents who have been started on antidepressants, including the SSRIs (www.fda.govcder/drug/antidepressants/SSRIPHA200410.htm). In 2007, the FDA expanded this warning to include young adults aged 18 to 24 years. Although the black-box warning does not prohibit providers from prescribing antidepressants, it is the strongest warning from the FDA to patients and providers regarding possible adverse events. The black-box warning has influenced pediatricians' prescribing practices.

Two medications that are not antidepressants, topiramate and ondansetron, have also been studied in adults with BN. Topiramate is an anticonvulsant medication with γ-aminobutyric acid/glutamate receptor antagonist activity. Topiramate has some appetite-suppressant and weight loss properties that have led to its use in obesity.[59,60] Topiramate has been studied in BN because of its appetite suppressant effects together with its mood stabilizing effects. Two RCTs have been conducted in BN with positive results.[61–63] However, side effects, including impaired concentration, memory function, and word finding, as well as peripheral paresthesias, make this medication more difficult to use. In addition, there are a few rare but potentially serious side effects associated with topiramate, including metabolic acidosis, predisposition to development of kidney stones, and a risk of glaucoma.[64] Topiramate has not been studied in adolescent populations with eating disorders, but has been FDA approved for safe use in children 10 years of age and older with partial onset or primary generalized tonic-clonic seizures.

Odansetron was studied in a single RCT in adult women with BN and found to be helpful in reducing the binge-purge frequency.[65] This serotonergic antagonist is used in the treatment of nausea and vomiting in other medical conditions, and was prescribed in this study to manage urges to binge eat or vomit. At present, this medication is not used routinely for the treatment of BN.

PHARMACOLOGIC TREATMENT OF EDNOS
BED

The success of antidepressant medications in decreasing symptoms in BN has led to the examination of the use of these medications in adults with BED. The class of antidepressant medications studied most extensively is the SSRIs. RCTs of fluoxetine, fluvoxamine, sertraline, citalopram, and escitalopram have been conducted in BED with many, but not all, of the studies finding that the SSRI was associated with statistically significant improvement in BED symptoms compared with placebo.[66–72] Limitations to this work include some inconsistent study findings, the high placebo response rates in all studies, the short-term nature of the improvement, and the puzzling fact that weight loss has not always been observed in studies with successful reduction in rates of

Table 1
Psychopharmacology of eating disorders in children and adolescents, demonstrated efficacy in adults, FDA approval for use in children and adolescents with other conditions, and side effects requiring particular caution

Medication	Eating Disorder for Which There is RCT-supported Evidence of Efficacy in Adults	Approved for use in Children and Adolescents with Other Conditions	Side Effects Requiring Particular Caution
Antidepressants			
MAOI	BN	No	Hypertension (with consumption of tyramine), hypotension
Tricyclic antidepressant	BN	No	Orthostatic hypotension, anticholinergic effects, QT prolongation, tachycardia
SSRI	BN, BED, NES	Yes	Increased risk of suicidal thinking or behavior
Bupropion	–	No	Seizures
Atypical Antipsychotic Medications			
Olanzapine	AN	No	Weight gain, orthostatic hypotension, QT prolongation, hyperglycemia, hyperlipidemia, tardive dyskinesia
Quetiapine	–	No	Weight gain, signs of metabolic syndrome, tardive dyskinesia
Other Medications Studied for Appetite or Binge Suppression			
Topiramate	BN, BED	Yes	Cognitive effects, paresthesia, metabolic acidosis, glaucoma
Sibutramine	BED	No	Hypertension, tachycardia
Orlistat	BED	Yes	Fecal leaking, incontinence
Atomoxetine (stimulants)	BED	Yes	Weight loss, appetite suppression, growth retardation, insomnia, cardiac effects

bingeing. A meta-analysis of the results of 6 RCTs studying the use of SSRIs in BED concluded that the SSRIs are more helpful than placebo at short-term reduction in binge-eating behavior.[73] However, there is little to suggest that medication is superior to CBT, because 2 controlled trials found that CBT alone is more effective than medication alone in reducing BED symptoms.[74,75]

Antiobesity medications such as sibutramine, topiramate, and zonisamide have also been studied in adults with BED and have been found to reduce binge-eating symptoms and reduce weight.[76–78] Orlistat, a medication that inhibits lipase activity in the gastrointestinal tract and thereby impedes fat absorption, has been found to improve weight loss in BED, but not to reduce binge eating.[79] Atomoxetine, a stimulant indicated for the treatment of attention-deficit/hyperactivity disorder (ADHD), has been studied in BED because of its known appetite suppressant effects. In a 10-week placebo-controlled trial, atomoxetine (n = 20) was superior to placebo (n = 20) in decreasing binge-eating frequency and increasing weight loss, but was not effective in improving depression symptoms.[80]

Although SSRIs and weight loss medications offer more benefit than placebo for BED symptoms, there is little evidence that medication is more effective than CBT for improving symptoms in BED. Together with medication studies having all been based on adult samples, this should make the clinician consider behavioral interventions before initiating any medications for children or adolescents with BED.

NES

There has been 1 controlled trial in NES in which 34 adults with NES were randomly assigned to receive sertraline or placebo for 8 weeks. Sertraline, flexibly dosed (50–200 mg) was associated with greater improvement in Clinical Global Impressions Scale and NES symptoms (including frequency of nocturnal awakenings and ingestions) than placebo.[81]

SUMMARY

There are no published RCTs of pharmacologic treatments for eating disorders specifically conducted in children and adolescents. This omission is particularly unfortunate because most eating disorders have their onset in adolescence, and identification of treatments that can help shorten course, improve recovery rates, and reduce rates of chronicity for these serious conditions is greatly needed. As is the case for other psychiatric conditions, extrapolation of findings from eating disorder treatment studies of adult subjects is often used to help guide treatment in children and adolescents, although this should not lessen the need for additional studies that specifically evaluate efficacy and safety of potential treatments in children and adolescents. **Table 1** summarizes the medications for which there is RCT-supported evidence of efficacy in adults with eating disorders, the medications for which there is FDA approval for use in children and adolescents with other conditions, and the side effects requiring particular caution.

For AN, there is no established effective pharmacologic treatment of patients of any age. Preliminary data suggest that olanzapine, and possibly other atypical antipsychotic medications, may be helpful for improving weight gain and some psychological symptoms, but further study is needed before this becomes a routinely prescribed treatment. Behavioral approaches should be the first line of psychological treatment. In children and adolescents, family-based treatment, in which the parents are empowered to help refeed their child with AN, has been examined in several randomized trials, and has been associated with short-term and longer-term success with weight restoration in younger patients.[82] The findings discussed earlier have led to treatment recommendations for children and adolescents that use behavioral approaches with family involvement whenever possible, and reserve medication treatments for cases in which other approaches are insufficient and/or in which comorbid conditions are significant.[83]

For BN, there is a greater evidence base supporting behavioral as well as pharmacologic treatments in adults. Specifically, CBT as well as antidepressant medications have been found to reduce frequency of binge-eating and purging behaviors. Fluoxetine 60 mg is FDA approved for use in BN. All of the RCTs have been conducted in adults. Nevertheless, uncontrolled data suggest that fluoxetine may be effective in adolescents with BN, and fluoxetine has been FDA approved for use in children with depression, which makes this medication the most likely choice for younger patients with BN. Practice guidelines, including those by The American Psychiatric Association[84] and National Institute for Health and Clinical Excellence (NICE),[85] suggest that CBT should be considered as a first-line psychological treatment of BN, with medication being considered for those who do not respond fully to the prescribed psychotherapy.

Little is known about BED treatment in children and adolescents but, in adults, the SSRIs and appetite suppressants have been found to be helpful. There has been little study of NES and possible treatments for this cluster of symptoms, but sertraline was found to be helpful in 1 small study of adults. For both BED and NES in children and adolescents, behavioral interventions should be attempted before medications are considered.

RCTs for children and adolescents with eating disorders are sorely needed to provide an evidence base to guide the treatment of younger patients with these serious conditions. Until then, medication should not be used as a primary treatment of eating disorders in this age group. In individual cases, such as in patients who have clinically significant comorbidity or in those who have not responded to behavioral or family-based treatment, medications that have been proved to be effective in adults, especially those known to have adequate safety profiles in children with other psychiatric disorders, may be tried, but should probably only be prescribed as an adjunct to multimodal treatment.

ACKNOWLEDGMENTS

The authors wish to thank Ana Fraser and Melanie Lipton for their editorial assistance with this manuscript.

REFERENCES

1. American Psychiatric Association. Diagnostic and Statistical Manual of Mental Disorders. Text Revision ed. 4th edition. Washington, DC: American Psychiatric Association; 2000.
2. American Psychiatric Association. Diagnostic and Statistical Manual of Mental Disorders version 5: proposed criteria. dsm5.org. Available at: http://www.dsm5.org/proposedrevisions/pages/eatingdisorders.aspx. Accessed January 1, 2010.
3. Hoek H, van Hoeken D. Review of the prevalence and incidence of eating disorders. Int J Eat Disord 2003;34(4):383–96.
4. Hudson JI, Hiripi E, Pope HG Jr, et al. The prevalence and correlates of eating disorders in the National Comorbidity Survey Replication. Biol Psychiatry 2007; 61(3):348–58.

5. Keski-Rahkonen A, Sihvola E, Raevuori A, et al. Reliability of self-reported eating disorders: optimizing population screening. Int J Eat Disord 2006;39(8):754–62.

6. Machado PP, Machado BC, Goncalves S, et al. The prevalence of eating disorders not otherwise specified. Int J Eat Disord 2007;40(3):212–7.

7. Rodriguez-Cano T, Beato-Fernandez L. Attitudes towards change and treatment outcome in eating disorders. Eat Weight Disord 2005;10(1):59–65.

8. Tanofsky-Kraff M, Yanovski S, Wilfley D, et al. Eating-disordered behaviors, body fat, and psychopathology in overweight and normal-weight children. J Consult Clin Psychol 2004;72(1):53–61.

9. Tanofsky-Kraff M, Faden D, Yanovski S, et al. The perceived onset of dieting and loss of control eating behaviors in overweight children. Int J Eat Disord 2005; 38(2):112–22.

10. Goossens L, Braet C, Decaluwé V. Loss of control over eating in obese youngsters. Behav Res Ther 2007;45(1):1–9.

11. Glasofer D, Tanofsky-Kraff M, Eddy K, et al. Binge eating in overweight treatment-seeking adolescents. J Pediatr Psychol 2007;32(1):95–105.

12. Levine M, Ringham R, Kalarchian M, et al. Overeating among seriously overweight children seeking treatment: results of the children's eating disorder examination. Int J Eat Disord 2006;39(2):135–40.

13. Goldschmidt A, Aspen V, Sinton M, et al. Disordered eating attitudes and behaviors in overweight youth. Obesity (Silver Spring) 2008;16(2):257–64.

14. Nattiv A, Loucks A, Manore M, et al. American College of Sports Medicine position stand. The female athlete triad. Med Sci Sports Exerc 2007;39(10):1867–82.

15. Nicholls D, Chater R, Lask B. Children into DSM don't go: a comparison of classification systems for eating disorders in childhood and early adolescence. Int J Eat Disord 2000;28(3):317–24.

16. Walsh BTBC, Fairburn CG, Halmi KA, et al. Defining eating disorders. In: Evans DL, Foa EB, Gur RE, et al, editors. Treating and preventing adolescent mental health disorders: what we know and what we don't know. New York: Oxford University Press, The Annenberg Foundation Trust at Sunnylands, and the Annenberg Public Policy Center of the University of Pennsylvania; 2005. p. 258–81.

17. Halmi K. The perplexities of conducting randomized, double-blind, placebo-controlled treatment trials in anorexia nervosa patients. Am J Psychiatry 2008; 165(10):1227–8.

18. Lacey J, Crisp A. Hunger, food intake and weight: the impact of clomipramine on a refeeding anorexia nervosa population. Postgrad Med J 1980;56(Suppl 1): 79–85.

19. Halmi K, Eckert E, LaDu T, et al. Anorexia nervosa. Treatment efficacy of cyproheptadine and amitriptyline. Arch Gen Psychiatry 1986;43(2):177–81.

20. Biederman J, Herzog D, Rivinus T, et al. Amitriptyline in the treatment of anorexia nervosa: a double-blind, placebo-controlled study. J Clin Psychopharmacol 1985;5(1):10–6.

21. Geller D, Biederman J, Stewart S, et al. Which SSRI? A meta-analysis of pharmacotherapy trials in pediatric obsessive-compulsive disorder. Am J Psychiatry 2003;160(11):1919–28.

22. Kaye W, Gwirtsman H, George D, et al. CSF 5-HIAA concentrations in anorexia nervosa: reduced values in underweight subjects normalize after weight gain. Biol Psychiatry 1988;23(1):102–5.

23. Kaye W, Gwirtsman H, George D, et al. Altered serotonin activity in anorexia nervosa after long-term weight restoration. Does elevated cerebrospinal fluid

5-hydroxyindoleacetic acid level correlate with rigid and obsessive behavior? Arch Gen Psychiatry 1991;48(6):556–62.

24. Attia E, Haiman C, Walsh B, et al. Does fluoxetine augment the inpatient treatment of anorexia nervosa? Am J Psychiatry 1998;155(4):548–51.

25. Holtkamp K, Konrad K, Kaiser N, et al. A retrospective study of SSRI treatment in adolescent anorexia nervosa: insufficient evidence for efficacy. J Psychiatr Res 2005;39(3):303–10.

26. Kaye W, Nagata T, Weltzin T, et al. Double-blind placebo-controlled administration of fluoxetine in restricting- and restricting-purging-type anorexia nervosa. Biol Psychiatry 2001;49(7):644–52.

27. Walsh B, Kaplan A, Attia E, et al. Fluoxetine after weight restoration in anorexia nervosa: a randomized controlled trial. JAMA 2006;295(22):2605–12.

28. Boachie A, Goldfield G, Spettigue W. Olanzapine use as an adjunctive treatment for hospitalized children with anorexia nervosa: case reports. Int J Eat Disord 2003;33(1):98–103.

29. Mehler C, Wewetzer C, Schulze U, et al. Olanzapine in children and adolescents with chronic anorexia nervosa. A study of five cases. Eur Child Adolesc Psychiatry 2001;10(2):151–7.

30. Mehler-Wex C, Romanos M, Kirchheiner J, et al. Atypical antipsychotics in severe anorexia nervosa in children and adolescents–review and case reports. Eur Eat Disord Rev 2008;16(2):100–8.

31. Powers P, Santana C, Bannon Y. Olanzapine in the treatment of anorexia nervosa: an open label trial. Int J Eat Disord 2002;32(2):146–54.

32. Barbarich N, McConaha C, Gaskill J, et al. An open trial of olanzapine in anorexia nervosa. J Clin Psychiatry 2004;65(11):1480–2.

33. Leggero C, Masi G, Brunori E, et al. Low-dose olanzapine monotherapy in girls with anorexia nervosa, restricting subtype: focus on hyperactivity. J Child Adolesc Psychopharmacol 2010;20(2):127–33.

34. Brambilla F, Garcia C, Fassino S, et al. Olanzapine therapy in anorexia nervosa: psychobiological effects. Int Clin Psychopharmacol 2007;22(4):197–204.

35. Bissada H, Tasca G, Barber A, et al. Olanzapine in the treatment of low body weight and obsessive thinking in women with anorexia nervosa: a randomized, double-blind, placebo-controlled trial. Am J Psychiatry 2008; 165(10):1281–8.

36. Powers P, Bannon Y, Eubanks R, et al. Quetiapine in anorexia nervosa patients: an open label outpatient pilot study. Int J Eat Disord 2007;40(1):21–6.

37. Bosanac P, Kurlender S, Norman T, et al. An open-label study of quetiapine in anorexia nervosa. Hum Psychopharmacol 2007;22(4):223–30.

38. Fisman S, Steele M, Short J, et al. Case study: anorexia nervosa and autistic disorder in an adolescent girl. J Am Acad Child Adolesc Psychiatry 1996;35(7): 937–40.

39. Newman-Tokor J. Risperidone in anorexia nervosa. J Am Acad Child Adolesc Psychiatry 2000;39(8):941–2.

40. Kaye W, Gendall K, Strober M. Nutrition, serotonin and behavior in anorexia and bulimia nervosa. Nestle Nutr Workshop Ser Clin Perform Programme 2001;5: 153–65, [discussion: 165–158].

41. Barbarich NC, McConaha CW, Halmi KA, et al. Use of nutritional supplements to increase the efficacy of fluoxetine in the treatment of anorexia nervosa. Int J Eat Disord 2004;35(1):10–5.

42. McKnight R, Park R. Atypical antipsychotics and anorexia nervosa: a review. Eur Eat Disord Rev 2010;18(1):10–21.

43. Walsh BT, Stewart JW, Roose SP, et al. A double-blind trial of phenelzine in bulimia. J Psychiatr Res 1985;19(2–3):485–9.
44. Shapiro JR, Berkman ND, Brownley KA, et al. Bulimia nervosa treatment: a systematic review of randomized controlled trials. Int J Eat Disord 2007;40(4): 321–36.
45. Goldstein DJ, Wilson MG, Ascroft RC, et al. Effectiveness of fluoxetine therapy in bulimia nervosa regardless of comorbid depression. Int J Eat Disord 1999;25(1): 19–27.
46. Alger SA, Schwalberg MD, Bigaouette JM, et al. Effect of a tricyclic antidepressant and opiate antagonist on binge-eating behavior in normoweight bulimic and obese, binge-eating subjects. Am J Clin Nutr 1991;53(4):865–71.
47. Walsh BT, Stewart JW, Roose SP, et al. Treatment of bulimia with phenelzine. A double-blind, placebo-controlled study. Arch Gen Psychiatry 1984;41(11):1105–9.
48. Rothschild R, Quitkin HM, Quitkin FM, et al. A double-blind placebo-controlled comparison of phenelzine and imipramine in the treatment of bulimia in atypical depressives. Int J Eat Disord 1994;15(1):1–9.
49. Horne RL, Ferguson JM, Pope HG Jr, et al. Treatment of bulimia with bupropion: a multicenter controlled trial. J Clin Psychiatry 1988;49(7):262–6.
50. Beumont PJ, Russell JD, Touyz SW, et al. Intensive nutritional counselling in bulimia nervosa: a role for supplementation with fluoxetine? Aust N Z J Psychiatry 1997;31(4):514–24.
51. Fichter MM, Leibl K, Rief W, et al. Fluoxetine versus placebo: a double-blind study with bulimic inpatients undergoing intensive psychotherapy. Pharmacopsychiatry 1991;24(1):1–7.
52. Fluoxetine Bulimia Nervosa Collaborative Study Group. Fluoxetine in the treatment of bulimia nervosa: a multicenter, placebo-controlled, double-blind trial. Arch Gen Psychiatry 1992;42(2):139–47.
53. Goldstein DJ, Wilson MG, Thompson VL, et al. Long-term fluoxetine treatment of bulimia nervosa. Fluoxetine Bulimia Nervosa Research Group. Br J Psychiatry 1995;166(5):660–6.
54. Kanerva R, Rissanen A, Sarna S. Fluoxetine in the treatment of anxiety, depressive symptoms, and eating-related symptoms in bulimia nervosa. Nord J Psychiatry 1995;49:237–42.
55. Romano SJ, Halmi KA, Sarkar NP, et al. A placebo-controlled study of fluoxetine in continued treatment of bulimia nervosa after successful acute fluoxetine treatment. Am J Psychiatry 2002;159(1):96–102.
56. Walsh BT, Sysko R, Parides MK. Early response to desipramine among women with bulimia nervosa. Int J Eat Disord 2006;39(1):72–5.
57. Sysko R, Sha N, Wang Y, et al. Early response to antidepressant treatment in bulimia nervosa. Psychol Med 2010;40(6):999–1005.
58. Kotler LA, Devlin MJ, Davies M, et al. An open trial of fluoxetine for adolescents with bulimia nervosa. J Child Adolesc Psychopharmacol 2003;13(3):329–35.
59. Eliasson B, Gudbjornsdottir S, Cederholm J, et al. Weight loss and metabolic effects of topiramate in overweight and obese type 2 diabetic patients: randomized double-blind placebo-controlled trial. Int J Obes (Lond) 2007;31(7):1140–7.
60. McElroy SL, Hudson JI, Capece JA, et al. Topiramate for the treatment of binge eating disorder associated with obesity: a placebo-controlled study. Biol Psychiatry 2007;61(9):1039–48.
61. Hedges DW, Reimherr FW, Hoopes SP, et al. Treatment of bulimia nervosa with topiramate in a randomized, double-blind, placebo-controlled trial, part 2: improvement in psychiatric measures. J Clin Psychiatry 2003;64(12):1449–54.

62. Hoopes SP, Reimherr FW, Hedges DW, et al. Treatment of bulimia nervosa with topiramate in a randomized, double-blind, placebo-controlled trial, part 1: improvement in binge and purge measures. J Clin Psychiatry 2003;64(11): 1335–41.

63. Nickel C, Tritt K, Muehlbacher M, et al. Topiramate treatment in bulimia nervosa patients: a randomized, double-blind, placebo-controlled trial. Int J Eat Disord 2005;38(4):295–300.

64. Schatzberg A, Cole J, DeBatistia C. Manual of clinical psychomarmacology. 4th edition. Washington, DC: American Psychiatric Association; 2003.

65. Faris PL, Kim SW, Meller WH, et al. Effect of decreasing afferent vagal activity with ondansetron on symptoms of bulimia nervosa: a randomised, double-blind trial. Lancet 2000;355(9206):792–7.

66. Arnold LM, McElroy SL, Hudson JI, et al. A placebo-controlled, randomized trial of fluoxetine in the treatment of binge-eating disorder. J Clin Psychiatry 2002; 63(11):1028–33.

67. Grilo CM, Masheb RM, Wilson GT. Efficacy of cognitive behavioral therapy and fluoxetine for the treatment of binge eating disorder: a randomized double-blind placebo-controlled comparison. Biol Psychiatry 2005;57(3):301–9.

68. Hudson JI, McElroy SL, Raymond NC, et al. Fluvoxamine in the treatment of binge-eating disorder: a multicenter placebo-controlled, double-blind trial. Am J Psychiatry 1998;155(12):1756–62.

69. Pearlstein T, Spurell E, Hohlstein LA, et al. A double-blind, placebo-controlled trial of fluvoxamine in binge eating disorder: a high placebo response. Arch Womens Ment Health 2003;6(2):147–51.

70. McElroy SL, Casuto LS, Nelson EB, et al. Placebo-controlled trial of sertraline in the treatment of binge eating disorder. Am J Psychiatry 2000;157(6): 1004–6.

71. McElroy SL, Hudson JI, Malhotra S, et al. Citalopram in the treatment of binge-eating disorder: a placebo-controlled trial. J Clin Psychiatry 2003;64(7):807–13.

72. Guerdjikova AI, McElroy SL, Kotwal R, et al. High-dose escitalopram in the treatment of binge-eating disorder with obesity: a placebo-controlled monotherapy trial. Hum Psychopharmacol 2008;23(1):1–11.

73. Reas DL, Grilo CM. Review and meta-analysis of pharmacotherapy for binge-eating disorder. Obesity (Silver Spring) 2008;16(9):2024–38.

74. Grilo CM, Masheb RM, Salant SL. Cognitive behavioral therapy guided self-help and orlistat for the treatment of binge eating disorder: a randomized, double-blind, placebo-controlled trial. Biol Psychiatry 2005;57(10):1193–201.

75. Ricca V, Mannucci E, Mezzani B, et al. Fluoxetine and fluvoxamine combined with individual cognitive-behaviour therapy in binge eating disorder: a one-year follow-up study. Psychother Psychosom 2001;70(6):298–306.

76. Appolinario JC, Bacaltchuk J, Sichieri R, et al. A randomized, double-blind, placebo-controlled study of sibutramine in the treatment of binge-eating disorder. Arch Gen Psychiatry 2003;60(11):1109–16.

77. Milano W, Petrella C, Casella A, et al. Use of sibutramine, an inhibitor of the reuptake of serotonin and noradrenaline, in the treatment of binge eating disorder: a placebo-controlled study. Adv Ther 2005;22(1):25–31.

78. Wilfley DE, Crow SJ, Hudson JI, et al. Efficacy of sibutramine for the treatment of binge eating disorder: a randomized multicenter placebo-controlled double-blind study. Am J Psychiatry 2008;165(1):51–8.

79. Golay A, Laurent-Jaccard A, Habicht F, et al. Effect of orlistat in obese patients with binge eating disorder. Obes Res 2005;13(10):1701–8.

80. McElroy SL, Guerdjikova A, Kotwal R, et al. Atomoxetine in the treatment of binge-eating disorder: a randomized placebo-controlled trial. J Clin Psychiatry 2007; 68(3):390–8.

81. O'Reardon JP, Allison KC, Martino NS, et al. A randomized, placebo-controlled trial of sertraline in the treatment of night eating syndrome. Am J Psychiatry 2006;163(5):893–8.

82. Lock J, Agras W, Bryson S, et al. A comparison of short- and long-term family therapy for adolescent anorexia nervosa. J Am Acad Child Adolesc Psychiatry 2005;44(7):632–9.

83. Couturier J, Lock J. A review of medication use for children and adolescents with eating disorders. J Can Acad Child Adolesc Psychiatry 2007;16(4):173–6.

84. American Psychiatric Association. Treatment of patients with eating disorders, third edition. American Psychiatric Association. Am J Psychiatry 2006;163:4–54.

85. National Institute for Clinical Excellence 2004. Eating disorders: core interventions in the treatment and management of anorexia nervosa, bulimia nervosa and related eating disorders. London: National Institute of Clinical Excellence. Available at: http://guidance.nice.org.uk/CG9/NICEGuidance/pdf/ English. Accessed 9/1/2010.

Pharmacotherapy for Obese Adolescents

Donald E. Greydanus, MD, Dr HC (ATHENS)[a],*, Lee A. Bricker, MD[b,c],
Cynthia Feucht, PharmD, BCPS[d,e]

KEYWORDS

• Obesity • Pharmacotherapy • Adolescents

Obesity is a well-known global phenomenon among children, adolescents, and adults.[1–10] Although pharmacotherapy can be effective in the management of obesity in some adults, its application to most adolescents is often limited to research protocols.[5,11–21] The precise safety, effectiveness, and long-term consequences of these medications for obese youth are presently unclear.[2] Use of such medications should only be part of a comprehensive program that emphasizes appropriate diet, exercise, and behavioral modification.[15,22–28]

Pharmacologic management is often used in obese youth who have not responded to changes in lifestyle or when medical complications develop (eg, obstructive sleep apnea or hypertension). Use of medication is considered before bariatric surgery.[3,7,15,21,28,29] Only modest weight loss is obtained with use of medication, such as 2 to 10 kg, and typically only during the first 6 months of use. At present, only a few agents have been approved by the FDA for use by those less than 18 years of age, including sibutramine and orlistat. Sibutramine was FDA approved for obese individuals 16 years of age and older, and orlistat still is for those 12 years and older.[5,6] Voluntary withdrawal of sibutramine was announced in October, 2010. This article discusses a variety of medications used for the treatment of obesity in adolescents.

OVER-THE-COUNTER HERBAL AGENTS

Various formulations of phenylpropanolamine (PPA), caffeine, and ephedrine are available that are adrenergic medications and recommended as products that will induce weight loss. However, they have limited, if any, effectiveness and should be avoided

[a] Department of Pediatrics and Human Development, Michigan State University College of Human Medicine, MSU/Kalamazoo Center for Medical Studies, 1000 Oakland Drive, Kalamazoo, MI 49009-1284, USA
[b] Michigan State University/Kalamazoo Center for Medical Studies, Kalamazoo, MI 49008-1284, USA
[c] Department of Internal Medicine, Clinics in Adult Endocrinology, Diabetes, and Metabolism, Michigan State University College of Human Medicine, East Lansing, MI, USA
[d] Borgess Ambulatory Care, 1701 Gull Road, Kalamazoo, MI 49048, USA
[e] Department of Pharmacy Practice, Ferris State University College of Pharmacy, Big Rapids, MI 49307, USA
* Corresponding author.
E-mail address: greydanus@kcms.msu.edu

Pediatr Clin N Am 58 (2011) 139–153
doi:10.1016/j.pcl.2010.10.007
0031-3955/11/$ – see front matter © 2011 Elsevier Inc. All rights reserved.
pediatric.theclinics.com

because they also have significant adverse cardiovascular effects.[2,5,30] PPA is a member of the phenethylamine family of drugs previously used as an appetite suppressant or decongestant. The FDA issued a public health advisory against PPA on November 6, 2000, because of reports of increased risk of hemorrhagic cerebrovascular accidents in 18- to 49-year-old female users; the FDA requested that pharmaceutical companies cease manufacturing and promoting any PPA-containing products.[31] The reasoning was that, although the risk for such adverse events was low, the event itself was serious.

Some Korean researchers have advocated the short-term safety and effectiveness of a traditional Korean herbal formula that is based on Taeumjowi-tang for children with an average age of 11 years.[32] This formulation is a popular herbal product in Korea that is recommended as a weight-loss product for children, adolescents, and adults.[32] It consists of a mixture of various roots, berries, nuts, seeds, and stalks, as noted in **Box 1**. One of its ingredients is *Ephedra sinica* (a species of ephedra or ma huang), and this contains alkaloids of pseudoephedrine and ephedrine.

Other supplement or herbal formulations have been produced that contain ephedrine (from ma huang) and caffeine (from kola nut, guarana, or green tea). Reports of sudden death as well as abuse potential have been noted with ephedrine, and, in 1997, the FDA advised against the use of herbal phen-fen (ephedra and *Hypericum perforatum*).[33] More than 800 adverse events related to ephedra had already been reported; in 2001 ephedra accounted for 64% of all adverse reactions gathered by poison control centers in relation to herbal products.[33] On April 12 2004, the FDA banned over-the-counter (OTC) dietary supplements containing ephedrine alkaloids (ephedra).[33] With the ban on ephedra products, many supplements changed their product components to be ephedra-free, using instead a variety of herbal supplements including *Citrus aurantium* (bitter orange) and caffeine. A variety of herbal products are marketed as weight-loss remedies but without proof of efficacy and safety; these include *Hoodia*, *Garcinia cambogia*, yerba mate, chitosan, chromium picolinate, and L-carnitine.[2,5,7,34]

Box 1
Components of the Korean formula based on Taeumjowi-tang

1. Seeds

   Coix lacryma-jobi (Job's tears, also found in the United States)

   Raphanus sativus (Japanese radish, also found in the United States)

   Pinus koraiensis (Korean pine, found in parts of Asia)

2. Roots

   Liriope platyphylla (flowering plant in Asia, especially China)

   Acorus calamus (plant called sweet flag found in North America, Europe, and Asia; many medicinal uses claimed)

   Pelargonium grandiflorum (Andrews) (large, flowery, shrubby plant native to South Africa and popular as a house plant)

3. Stalks (*E sinica*; see text)

4. Berries (*Schisandra chinensis*; woody vine with clusters of red berries, found in China, Russia, and Korea)

5. Nuts (*Castanea crenata*) (Japanese or Chinese chestnut)

NORADRENERGIC PRODUCTS

Amphetamines can lower weight, but may lead to severe cardiac and mental health problems, including addiction; amphetamine products are neither recommended nor approved for use as weight-loss products. In addition, several noradrenergic medications have been marketed. Phentermine received FDA approval in 1959 as an appetite-suppressing drug, even though there are limited studies attesting to its efficacy as a weight reduction product. This sympathomimetic amine has limited use in adolescents because of its schedule IV US Drug Enforcement Administration (DEA) classification, its potential for addiction, its structure and side effects being similar to those of amphetamine, and the lack of evidence for safety as well as long-tem efficacy. Its link with fen-phen, as noted elsewhere, has led to its highly restricted use as a weight-loss product in adolescents.

Several phentermine products are available, including Ionamin and Adipex P; they have been recommended for those individuals with a body mass index (BMI, calculated as weight in kilograms divided by the square of height in meters) greater than 30 kg/m^2 or greater than 27 kg/m^2 in the presence of other risk factors, such as diabetes mellitus, hypertension, and other diseases. These products should only be used for short periods, such as up to 12 weeks, in patients more than 16 years of age, and in combination with other traditional weight-loss measures (such as diet and exercise plans).

Several other schedule III noradrenergic drugs have been approved by the FDA for short-term use to induce weight loss, and these include phendimetrazine (Bontril) and benzphetamine (Didrex).[2] Diethylpropion is approved for adolescents more than 16 years of age and benzphetamine is FDA approved in adolescents 12 years of age and older; both these products are for short-term use only. Diethylpropion (Tenuate) is a schedule IV noradrenergic agent that is FDA approved for short-term weight loss in adults.[17] All these sympathomimetic amines have various side effects, including cardiovascular effects (hypertension, valvular disease), sleep dysfunction (insomnia, restlessness), and gastrointestinal complaints (nausea, constipation, diarrhea).[7] Noradrenergic products should be avoided in patients with cardiovascular disease, moderate-to-severe hypertension, pulmonary hypertension, hyperthyroidism, and patients with a history of drug abuse.

SEROTONINERGIC AGENTS

Serotoninergic drugs stimulate serotonin release from nerve endings, inhibit serotonin reuptake, or do both, resulting in enhanced serotonin effect at the central nervous system postsynaptic nerve ending. Fenfluramine induces satiety, reducing hunger, carbohydrate craving, and bingeing. Historically, it was manufactured as Pondimin (mixed dextro- and levofenfluramine) and also Redux (dexfenfluramine).

The popular phen-fen diet (phentermine and fenfluramine) was considered effective in inducing weight loss, with sustained benefit noted for as long as 3.5 years with continued use; however, when this agent was stopped, weight gain resumed.[2,22] These drugs were used for longer periods of time in the 1990s and, at least in some studies, were associated with cardiac valvulopathy. The FDA withdrew fenfluramine from the market on September 15, 1997, based on research indicating that 30% of patients taking these products had abnormal echocardiograms despite absence of symptoms.[35] Fenfluramine and dexfenfluramine have both been associated with rare cases of pulmonary hypertension. The FDA did not direct that phentermine itself be removed from the market.

MIXED NORADRENERGIC-SEROTONERGIC PRODUCTS

The FDA had approved the use of sibutramine (Meridia) for obesity management in adults.[17,20,36,37] Sibutramine is classified as a DEA schedule IV drug. It inhibits the reuptake of serotonin and norepinephrine and, to some degree, inhibits dopamine as well. Thus, brain concentrations of these neurotransmitters are increased, leading to various effects, including appetite reduction. Sibutramine is a centrally acting agent that seems to be well tolerated in most adult patients, with a 5% to 10% loss of initial body weight; this weight loss is reported to be sustained in 8 of 10 research trials.[5] Sibutramine is prescribed at a dose of 10 mg (5–15 mg) per day for up to 2 years. Although no valvulopathy has been identified, clinicians should understand that there is a dose-related increase in blood pressure and pulse that can be of clinical significance for some patients.[20,37–40]

The FDA had approved sibutramine for patients 16 years and older and research trials have reported some limited weight loss in adolescents, averaging 3 kg more than control subjects with a BMI reduction up to 5.6 kg/m^2; however, weight loss beyond 6 months of use has not been reported.[4,6,14,20,26–28,38–41] This medication may also be of use for children with hypothalamic obesity and exogenous obesity.[42]

Box 2 provides a list of potential side effects and contraindications for use of sibutramine. Drug interactions may occur because sibutramine is metabolized by the

---

Box 2
Sibutramine (Meridia) side effects and contraindications

Side effects

1. Anxiety
2. Asthenia
3. Constipation
4. Depression
5. Dizziness
6. Dry mouth
7. Headache
8. Insomnia
9. Nausea
10. Increase in both blood pressure and pulse (usually a minor increase)

Contraindications: do not use in those with:

1. Heart disease
2. Poorly controlled hypertension
3. Substance abuse disorders
4. Severe renal or hepatic dysfunction
5. Narrow-angle glaucoma
6. Anorexia or bulimia nervosa
7. Patients taking serotonergic medications, such as triptans, tramadol, selective serotonin reuptake inhibitors (SSRIs), and others
8. Do not use during or within 2 weeks of monoamine oxidase inhibitors

cytochrome P-450 3A4 substrate. Clinicians should exercise caution when adding agents that can increase (ie, verapamil, clarithromycin, nefazadone,) or decrease sibutramine effect (ie, phenytoin, rifampin, carbamazepine). The FDA and the manufacturer announced a voluntary withdrawal of sibutramine from the market on October 8 2010 because of the risks of serious cardiovascular events (http://www.fda.gov/Safety/MedWatch/SafetyInformation/SafetyAlertsforHumanMedicalProducts/ucm228830.htm).

LIPASE INHIBITOR

Orlistat (Xenical) is a lipase (gastric and pancreatic) inhibitor and has been effective in reducing weight in adult as well as adolescent clinical trials because of its ability to induce dose-dependent fat malabsorption.[5,14,17,20,25,43,44] Orlistat blocks approximately 30% of dietary fat with the 120 mg prescription dose and 25% with the 60-mg dose.[44,45] Orlistat is used in adolescents as well as adults.[15,25] Orlistat is given in a dosage of 120 mg 3 times a day with meals. An OTC formulation (Alli) containing half the prescription dose has been approved by the FDA for use in a weight-loss program that also includes appropriate dietary counseling.[44] It was approved by the FDA in 2003 for use in weight management of obese youth 12 years of age and older.[6]

Using this lipase inhibitor can also lead to improved blood pressure, glucose and lipid levels, and insulin sensitivity.[5,15,45] One 16-week research study of adults who combined orlistat with a low-fat, reduced-calorie diet reported that the subjects taking orlistat lost 1.15 kg more than those taking placebo.[46] Some investigators have reported a BMI lowering of up to 4.09 kg/m^2 for patients taking orlistat.[20] However, some research notes no weight reduction benefit from this medication when given to obese adolescents.[47]

Reported side effects with orlistat include flatulence, steatorrhea, malabsorption, fecal urgency, fecal incontinence, abdominal pain, gastric upset, dyspepsia, and reduced absorption of fat-soluble vitamins (A, D, E, and K).[7,44,48] A daily multivitamin that contains fat-soluble vitamins is recommended for those taking this drug. Orlistat is contraindicated in patients with cholestasis and chronic malabsorption syndrome. Its effect on growth is not known and its gastrointestinal side effects have lowered its acceptance by adolescents. Orlistat can also increase the anticoagulant effect of warfarin because of reduced vitamin K absorption, and it can interfere with the absorption of various medications.[46]

Acarbose (Precose) is another medication that inhibits intestinal α-glucoside hydrolase and pancreatic α-amylase. The physiologic effects include a lowering of postprandial blood glucose concentrations, and acarbose may be useful for obese children as well as youth with hyperinsulinemia. It can be used to manage postprandial glucose increases in those with type 2 diabetes mellitus. The initial oral dosage is 25 mg 3 times a day and this is gradually increased as tolerated; adults are maintained on 50 to 100 mg 3 times a day. Side effects include gastrointestinal upset, diarrhea, and flatulence; there can also be symptomatic reduction in blood glucose if acarbose is used with insulin or a sulfonylurea.

METFORMIN

Metformin (Glucophage, Glumetza, Fortamet, Riomet) is a biguanide that has been FDA approved since 1994 to manage type 2 diabetes mellitus. It is a glucose-sensitizing drug that increases the sensitivity of various tissues (muscle, liver, fat) to the uptake and action of insulin. It lowers hepatic gluconeogenesis and improves cell membrane movement of glucose in skeletal muscle and adipose tissue.[5] Metformin has also been used for polycystic ovary syndrome (PCOS), which is associated with hyperinsulinemia and hyperandrogenism. Metformin improves insulin sensitivity by lowering levels of insulin and reducing PCOS symptoms, including menstrual cycle irregularity, increased androgen levels, and unpredictable ovulation.[49–51]

Metformin is prescribed for adults with morbid obesity and with the metabolic syndrome; it has also been used for weight reduction in nonobese patients.[5,7,52] An Australian study reported an average loss of 4.35 kg in 6 months in male pediatric patients (9–18 years old) taking 1 g of metformin twice a day.[53] Dosing in adolescents aged 10 to 16 years is 500 mg of metformin twice a day orally for obesity, and this is increased by 500 mg a week to a maximum of 2 g per day if managing type 2 diabetes mellitus. More research is needed to pinpoint its efficacy in overweight adolescents.[20,29,52] Side effects, listed in **Box 3**, are typically dose related and tend to improve with time. Lactic acidosis is noted in 1 in 30,000 patients on this medication, with 50% mortality, and lactic acidosis is more common in those with renal insufficiency.

RIMONABANT

Rimonabant is a CB1-selective cannabinoid receptor antagonist/inverse agonist that had been used in European studies in association with a diet and exercise strategy for weight loss in obese adults.[7,21,54,55] Effects of rimonabant include appetite reduction (dose dependent), lower triglycerides, and an increase in high-density lipoprotein with no effect on low-density lipoprotein levels.[56] It is also used in various countries for management of drug addiction, including nicotine addiction.[57,58] These endocannabinoids are key modulators during conditions of stress, anxiety, depression, phobias, and posttraumatic stress disorder.[58]

Rimonabant received an initial letter of approval from the FDA in 2006 for obesity treatment in adults but not as a smoking cessation product because of concerns with

---

Box 3
Side effects and contraindications for metformin

Side effects

1. Abdominal discomfort
2. Diarrhea
3. Emesis
4. Flatulence
5. Indigestion
6. Diarrhea
7. Lactic acidosis
8. Vitamin B_{12} malabsorption

Contraindications

1. Avoid in patients with congestive heart failure who require pharmacologic management
2. Do not use in critically ill patients
3. Do not use in those with liver disease or hypoxia
4. Avoid in patients with renal insufficiency (serum creatinine >1.4 mg/dL in women and >1.5 mg/dL in men)

safety. Studies note a relative risk of 1.5 to 2.5 for psychiatric problems, such as depression and increased suicide ideation, for patients in 4 trials of rimonabant used for obesity management.[58] The FDA Endocrinologic and Metabolic Drugs Advisory Committee voted unanimously on June 13 2007 to not approve rimonabant as a treatment of obesity, because of the high risk for serious psychiatric sequelae, high drop-out rates from studies, and what they considered was a clear need for more long-term data.[58]

POTENTIAL NEW PHARMACOLOGIC APPROACHES

A large and growing array of new approaches to pharmacologic management of obesity are being investigated (**Box 4**). These approaches include several agents originally directed at other diseases, including seizure disorders and diabetes. None has been proved effective or safe with adults or adolescents; however, many bear watching for release in the future.

Antidepressants

The antidepressant, fluoxetine (Prozac), is an SSRI known to have the side effect of limited weight loss.[59] Other antidepressants with anorexic effects include sertraline (Zoloft, another SSRI) and bupropion (Wellbutrin). However, these antidepressants are approved for treating mental health disorders (such as depression) in adults and not obesity itself.[2,60]

Antiseizure Medications

Some antiepilepsy medications have shown interesting properties in the battle against obesity. Bray and colleagues[61] studied the antiseizure agent topiramate after researchers noted that several patients using it were losing weight. They studied 385 subjects and noted that drug-treated patients lost significantly more weight at

---

Box 4
Medications or chemicals studied but not proved beneficial or safe in obesity treatment

1. Amylin
2. Bupropion (antidepressant)
3. Cholecystokinin
4. Ciliary neurotrophic factor
5. Dipeptidyl-peptidase IV (DPP-IV) inhibitors
6. Ghrelin
7. Glucagonlike peptide-1 (incretin mimetics: exenatide and liraglutide)
8. Leptin (neuropeptide produced by adipose tissue)
9. Neuropeptide Y
10. Oxyntomodulin
11. SSRIs (fluoxetine, sertraline)
12. Somatostatin receptor analogue: octreotide (for hypothalamic obesity)
13. Synthetic β-3 agonists
14. Topiramate (anticonvulsant)
15. Zonisamide (anticonvulsant)

24 weeks than did placebo-treated subjects. Adverse events, including somnolence and difficulty in concentration, were dose related, occurred early, and usually resolved. Other antiseizure medications have also been found potentially useful in obesity management, including zonisamide, phenytoin, carbamazepine, and valproate.[17,62] The long-term value of these drugs in management of obesity remains of interest and concern.

Ciliary Neurotrophic Factor

Ciliary neurotrophic factor (CNTF) is a neuroprotective polypeptide hormone with actions largely limited to the central nervous system, where it seems to stimulate neurotransmitter production. It has had some salutary effects in animal models of amyotrophic lateral sclerosis but has had no clinical effect in patients.[63] However, it has been shown to induce marked weight loss in some patients with amyotrophic lateral sclerosis. It mimics the actions of leptin while overcoming resistance to it, and it has several other inflammation-related effects that may foreshadow a new obesity management strategy. CNTF has long-lasting effects that act through pro-opiomelanocortin neurons involved in producing anorexia in mice.[64–66] If studies confirm clinical usefulness, CNTF may not require ongoing administration to maintain its effectiveness.

Gut Hormones, Leptin, and the Hypothalamus

The hypothalamus has long been known to play a crucial role in appetite regulation, in concert with a group of hormones mostly arising from the gastrointestinal tract. These agents have a variety of effects on food intake and satiation, and the increasing understanding of them offers some promise of newer and more effective means of managing obesity.[67,68] Roth and Reinehr[68] recently reviewed this topic and discussed the major hormones currently known to be involved in energy homeostasis.

Leptin is a true hormone, a 167-amino-acid polypeptide produced by adipocytes in proportion to their mass.[69,70] Leptin has an important signaling mechanism, informing brain centers about the state of the body's nutrient sufficiency. Total aleptinemia is rare and is associated with hypogonadotropic hypogonadism and severe insulin resistance, although such patients do not develop diabetes. Exogenously administered leptin shows beneficial effects in this setting.[71] However, in most obese individuals, serum leptin levels are increased and the problem is one of resistance to leptin at the hypothalamic level rather than hormone insufficiency.

The role of leptin is physiologically relevant, although increasing degrees of obesity are paradoxically associated with decreasing effectiveness in moderating nutrient intake. Nonetheless, the defect may sometimes be overcome by exogenous administration of leptin in selected patients,[72] in whom it is anorexigenic, crossing the blood-brain barrier and inhibiting appetite.[73]

Leptin has stimulated interest in the signaling mechanisms between adipose tissue and the brain that regulate feeding and energy balance. Although obese mice lose excess fat when injected with leptin, the effect of leptin administration to obese human subjects has not proved helpful. Leptin levels correlate with fat stores, but seem to have limited application as a therapeutic tool for human obesity management, because apparent resistance to leptin worsens as obesity becomes more severe.

Gastrointestinal Hormones and Antagonists

Several peptides are released from the gastrointestinal tract in response to nutrient intake and they may play a role in appetite regulation. Amylin is a peptide cosecreted by pancreatic islet cells along with insulin and is a physiologic moderator of the latter hormone. Amylin normally acts to limit postprandial hyperglycemia, working by reducing prandial glucagon release, slowing gastric emptying, and apparently exerting a direct central effect on appetite.

An injectable amylin analogue, pramlintide, has shown usefulness in the management of diabetes.[74,75] It also has shown promise in managing obesity and is being actively studied for that purpose.[76,77] Nausea has been a frequent side effect of its use in both diabetes and in obesity management, although this effect, and a degree of injection-site irritation, tends to lessen with time in many patients. Its long-term value in moderating obesity is currently being studied.

Incretin mimetics, specifically exenatide and liraglutide, are glucagonlike peptide (GLP-1) analogues of gastrointestinal hormones that moderate the effects of prandial glucagon excursions, limiting hyperglycemia, and stimulating insulin secretion in a glucose-dependent manner.[78] GLP-1 also signals satiety, suppressing food intake and bringing about improved glycemic control and weight loss in patients with type 2 diabetes, a loss that may be impressive and sustained.[79]

Native GLP-1 is rapidly destroyed in a physiologic setting by the enzyme DPP-IV, such that its use as a pharmacologic agent requires its continuous intravenous administration.[80] The incretin mimetics are pharmacologic agents with GLP-1–like activity and with molecular structures similar to native GLP-1, but their slight structural differences from native GLP-1 render them resistant to the hydrolytic effects of DPP-IV. They were developed to remediate the deficient native secretion of GLP-1 found in type 2 diabetes.

Whether this form of management will show permanent weight-loss effectiveness in those who use it on a continuing basis remains to be seen. Nausea is an early, limiting side effect in a substantial subset of patients with diabetes, but the symptom abates with time in some affected people. Use of incretin mimetics in obese patients without diabetes remains a subject of debate and is not well studied. Use of exenatide in adolescent patients may be a valuable therapeutic adjunct.[81]

Another class of pharmacologic agents directly inhibits DPP-IV, as opposed to resisting its hydrolytic effects, as is the case with the mimetic agents. These agents include sitagliptin, vildagliptin, and saxagliptin, which can be taken orally. They have proved effective in management of type 2 diabetes and its associated dyslipidemias, but their effects in promoting weight loss have proved more modest.[82,83]

Oxyntomodulin is a naturally occurring peptide produced in the colonic oxyntic mucosa. It has an appetite-suppressing capacity. It is structurally related to glucagon and GLP-1 with actions similar to those of GLP-1 and peptide YY (PYY). Injected subcutaneously, oxyntomodulin has been associated with a significant weight loss compared with placebo in a 4-week period.[84]

PYY is another peptide group released principally by L-cells of the gastrointestinal tract.[85,86] These hormones are structurally similar to other pancreatic peptides mediating effects through several subtypes of PYY receptors, including neurons in the Y2R receptor in the arcuate nucleus of the hypothalamus, an area of the brain involved with appetite control. In response to nutrient ingestion, PYY levels increase, peaking at a level proportional to ingested calories. Such data, including inhibition of food intake in rodents with peripheral administration of PYY, suggest that PYY may function as a physiologic appetite regulator. Its anorexigenic effects in human obesity remain unimpressive. However, PYY levels have been shown to be increased in adolescent girls with anorexia nervosa.[87]

Ghrelin, in contrast with all other known hormones arising from the gastrointestinal tract, uniquely signals the brain that hunger is present and promotes eating. It also stimulates production of growth hormone and shows a variety of other effects, including antiinflammatory properties.[88] Ghrelin is present in higher concentrations before anticipated meals, and levels decrease after eating; it has a leptinlike effect, with decreasing postprandial levels inducing satiation.[89] Thus, development of an effective agent able to antagonize or suppress ghrelin (other than food itself) could prove therapeutically useful.

Obestatin, a peptide hormone in human plasma, shows a ghrelin-inhibiting property and is being actively studied.[90–94] The hormone shows promise as a means of increasing lean body mass in cachexia. Evidence is developing that combined approaches may have greater efficacy in managing obesity than monotherapy in some settings. Pramlintide and the leptin analogue, metreleptin, have shown effectiveness when given together,[77,95] as has a combination of PYY and oxyntomodulin. Octreotide is a somatostatin receptor analogue that has caused weight loss in pediatric patients with hypothalamic obesity.[7]

SUMMARY

Pharmacologic therapy for obesity is recommended only in conjunction with a comprehensive weight-loss program that involves diet, exercise, and behavioral modification. Phentermine is a sympathomimetic amine that, in 1959, was the first FDA-approved product for short-term weight loss in adults. Additional amines, including diethylpropion, benzphetamine, and phendimetrazine, were then approved for short-term use in adults. To date, the only drug that is FDA approved for long-term use in obese adults is orlistat (lipase inhibitor); orlistat is FDA approved for those 12 years of age and older.

Sibutramine (a mixed noradrenergic-serotonergic product) was previously approved but was voluntarily withdrawn from the market in October 2010 because of the risk of serious cardiovascular events.

Other agents being studied for use in obese adults include metformin (a biguanide used to treat diabetes mellitus type 2 and metabolic syndrome in adolescents as well as adults) and rimonabant (a CB1-selective cannabinoid receptor antagonist). A variety of other agents are being studied, including antidepressants, anticonvulsants, and various gastrointestinal hormones (see **Box 4**). Herbal products are advocated by some for use as weight-loss agents. However, the safety record is poor for some, as noted with ephedra, which is no longer available. Many products now contain caffeine, C aurantium, and a variety of other supplements and herbs. A lack of standardization and supportive research, and the potential for side effects make these products undesirable as a treatment alternative. The role of bariatric surgery, with or without the use of pharmacology, remains for further research to elucidate.[96]

REFERENCES

1. Reddy V. Obesity. In: Greydanus DE, Patel DR, Pratt HD, editors. Behavioral pediatrics. 3rd edition. New York: Nova Science Publishers; 2009. p. 405–15, chapter 24.
2. Yanovski SZ, Yanovski JA. Obesity. N Engl J Med 2002;346(8):591–602.
3. Kirk S, Scott BJ, Daniels SR. Pediatric obesity epidemic: treatment options. J Am Diet Assoc 2005;105(5 Suppl 1):S44–51.
4. Godoy-Matos A, Carraro L, Vieira A, et al. Treatment of obese adolescents with sibutramine: a randomized, double-blind, controlled study. J Clin Endocrinol Metab 2005;90:1460–5.
5. Rowlett JR. Obesity in the adolescent. In: Greydanus DE, Patel DR, Pratt HD, editors. Essential adolescent medicine. New York: McGraw-Hill Medical Publishers; 2006. p. 651–65, chapter 31.

6. Barlow SE and the Expert Committee. Expert committee recommendations regarding prevention, assessment, and treatment of child and adolescent overweight and obesity: summary report. Pediatrics 2007;120(Suppl 4):S164–92.

7. Skelton JA, Rudolph CD. Overweight and obesity. In: Kliegman RM, Behrman RE, Jenson HB, et al, editors. Nelson textbook of pediatrics. 18th edition. Philadelphia: Saunders/Elsevier; 2007. p. 232–42, chapter 44.

8. Eneli I, Davies HD. Epidemiology of childhood obesity. In: Davies HD, editor, Obesity in childhood and adolescence, vol. 1. Westport (CT): Praeger Publishers; 2008. p. 3–23, chapter 1.

9. Jones KL. Role of obesity in complicating and confusing the diagnosis and treatment of diabetes in children. Pediatrics 2008;121(2):361–8.

10. Kiess W, Boettner A. Obesity in the adolescent. Adolesc Med 2002;13:181–90.

11. Atkinson RL, Hubbard VS. Report on the NIH Workshop on Pharmacologic Treatment of Obesity. Am J Clin Nutr 1994;60(2):153.

12. Bray GA, Tartaglia L. Medicinal strategies in the treatment of obesity. Nature 2000;404:672–7.

13. Jensen MD. Medical management of obesity. Semin Gastrointest Dis 1998;9: 156–62.

14. Freemark M, Kiess W. Anti-obesity medication use in adolescents: risks and benefits. Pediatr Endocrinol Rev 2004;2(Suppl 1):168–70.

15. McDuffie JR, Calis KA, Uwaifo GI, et al. Efficacy of orlistat as an adjunct to behavioral treatment in overweight African American and Caucasian adolescents with obesity-related co-morbid conditions. J Pediatr Endocrinol Metab 2004;17: 307–19.

16. Molnar D. New drug policy in childhood obesity. Int J Obes (Lond) 2005; 29(Suppl 2):S62–5.

17. Snow V, Barry P, Fitterman N, et al. Pharmacologic and surgical management of obesity in primary care: a clinical practice guideline from the American College of Physicians. Ann Intern Med 2005;142:525–31.

18. Joffe A. Pharmacotherapy for adolescent obesity: a weighty issue. JAMA 2005; 293:2932–4.

19. Lean M, Finer N. ABC of obesity. Management: part II—drugs. BMJ 2006;333: 794–7.

20. Dunican KC, Desilets AR, Montalbano JK. Pharmacotherapeutic options for overweight adolescents. Ann Pharmacother 2007;41:1445–55.

21. Eneli I, Mantinan KD. Managing the overweight child. In: Fitzgerald HE, Mousouli V, editors, Obesity in childhood and adolescence, vol. 2. Westport (CT): Praeger Publishers; 2008. p. 191–225, chapter 9.

22. Hofmann AD. Obesity. In: Hofmann AD, Greydanus DE, editors. Adolescent medicine. 3rd edition. Stamford (CT): Appleton & Lange; 1997. p. 663–82, chapter 30.

23. Greydanus DE, Bricker LA, Patel DR. The benefits of sports participation in childhood and adolescence to prevent obesity in adolescents and adults. Asian J Paediatric Practice 2006;9(4):1–7.

24. Greydanus DE, Bhave S. Obesity in the adolescent. Indian Pediatr 2004;41(6): 545–50.

25. Chanoine JP, Hampl S, Jensen C, et al. Effect of orlistat on weight and body composition in obese adolescents: a randomized controlled trial. JAMA 2005; 293:2873–83.

26. Berkowitz RI, Wadden TA, Tershakovec, et al. Behavioral therapy and sibutramine for the treatment of adolescent obesity. A randomized controlled trial. JAMA 2003;289:1805–12.

27. Berkowitz RI, Fujioka K, Daniels SR, et al. Effects of sibutramine treatment in obese adolescents: a randomized trial. Ann Intern Med 2006;145:81–90.
28. Reisler G, Tauber T, Afriat R, et al. Sibutramine as an adjuvant therapy in adolescents suffering from morbid obesity. Isr Med Assoc J 2006;8:30–2.
29. Webb E, Viner R. Should metformin be prescribed to overweight adolescents in whom dietary/behavioural modifications have not helped? Arch Dis Child 2006; 91:793–4.
30. Silverstone T. Appetite suppressants. A review. Drugs 1992;43(6):820.
31. US Food and Drug Administration [homepage on the Internet] [cited 2008 March 6]. Food and Drug Administration Science Background Safety of Phenylpropanolamine; [about 2 Screens]. Available at: http://www.fda.gov.cder/drug/infopage/ppa/science.htm. Accessed November 15, 2010.
32. Yoo JH, Lee EJ, Kwak CK, et al. Clinical trial of herbal formula on weight loss in obese Korean children. Am J Chin Med 2005;33:713–22.
33. Seamon M, Clauson K. Ephedra: yesterday, DSHEA, and tomorrow-a ten year perspective on the dietary supplement health and education act of 1994. J Herb Pharmacother 2005;5:67–86.
34. Greydanus DE, Patel DR. Sports doping in the adolescent athlete: the hope, hype, and hyperbole. Pediatr Clin North Am 2002;49:829–55.
35. US Food and Drug Administration [homepage on the Internet] [cited 2008 March 6]. FDA Announces Withdrawal Fenfluramine and Dexfenfluramine (Fen-Phen); [about 2 Screens]. Available at: http://www.fda.gov/cder/news/phen/fenphenpr 81597.htm. Accessed November 20, 2010.
36. Sibutramine for obesity. Med Lett Drugs Ther 1998;40:32.
37. Early JL, Apovian CM, Aronne LJ, et al. Sibutramine plus meal replacement therapy for body weight loss and maintenance in obese patients. Obesity (Silver Spring) 2007;15:1464–72.
38. Violante-Ortiz R, Rel-Rio-Navarro BE, Lara-Esqueda A, et al. Use of sibutramine in obese Hispanic adolescents. Adv Ther 2005;22:642–9.
39. Garcia-Morales LM, Berber A, Macias-Lara CC, et al. Use of sibutramine in obese Mexican adolescents: a 6 month, randomized, double-blind, placebo- controlled, parallel-group trial. Clin Ther 2006;28:770–82.
40. Daniels SR, Long B, Crow S, et al. Cardiovascular effects of sibutramine in the treatment of obese adolescents: results of a randomized, double-blind, placebo-controlled study. Pediatrics 2007;120:e147–57.
41. Doggrell SA. Sibutramine for obesity in adolescents. Expert Opin Pharmacother 2006;7:2435–8.
42. Danielsson P, Janson A, Norgren S, et al. Impact sibutramine therapy in children with hypothalamic obesity or obesity with aggravating syndromes. J Clin Endocrinol Metab 2007;92:4101–6.
43. Davidson MH, Hauptman J, DiGirolamo M, et al. Weight control and risk factor reduction in obese subjects treated for 2 years with orlistat: a randomized trial. JAMA 1999;281:235–42.
44. Orlistat OTC for weight loss. Med Lett Drugs Ther 2007;49:49.
45. Orlistat for obesity. Med Lett Drugs Ther 1999;41:55.
46. Anderson JW. Low-dose orlistat effects on body weight of mildly to moderately overweight individuals: a 16 week, double-blind, placebo-controlled trial. Ann Pharmacother 2006;40:1717.
47. Maahs D, de Serna DG, Kolotkin RL, et al. Randomized, double-blind, placebo-controlled trial of orlistat for weight loss in adolescents. Endocr Pract 2006;12: 18–28.

48. Ozkan B, Bereket A, Turan S, et al. Addition of orlistat to conventional treatment in adolescents with severe obesity. Eur J Pediatr 2004;163(12):738–41.
49. Nestler JE. Metformin for the treatment of polycystic ovary syndrome. N Engl J Med 2008;358(1):47–54.
50. Hoppin AG, Katz ES, Kaplan LM, et al. Case 31-2006: a 15-year-old girl with severe obesity. N Engl J Med 2006;355(15):1593–602.
51. Harborne L, Fleming R, Lyall H, et al. Metformin or antiandrogen in the treatment of hirsutism in polycystic ovary syndrome. J Clin Endocrinol Metab 2003;88: 4116–23.
52. Freemark M. Pharmacotherapy of childhood obesity: an evidence-based, conceptual approach. Diabetes Care 2007;30:395–402.
53. Srinivasan S, Ambler GR, Baur LA, et al. Randomized, controlled trial of metformin for obesity and insulin resistance in children and adolescents: improvement in body composition and fasting insulin. J Clin Endocrinol Metab 2006;91(6): 2074–80.
54. Pagotto U, Pasquali R. Fighting obesity and associated risk factors by antagonizing cannabinoid type 1 receptors. Lancet 2005;365:1363–4.
55. Pi-Sunyer FX, Arrone LJ, Heshmati HM, et al. Effect of rimonabant, a cannabinoid-1-receptor blocker on weight and cardiometabolic risk factors in overweight or obese patients. JAMA 2006;295:761–75.
56. Huestis MA, Gorelick DA, Heishman SJ, et al. Blockage of effects of smoked marijuana by the CB1-selective cannabinoid receptor antagonist SR141716. Arch Gen Psychiatry 2001;58(4):322–8.
57. Maldonado R, Valverde O, Berrendero F. Involvement of the endocannabinoid system in drug addiction. Trends Neurosci 2006;29(4):225–32.
58. US Food and Drug Administration [homepage on the Internet] [cited 2008 March 6]. FDA Briefing Document; NDA 21-888 (rimonabant); [about 84 screens]. Available at: http://www.fda.gov/ohrms/dockets/ac/07/briefing/2007-4306b1-fda-backgrounder.pdf.
59. Fluoxetine (Prozac) and other drugs for treatment of obesity. Med Lett Drugs Ther 1994;36(936):107.
60. Greydanus DE, Calles J, Patel DR. Pediatric and adolescent psychopharmacology: a primer for the pediatrician. Cambridge (UK): Cambridge University Press; 2008. p. 300.
61. Bray GA, Hollander P, Klein S, et al. A 6-month randomized, placebo-controlled, dose-ranging trial of topiramate for weight loss in obesity. Obes Res 2003;11(6): 722–33.
62. McElroy SL, Guerdjikova AI, Martens B, et al. Role of antiepileptic drugs in the management of eating disorders. CNS Drugs 2009;23(2):139–56.
63. Bongioanni P, Reali C, Sogos V. Ciliary neurotrophic factor (CNTF) for amyotrophic lateral sclerosis or motor neuron disease. Cochrane Database Syst Rev 2004;3:CD004302.
64. Matthews VB, Febbraio MA. CNTF: a target therapeutic for obesity-related metabolic disease? J Mol Med 2008;86(4):353–61.
65. Gloaguen I, Costa P, Demartis A, et al. Ciliary neurotrophic factor corrects obesity and diabetes associated with leptin deficiency and resistance. Proc Natl Acad Sci U S A 1997;94(12):6456–61.
66. Kokoeva MV, Yin H, Flier JS. Neurogenesis in the hypothalamus of adult mice: potential role in energy balance. Science 2005;310(5748):679–83.
67. Suzuki K, Simpson KA, Minnion JS, et al. The role of gut hormones and the hypothalamus in appetite regulation. Endocr J 2010;57(5):359–72.

68. Roth CL, Reinehr T. Roles of gastrointestinal and adipose tissue peptides in child-hood obesity and changes after weight loss due to lifestyle intervention. Arch Pediatr Adolesc Med 2010;164(2):131–8.
69. Considine RV, Sinha MK, Heiman ML, et al. Serum immunoreactive-leptin concentrations in normal-weight and obese humans. N Engl J Med 1996;334:292–5.
70. Montague CT, Farooqi IS, Whitehead JP, et al. Congenital leptin deficiency is associated with severe early-onset obesity in humans. Nature 1997;387(6636): 903–8.
71. Farooqi IS, Matarese G, Lord GM, et al. Beneficial effects of leptin on obesity, T cell hyporesponsiveness, and neuroendocrine/metabolic dysfunction of human congenital leptin deficiency. J Clin Invest 2002;110:1093–103.
72. Heymsfield SB, Greenberg AS, Fujioka K, et al. Recombinant leptin for weight loss in obese and lean adults: a randomized, controlled, dose escalation trial. JAMA 2000;283:1567–8.
73. Ahima RS, Flier JS. Leptin. Annu Rev Physiol 2000;62:413–37.
74. Fineman MS, Koda JE, Shen LZ, et al. The human amylin analog, pramlintide, corrects postprandial hyperglucagonemia in patients with type 1 diabetes. Metabolism 2002;51:636–41.
75. Hirsch IB, Blonde L, Buse J, et al. Consensus development conference on pramlintide in the management of type 1 and type 2 diabetes. Lakeville (CT): The Diabetes Education Group; 2006.
76. Dunican KC, Adams NM, Desilets AR. The role of pramlintide for weight loss. Ann Pharmacother 2010;44(3):538–45.
77. Ravussin E, Smith SR, Mitchell JA, et al. Enhanced weight loss with pramlintide/metreleptin: an integrated neurohormonal approach to obesity pharmacotherapy. Obesity (Silver Spring) 2009;17(9):1736–43.
78. Parkes DG, Pittner R, Jodka C, et al. Insulinotropic actions of exendin-4 and glucagon-like peptide 1 in vivo and in vitro. Metabolism 2001;50:583–9.
79. Riddle MC, Henry RR, Poon TH, et al. Exenatide elicits sustained glycaemic control and progressive reduction of body weight in patients with type 2 diabetes inadequately controlled by sulphonylureas with or without metformin. Diabetes Metab Res Rev 2006;22(6):483–91.
80. Nauck MA, Kleine N, Orskov C, et al. Normalization of fasting hyperglycaemia by exogenous glucagon-like peptide 1 (7–36 amide) in type 2 (non-insulin-dependent) diabetic patients. Diabetologia 1993;36:741–74.
81. Raman VS, Mason KJ, Rodriguez LM, et al. The role of adjunctive exenatide therapy in pediatric type 1 diabetes. Diabetes Care 2010;33(6):1294–6.
82. Colagiuri S. Diabesity: therapeutic options. Diabetes Obes Metab 2010;12(6): 463–73.
83. Niswender K. Diabetes and obesity: therapeutic targeting and risk reduction – a complex interplay. Diabetes Obes Metab 2010;12(4):267–87.
84. Wynne K, Park AJ, Small CJ, et al. Subcutaneous oxyntomodulin reduces body weight in overweight and obese subjects: a double-blind, randomized, controlled trial. Diabetes 2005;54(8):2390–5.
85. Batterham RL, Bloom SR. The gut hormone peptide YY regulates appetite. Ann N Y Acad Sci 2003;994:162–8.
86. Gantz I, Erondu N, Mallick M, et al. Efficacy and safety of intranasal peptide YY3-36 for weight reduction in obese adults. J Clin Endocrinol Metab 2007; 92(5):1754–7.
87. Misra M, Miller KK, Tsai P, et al. Elevated peptide YY levels in adolescent girls with anorexia nervosa. J Clin Endocrinol Metab 2006;91(3):1027–33.

88. Ueno H, Shiiya T, Nakazato M. Translational research of ghrelin. Ann N Y Acad Sci 2010;1200:120–7.
89. Inui A, Asakawa A, Bowers CY, et al. Ghrelin, appetite, and gastric motility: the emerging role of the stomach as an endocrine organ. FASEB J 2004;18(3): 439–56.
90. Zhang JV, Ren PG, Avsian-Kretchmer O, et al. Obestatin, a peptide encoded by the ghrelin gene, opposes ghrelin's effects on food intake. Science 2005; 310(5750):996–9.
91. Hassouna R, Zizzari P, Tolle V. The ghrelin/obestatin balance in the physiological and pathological control of GH secretion, body composition and food intake. J Neuroendocrinol 2010;22:793–804.
92. Verhagen LA, Egecioglu E, Luijendijk MC, et al. Acute and chronic suppression of the central ghrelin signaling system reveals a role in food anticipatory activity. Eur Neuropsychopharmacol 2010;20. [Epub ahead of print].
93. Germain N, Galusca B, Grouselle D, et al. Ghrelin and obestatin circadian levels differentiate bingeing-purging from restrictive anorexia nervosa. J Clin Endocrinol Metab 2010;95(6):3057–62.
94. Ashitani J, Matsumoto N, Nakazato M. Ghrelin and its therapeutic potential for cachectic patients. Peptides 2009;30(10):1951–6.
95. Field BC, Wren AM, Peters V, et al. PYY3-36 and oxyntomodulin can be additive in their effect on food intake in overweight and obese humans. Diabetes 2010;59(7): 1635–9.
96. Nandagopal R, Brown RJ, Rother KI. Resolution of type 2 diabetes following bariatric surgery: implications for adults and adolescents. Diabetes Technol Ther 2010;12(8):671–7.

Psychopharmacology of Depression in Children and Adolescents

Susan M. Smiga, MD[a],*, Glen R. Elliott, PhD, MD[b]

KEYWORDS

- Depressive disorders • Children • Adolescents
- Psychopharmacology

By the mid-1980s, the revised third edition American Psychiatric Association's *Diagnostic and Statistical Manual of Mental Disorders* (DSM-IIIR)[1] formally acknowledged that depression could occur in younger individuals and even modified some criteria to accommodate the variations in the syndrome in that age group, for example, allowing an "irritable" mood instead of a "depressed" mood. Developmental variations in symptom presentation are not easily incorporated into a diagnostic system, but DSM-IV[2] did attempt to broaden the definition by shortening the chronicity of symptoms for children to meet criteria for dysthymia. A substantial, though still incomplete, body of knowledge regarding the occurrence, course, and treatment of depression in childhood and adolescence has continued to evolve.[3–7]

The prevalence of major depression is lower in prepubertal children (2.8%) and more common in adolescents (5.6%),[8] who may have a lifetime prevalence of 25%[9] Although no completely satisfactory studies of prevalence rates of depression in the young are available, in the United States the likelihood of having major depression does increase markedly with age. Depression occurs in about 9 per 1000 preschool children, 20 per 1000 school-age children, and nearly 50 per 1000 adolescents, which is a similar rate to that in adults.[10] With early adolescence comes a distinct and rather rapid change in the sex distribution of depression from the 1:1 male/female ratio observed in preadolescent children to the 1:2 male/female ratio typical in adult populations.[11] Although the age at which this occurs roughly coincides with the onset of puberty, researchers have offered a range of biological, psychological, and social explanations for the change, none of which is clearly superior to the others.

[a] Pediatric-Psychiatry Collaborative Programs, Department of Psychiatry, Dartmouth Hitchcock Medical Center, One Medical Center Drive, Lebanon, NH 03766, USA
[b] Children's Health Council, 650 Clark Way, Palo Alto, CA 94304, USA
* Corresponding author.
E-mail address: susan.m.smiga@dartmouth.edu

Pediatr Clin N Am 58 (2011) 155–171
doi:10.1016/j.pcl.2010.11.007
0031-3955/11/$ – see front matter © 2011 Elsevier Inc. All rights reserved.

Certain subpopulations of children and adolescents have far higher rates of depression than those cited above. For example, one study of pediatric neurology inpatients undergoing evaluations for unexplained headaches reported a 40% incidence of depression, whereas the incidence among general pediatric inpatients was around 7%.[12] Children with chronic illnesses or frequent somatic complaints may also be at increased risk. Individuals with developmental delays and other special needs are another important population with notable rates of depression that too often is overlooked.[13]

Models of depression based on behavioral, cognitive, psychodynamic, and family theory often can help clinicians to pinpoint key aspects of the clinical picture that may be amenable to change, but they do not offer definitive explanations for its etiology. In young children, especially those younger than 6 to 7 years, the most common cause of marked depression appears to be severe neglect or abuse. Therefore, the evaluation of any young child who presents with severe depression must include a careful assessment of his or her psychosocial environment for these potential contributing factors.

Biological models of depression invoke no special mechanisms for the young,[3,14] but efforts to establish continuity of underlying biological factors across the age range have been far from satisfactory. The development of new, safe technologies for exploring brain structure and function in young individuals is creating great excitement about possible advances in the understanding of the biological underpinnings of depression.[15] Despite these advances, no biological test yet known is useful in making the diagnosis of an affective disorder in children or adolescents.

Parental and environmental influences on the development of depression in children and adolescents are readily evident and probably multifactorial.[16,17] Some forms of depression certainly have strong genetic components. For instance, monozygotic twins reared together have a 76% concordance for affective disorders. The fact that this drops to 67% for monozygotic twins reared separately and remains at 19% for dizygotic twins reared together underscores the concomitant importance of nongenetic influences. From 10% to 15% of adolescents whose parents are depressed are themselves depressed, while many more exhibit nondiagnostic symptoms that may be related to depression, including rebellion, withdrawal, defiance, and ongoing family conflicts; such outcomes may, of course, reflect either biological or psychological factors.[18,19]

The diagnostic criteria for depression in young individuals rely on the same set of symptoms as in adults, with slight variations. It is important to understand that children or teens who present with symptoms of depression may be suffering from any number of disorders or situational stressors, and that even subclinical depression often has a negative impact on a child's function and development. Children with frequent somatic complaints such as headaches, stomach aches, breathing difficulties, or chest pain may have underlying mental health issues, including depression or anxiety.

Because primary care providers are far more likely to have regular contact with children and teens than do mental health professionals, they have an essential role in recognizing depression in those they treat; they also need to be able both to facilitate access to appropriate mental health services and to initiate pharmacological management when indicated. Many factors, ranging from deficits in knowledge, skills, attitude, or fear can cause many primary care providers to miss the diagnosis and to undertreat these patients.

Numerous recent publications in pediatrics have highlighted the focus on depression in children and the responsibilities in primary care to address the needs of this population. A systematic review conducted for the United States Preventative Task Force evaluated models for screening for depression in primary care, and supported that screening tools can accurately identify youth at risk and that treatment improves outcome.[20] A second publication offers strategies for primary care practices to prepare themselves to meet the mental health needs of their patients,[21] and a third defines the American Pediatric Academy proposed competencies requisite for providing for mental health and substance abuse treatment in primary care.[22]

This article is intended to help primary care providers prepare themselves and their practices to screen effectively for depression in children and teens, and to respond appropriately in supporting these youths to obtain effective services including psycho-pharmacological management.

DIAGNOSIS

Recognizing depression and making an accurate diagnosis is the first step toward developing a treatment plan. Depression can be a primary disorder; or it may be secondary to a medical condition, be substance induced, or occur in response to a specific stressor (eg, parental divorce, death of a family member, abuse). The latter is commonly labeled as an adjustment disorder and does not constitute a major psychiatric disorder, although it still can markedly impair a child's ability to function and require interventions. Evidence suggests that depression seldom occurs by itself in children and adolescents.[23–26] A young patient may display behaviors that warrant simultaneous diagnoses of affective, anxiety, or personality disorder, drug abuse, family conflicts, gender identity disorder, and others. Furthermore, depressive signs and symptoms are common features of many behavioral disturbances, such as "not being able to concentrate." Identification and clarification of concurrent diagnoses may require repeated assessments over time. Such an effort is vital, because a comorbid diagnosis such as substance abuse or trauma can alter markedly both the course of the depression and the long-term prognosis of the patient.[25,26]

At all ages, prominent features of the primary psychiatric depressive disorders include alterations in mood—either depression or irritability—with concomitant changes in sleep, interest in activities, feelings of guilt, loss of energy, impaired concentration, changes in appetite, psychomotor processing (retardation or agitation), and suicidal ideation. Compared with depressed prepubescent children, depressed adolescents may be more likely to experience anhedonia, defined as a profound lack of enjoyment in life and activities, hypersomnia, significant weight gain, and hopelessness. Co-occurrence of depression and substance abuse is common in teens. Often the substance use is noted as a likely cause of the depression; however, there is also significant data to suggest that depression in adolescence may be a predisposing factor for later substance abuse disorders, even in the absence of persistent mood disturbance.[27] Psychosis, although rare, can occur as part of a depressive episode and may suggest a higher likelihood of developing bipolar illness at a later age.[28]

One confusing aspect of depression in children and adolescents is that their symptoms may be less persistent and consistent over time than is the case for adults. Thus, parents not uncommonly will report that their child is sullen and irritable around the home yet seems happy and friendly with peers. Some incorrectly interpret this inconstancy of mood as proof that the child must not be "really" depressed. It is important to ask about mood states in a variety of circumstances, especially how the child feels when alone and not under specific demands, such as when doing homework or in the company of peers. Younger children, and even some teens, can be quite concrete in their thinking and may lack the vocabulary to describe feeling "depressed." These children may think of the feeling as "sad," "bored," "down," or "irritable." Parents and teachers often may report that the child is not clearly depressed so much as irritable, short-fused, or angry; moreover, some children describe similar mood states rather than depression. Using several descriptors can help avoid missing a persistent impairment of mood. One acronym that captures criteria for major depression is SIGE-CAPS (**Box 1**), with the requirement that 5 of 9 of these symptoms be present for at least 2 solid weeks "most days, most of the day" to meet diagnostic criteria.

Changes such as deteriorating school performance, a notable loss of friends, or a significant curtailment of previously enjoyable activities are relatively late indicators of major depression. Subtler, early signs may be decreased initiative in contacting friends and a withdrawal from family routines. Of course, such behaviors may also be well within the scope of normal behavior or indicative of other mental health disorders. Family history of depression can be a helpful clue, when present, but the inheritance patterns differ markedly among various subtypes of affective disorders.

A diagnosis of dysthymia requires fewer symptoms than major depression but of a longer duration. The requirement that symptoms be present for at least 1 year in children and teens with no period of more than 2 months symptom-free connotes a chronicity and pervasiveness that can have very serious consequences on the youth's development. Though considered to be a "milder" form of depression, dysthymia has significant long-term costs to the development of the child. Furthermore, 70% of youth with dysthymia go on to have a major depressive episode.[29]

Even if the specific diagnosis is unclear, it often may be best for clinicians to assume that the depressive symptoms are important, whether or not they are primary. Efforts to intervene with the depression may help clarify other problems, but clinicians should not conclude that depression necessarily is the only or even the most important reason a patient might have signs and symptoms of depression. Subclinical depression that does not meet full criteria for diagnosis still has significant negative impact on function, and early treatment may prevent the development of a full-blown major depressive episode and lessen impact on function and development.

One useful way of screening populations for mood disorders and suicide risk is to use structured measures, of which several are readily available. These measures typically are self-administered, take little time, and are easy to score. Moreover, they can be useful for initial screening and for monitoring treatment response. Some data suggest that children, or at least teens, may be more likely to endorse symptoms on a pen-and-paper questionnaire than in face-to-face direct inquiry. There are multiple screening tools that are valid and reliable for screening for adolescent depression available in the public domain. Several available tools include the K-SAD, PHQ 9 modified for adolescents, and the Columbia Depression Scale.[30]

Box 1
Signs and symptoms of major depression: SIGE-CAPS

Sleep: insomnia or hypersomnia

Interest: markedly decreased interest or pleasure in most activities

Guilt: or feelings of worthlessness

Energy: fatigue or loss of energy

Concentration: diminished ability to think or concentrate, indecision

Appetite: increased or decreased or weight change (5% body weight in a month)

Psychomotor agitation or retardation: observable by others

Suicidality: recurrent thoughts of death or suicide

TREATMENT OPTIONS

Once a clinician has diagnosed a depressive disorder in a child or adolescent, educating the patient and family about the disorder and treatment options is the first step toward planning an effective intervention. Deciding what level of care, for example, outpatient or inpatient, and what modality of treatment is indicated, for example, psychotherapy and/or pharmacotherapy, as well as developing a crisis plan are important components of this early assessment and intervention. It is important to determine what part of the care and management will be provided within the primary care setting.

Having these resources handy and up to date facilitates better care and alleviates provider stress related to acute situations when patients present with depression. If a provider or practice is committed to screening and treating depression in youth, knowing the resources is essential.

Typical treatment options for youth fall into 2 broad categories: pharmacologic and nonpharmacologic.[31,32] Many published guidelines exist that can assist in decision making, which were developed in part in response to the concern raised when the "black-box" warning was issued by the Food and Drug Administration (FDA) in 2003. These guidelines include the practice parameters by the American Academy of Child and Adolescent Psychiatry (AACAP)[33] and the updated Texas Children's Medication Algorithm Project (CMAP).[34] Both the United Kingdom and Canada have drafted similar documents with similar recommendations.[30,35] Several variables often influence, if not dictate, the clinician's decision about treatment, including the severity of symptoms and impact on function, duration of symptoms, family and patient preference, family history of medication responsiveness, and suicide risk. In less complicated, first episodes with mild or moderate symptoms and impairment, active monitoring may be indicated for 1 month.[33,35] The availability and a patient's willingness and capacity to access specific interventions or therapy may warrant a course of therapy before introducing medication. Practice guidelines that provide stepwise systematic approaches to treatment, often in a stage-of-treatment model, and some treatment algorithms are available to assist clinicians in making these choices.[36,37] A recent article suggests that use of these algorithms improves outcome.[37]

There is a growing body of evidence to assist the clinician in making decisions about rank ordering the interventions or sequencing them. One, a multisite study funded by the National Institute of Mental Health (NIMH) called the Treating Adolescent Depression Study (TADS), compared the use of a selective serotonin reuptake inhibitor (SSRI) alone, cognitive behavioral therapy (CBT) alone, or the two in combination.[38] The findings indicated that the combination of CBT and fluoxetine offered the highest treatment response rates. Fluoxetine alone had significant response rates, whereas CBT alone did not.

A second NIMH-funded multisite study in progress, called Treatment of Resistant Depression in Adolescents (TORDIA), looked at the sequencing of treatments for individuals who do not respond to an initial SSRI trial. The comparison groups include a second SSRI, an antidepressant from a different class, or adding CBT. The advantage of these 2 studies is that they compare 2 active treatment arms rather than active treatment to placebo and are designed to more accurately mirror real-world patient populations and practices. There were no differences in the response rates for either medication switch; however, the addition of CBT led to greater response than medication switch alone.[39]

The response rate for children and adolescents with major depressive disorder during the acute phase of treatment to a first antidepressant is 50% to 60%,[40] and the response for those who fail a first trial is 40% to 50% when tried on a second agent.[33] Because mood disorders tend to be recurring and relapsing conditions, even when a patient responds well to medication, several issues remain to be addressed. It is important to explore whether other adjunctive therapy is needed. Some patients do well once the depression has lifted and return readily to their activities. For others, the disruption to self-esteem and interference with other critical tasks of development are more profound and less easily dispelled. School performance may suffer, as may peer relationships. Especially in adolescents, for whom self-image is crystallizing, effects on self-confidence and self-esteem may be profound and enduring. Specific inquiry into such areas of function can help the patient and family identify additional services that may be of help in completing the return to full function.

Tailoring individual needs to available resources is a common challenge in designing a treatment program for depressed patients. Ongoing contact with the patient is vital for success. Helping the child or adolescent feel supported while fostering individual responsibility requires a delicate balance, especially early in treatment. Parents must be recruited as allies, even as their contributions in the environment in which their child is failing to thrive is acknowledged and altered. When chronic conflict within the family is a prominent part of the clinical picture, these dual perspectives sometimes are maintained best if patients and parents work with different individuals who can coordinate the treatment with each other.

In the case of depression, patients or families who do not want to use medications have clear, research-based options. Cognitive-based and other time-limited therapies have proven efficacy[3,23,41–47]; however, availability of these options varies markedly across the United States. Further, these types of interventions have focused almost exclusively on adolescents; their efficacy for younger patients remains unclear. Typical models include CBT and interpersonal therapy (IPT).[48] Where family conflict seems to play a major contributing role, referral for family therapy should be considered. If an adolescent resists individual therapy, some adolescents may be more open to services delivered in a groups setting or that are school based.

Primary care providers generally will prescribe from 2 main categories of antidepressants: an SSRI and/or a serotonin-norepinephrine reuptake inhibitor (SNRI). The tricyclic antidepressants (TCAs) and monoamine oxidase inhibitors (MAOIs) are rarely used, even by child psychiatrists, given their higher risk profile for adverse effects and toxicity, especially in overdose and lack of demonstrated efficacy.[49,50] Both the ready availability of less toxic alternatives and research suggesting that TCAs are not effective in treating depression in adolescents have resulted in a significant decrease in their use.[51] No TCAs are FDA endorsed for depression in children or teens. Some MAOIs are FDA endorsed for depression in youth older than 16 years, but they are rarely if ever used as a first-line choice.

The first relatively convincing evidence that an antidepressant can effectively treat depression in children and adolescents was published in 1997[52,53] and looked at fluoxetine, an SSRI. Evidence for such benefits has accrued only over the past few years,[3,52–57] and these studies seem to confirm that, at least for some SSRIs, antidepressants can be safe and effective for treating depression in both children and adolescents. FDA-endorsed SSRIs for depression include fluoxetine for children 8 years and older[38,52] and escitalopram[58,59] in adolescents 12 years and older. Citalopram and sertraline, which have some, though mixed, support from randomized controlled trials (RCTs), are also reasonable alternatives despite lack of FDA endorsement.

Paroxetine, however, is relatively contraindicated, due to its short half-life and associated withdrawal symptoms and higher association with suicidal ideation during treatment. Fluoxetine has the benefit of a very long half-life, so mixed compliance is less likely to lead to subtherapeutic levels; it does, however, have significant cytochrome-P450 interactions, and is a potent inhibitor of the 2D6 enzyme thus having potential for significant D-D interactions. Citalopram and escitalopram have limited cytochrome-P450 effects so may be advantageous for youth on multiple other medications.[60] Considering the cost of the specific medication is critical when this may preclude a family being able to afford the recommended treatment.

Because side effects can vary widely across patients, clinicians need to be prepared for the paradoxical or unexpected effects. Common side effects fall into several organ systems, predominantly central nervous system, gastrointestinal, and sexual. Central nervous system effects include agitation or restlessness, sleep (insomnia or sedation), headaches, tremor, and apathy. Gastrointestinal changes include changes in appetite, weight gain or loss, nausea, and occasionally diarrhea. Sexual effects that may be of particular importance to adolescents and yet difficult for them to discuss relate to sexual function. Most SSRIs have a notable incidence of anorgasmia that can affect both males and females. The effect is dose-related and reversible, but it is wise to mention this possibility even to adolescents who state that they are not sexually active. Many of these side effects also occur commonly as concomitants of depression, so patients should be urge to report any abrupt onset of such symptoms timed with starting or changing the dose of medication. Other postmarketing adverse events that may present to the pediatrician include epistaxis, purpura, enuresis, sinusitis, diaphoresis, and diastolic hypertension.

Although the SSRIs typically are well tolerated and previously were thought to require little or no monitoring for safety, recent controversy has raised significant concerns regarding their potential for inducing suicidal thoughts, behaviors, and violence.[61] A review of 24 studies using SSRIs prescribed to teens looked at adverse event reporting, and noted a twofold increase—from 2% to 4%—reporting suicidal ideation or behaviors.[62] Although there is a slight increase in the risk of suicidality among youth in the acute phase of treatment with an antidepressant, there is a lack of evidence to prove causality.[63] This finding led to the addition in October 2004 of a black-box warning on all antidepressants prescribed to children or adolescents. Patient and family education must include warnings about possible new-onset suicidal ideation that may or may not be related to such adverse side effects as behavioral activation, akathesia, mania, or acute delirium.[64] The FDA recommendations include weekly visits for the first month after initiating a trial of all antidepressants, followed by every other week for 2 more visits. Patients should be reevaluated again for response and adverse effects at least at 12 weeks and then as needed. Despite these recommendations, large-scale reviews of actual practice have indicated that fewer than 5% of youth experience this level of supervision; in fact, approximately 40% of children do not even have 3 visits in the 3 months following starting on an antidepressant.[65] These warnings may have contributed to a decrease in prescribing from 2003 to 2005 with a concomitant increase in completed suicides.[66]

Pediatricians who find the aforementioned information intimidating should be aware that studies that specifically measured suicidal thinking and behaviors before and during treatment actually showed no change or even a decrease in suicidal thinking and behaviors with use of SSRIs. In addition, in the TADS, suicidal ideation dropped from 29% to 10% with treatment, though suicide-related events were higher (7% vs 4%).[38] Also, no completed suicides have occurred in more than 4000 pediatric subjects in trials with antidepressants (2200 with SSRIs), even with this being a potentially higher than average-risk population. Because it is commonly observed that energy and motivation may improve earlier in treatment than depressed mood leaving patients more vulnerable to act on previous suicidal thoughts, and that depression carries its own inherent risks, closer monitoring early in a trial of antidepressants is now recommended. A useful resource for practitioners and for parents can be found at medguide.org or parentmedguide.org, respectively.

Although suicide rates are fortunately much lower than rates of mood disorders, suicide remains the third leading cause of death in older adolescents and the fifth leading cause of death in children between 5 and 14 years of age.[47,67] In general, completed suicides escalate rapidly during the adolescent years.[47,68] Some studies suggest that as many as 25% of adolescents have seriously considered committing suicide, and perhaps 9% of adolescents attempt suicide at least once. Whereas males predominate in completed suicides, females are greatly overrepresented among those who survive a suicide attempt. Alarmingly, trends in the suicide method used by females has recently shifted to use of more lethal methods such as hanging, which were previously used more by males and may likely contribute to the observed increased death rates for females by suicide.[69]

Because it is a true emergency and often offers the first access to a depressed child or adolescent, an active suicide attempt or threat of suicide demands a careful assessment.[68] Although efforts are under way to standardize suicide assessment of youth, as yet no system has achieved widespread use. Common features among assessment tools suggest some key factors that clinicians can consider in evaluating the risk of a particular child or adolescent for completing a suicide, and are captured by the acronym "Sad Persons" (**Box 2**).[70]

Developmental influences can potentiate risk of suicide ideation and attempts, as children and teens may be more apt to react to "minor" stressors such as rejection by a peer, a poor grade, or teasing with self harm. Severe suicidal intent tends to be an acute problem that typically abates rapidly, if the individual receives the necessary support during the crisis, so accurate assessment and appropriate intervention literally can be lifesaving.[71]

Box 2
Sad Persons scale, modified

The score is calculated from 10 yes/no questions, with points given for each affirmative answer as follows:

- S: Male sex → 1
- A: Age <19 or >45 years → 1
- D: Depression or hopelessness → 2
- P: Previous suicidal attempts or psychiatric care → 1
- E: Excessive ethanol or drug use → 1
- R: Rational thinking loss (psychotic or organic illness) → 2
- S: Single, widowed or divorced → 1
- O: Organized or serious attempt → 2
- N: No social support → 1
- S: Stated future intent (determined to repeat or ambivalent) → 2

This score is then mapped onto a risk assessment scale as follows:

- 0–5: May be safe to discharge (depending on circumstances)
- 6–8: Probably requires psychiatric consultation
- >8: Probably requires hospital admission

Knowledge about general strategies for evaluating and intervening with young, suicidal patients is necessary for all primary care providers. It is important for clinicians to identify both immediate factors leading up to the suicide attempt and acute or chronic mental disorders, including depression that might promote suicidality. Perhaps the most important intervention is to ask: asking if someone is suicidal does not make him or her more likely to commit suicide. Quite to the contrary, those who harbor such thoughts often are terrified to reveal such ideas spontaneously but will discuss the issue freely if invited to do so. If suicidal ideation is suspected, it is crucial to seek an explicit exploration of intention and access to possible suicidal means. A study of emergency room suicide evaluations indicated that most physicians fail even to ask if there are guns in the house.[72] If suicidal intent seems high, hospitalization may well be needed; otherwise, the family needs to be recruited in a frank discussion of who will be with the child or adolescent and what steps can be taken to ensure safety. Serious suicidal intent is the most frequent justification for inpatient care for children or adolescents; the intent is both to protect the individual and to begin establishing contributing factors.[71]

Essentially all antidepressants can induce mania in susceptible individuals; thus, awareness of the risk of bipolar illness is important when initiating a trial of antidepressants for depression. All patients and families should be advised of the possibility of a manic response, particularly those with a family history of bipolar illness. A medication-induced manic state does not automatically lead to a diagnosis of bipolar illness to the child, because some individuals will become manic only when on an antidepressant. More controversial is whether a drug-induced manic state has any long-term adverse consequences for young patients who are at risk for developing bipolar affective disorder.[73] To date, no compelling evidence exists to suggest that an antidepressant trial should be avoided even when a strong suspicion of a bipolar affective disorder exists; however, emergence of manic symptoms after initiation of an antidepressant, usually between the first and fourth weeks, should result in prompt cessation of the medication and diagnostic and clinical reassessment. Early indicators of this switch to mania may include elated mood, decreased need for sleep, grandiosity, hypersexuality, racing thoughts, and pressured speech.

Another concern when prescribing SSRIs is the serotonin syndrome, which can occur when a patient is on high doses of an SSRI or is taking several medications that, together, increase total brain serotonin concentrations. Though relatively rare, this potentially lethal syndrome often resembles flu-like symptoms or sepsis, with fever, disorientation, confusion, agitation, tremor, muscle twitching and myoclonus, excess salivation, and ataxia; its presence constitutes a medical emergency. There have been no reports of long-term adverse effects from SSRIs, and "routine" monitoring of major organ functioning is not required. However, because many are metabolized through the cytochrome P450 enzyme system, interactions with other medications must be considered.[74]

Discontinuation syndrome, especially relevant with SSRIs with shorter half-lives, such as paroxetine and fluvoxamine, also can be important. In general, a slow taper of several weeks is appropriate and minimizes likelihood of problems, regardless of the SSRI being used.

Because SSRIs are generally the first-line pharmaceutical agent for treating depression in youth at this time and a patient may respond to a different drug in the same class, a reasonable standard of practice for physicians caring for children and adolescents is to develop familiarity with at least 2 or 3 of the SSRIs. In the absence of marked side effects, an adequate trial typically would be 8 to 10 weeks at a usual therapeutic dose for that medication. After a failure of 2 SSRIs, most treatment guidelines recommend switching to a non-SSRI. Often this is the point at which many primary care physicians will seek a consultation from a child and adolescent psychiatrist. Of course, sudden deterioration, suicidal ideation, psychotic ideation, comorbid substance abuse, or unusual responses to or side effects from treatment interventions also suggest the need for such a consultation.

Newer antidepressants that are not SSRIs such as bupropion, venlafaxine, desvenlafaxine, mirtazapine, and duloxetine are less well studied in young patients but may offer additional treatment options. It must be emphasized that the research base remains small, especially in terms of possible long-term consequences of using antidepressants of any type for this age range. Nevertheless, some of the newer agents may be particularly useful when certain comorbidities are present, for example, prescribing bupropion when patients also have attention-deficit/hyperactivity disorder (ADHD) or venlafaxine when anxiety also is present. Venlafaxine has been studied in 3 RCTs that did not show efficacy in nontreatment-resistant pediatric patients; however, venlafaxine was effective in the TORDIA study for treatment-resistant teens[75]; pooled analysis of 2 identical studies did show effectiveness for teens but not for children.[52] Mirtazapine is a serotonin receptor-2 antagonist. Two pediatric RCTs have been conducted, neither of which showed superiority over placebo.[37] In a single, open-label trial with bupropion, adolescents with and without ADHD had reduced depressive symptoms after 2 weeks.[76] Duloxetine is a relatively newly available SNRI for which no RCT with minors exists. **Box 3** provides a summary of available antidepressant medications and the recommended dosing strategies.

GENERAL GUIDELINES FOR ANTIDEPRESSANT USE

The initial phase of pharmacologic management is called the acute phase and consists of the first 6 to 12 weeks, with a goal to achieve remission of symptoms. If a medication trial seems appropriate, dosing generally should start low and build reasonably slowly—a guideline that contradicts the understandable urge to provide

---

Box 3
Antidepressants used to treat depression in children and adolescents

- Selective serotonin reuptake inhibitors

  Fluoxetine (Prozac) 5–60 mg/d[a]

  Escitalopram (Lexapro) 5–20 mg/d[a]

  Sertraline (Zoloft) 25–200 mg/d

  Fluvoxamine (Luvox) 12.5–300 mg/d

  Citalopram (Celexa) 5–40 mg/d

  Paroxetine (Paxil) 5–40 mg/d

- Other antidepressants

  Bupropion (Wellbutrin SR) 37.5–400 mg/d

  Venlafaxine (Effexor XR) 37.5–225 mg/d

  Desvenlafaxine (Pristiq) 50–400 mg/d

  Mirtazapine (Remeron) 15–45 mg/d

  Duloxetine (Cymbalta) 20–60 mg/d

[a] FDA endorsed for depression age ≥8 and ≥12 years old, respectively; available in liquid form.

prompt relief. Raising the dose too quickly enhances the likelihood of side effects that may derail treatment; however, going too slowly may lead the patient and family to grow impatient and terminate care. It must be emphasized that, typically, side effects to antidepressants occur early whereas therapeutic responses are delayed. Clear benefits often occur only after a minimum of 2 to 4 weeks at an adequate dose. Most SSRIs can be raised to therapeutic doses within 1 week, if there are no significant side effects. After 4 to 6 weeks at this dose, response should be assessed for further titration.[77] For those patients with especially severe symptoms or comorbid anxiety, titrating to higher maximum therapeutic doses may be needed. In a secondary study of an RCT with fluoxetine, youth who had not responded to 20 mg were more likely to respond to 40 to 60 mg than to continuation at 20 mg. These results did not achieve significance, due to being underpowered, but suggest aggressive titration for partial responders.[78]

Early side effects may subside over the course of a few weeks. Most research has been conducted as short-term studies and has only looked at efficacy during the acute phase. Meta-analysis of these studies indicates that the benefit of antidepressant use outweighs the risks in this population.[63]

Patients and families almost certainly will want to know how long to continue the medication. For individuals who have responded positively to medication, the general recommendation is to continue at the same dose for 6 to 9 months. This period is known as the continuation phase and is geared to preventing relapse.[36] For individuals at high risk for recurrence (eg, those who have had multiple prior episodes) or have had severe impairment during the previous episode (suicide attempt, poor functioning, prolonged recovery), medication may be continued for 1 to 2 years or longer; this is called the maintenance phase, and the goal is to prevent recurrence. There is increasing evidence derived directly from the pediatric literature to support this extended treatment. One early study found that, despite extended pharmacologic treatment with fluoxetine, relapse rates were high (42% on fluoxetine vs 69.2% on placebo).[79] In a small study, depressed youth who responded to sertraline in acute-phase treatment and did not relapse during 24 weeks of continuation were randomized for 52 weeks to either continued sertraline or placebo; 38% of the teens maintained on sertraline remained well, compared with 0% on placebo.[80]

Discontinuation should be scheduled to minimize disruption and to avoid confusion. For example, it seldom is wise to stop a medication just as a family is preparing for a major move or a student is preparing for an important examination. A slow taper typically is best.

In cases of recurrent severe depression in adults, a life-long course is recommended, though in adolescents a trial off medication may be considered after a significant developmental period; for example, for a prepubertal child a trial off medication in adolescence may be considered. These decisions may be less about age than about changes in the individual's environment that seem likely to be contributory to the problem, or the acquisition of skills that might help increase the individual's coping strategies. In general, the dose needed for acute remission of symptoms is that recommended for maintenance.

If a patient has unacceptable side effects or fails to respond to an adequate dose over a reasonable interval (typically 8–10 weeks), 2 distinct strategies are suggested. The first is switching to an alternative agent; the second is augmenting the first agent (generally reserved for partial responders; 50% reduction in symptoms but not remission). When making a switch for drugs within the same class, it is possible to switch rapidly from one to the other, but a slow taper or cross-taper also works well and is generally preferred.[81]

Support for augmentation draws heavily from the adult literature, including the Sequential Treatment Alternatives to Relieve Depression (STAR*D) trial.[82] Augmentation may involve the addition of a second antidepressant, thyroid hormone, stimulant, buspirone, lithium, or an atypical antipsychotic. Data for teens are quite limited; however, a recent case series of 10 adolescents who had failed treatment with fluoxetine alone did improve with the addition of quetiapine.[83] Lithium may have a role as primary antidepressant in youth who do not respond to standard antidepressants, though this has been evaluated only as augmentation of TCA.[84]

Lithium is effective for both the acute manic and depressive phase of bipolar disorder and for prevention of recurrences. Levels are always done as a "trough," preferably 12 hours after a dose and 5 days after a dose change. The therapy starts at 300 mg per day. The therapeutic window is quite narrow, and toxicity is a major concern, especially in overdose; tolerance changes with marked alteration of fluid and salt intake. Side effects include dermatologic changes, specifically acne, hypothyroidism, tremor, benign leukocytosis, reversible conduction delays (reversible), and diabetes insipidus with associated polyuria and polydypsia.

For a youth with psychotic symptoms, treating the underlying depression may be sufficient; however, adding an antipsychotic may be necessary at least until the mood symptoms are adequately treated. Of the newer antipsychotics, olanzapine and risperidone both have FDA endorsements for use in individuals older than 18 years for mania, and risperidone and aripiprazole have endorsement for younger autistic children with aggressive behaviors. The main concerns for these medications include significant weight gain and metabolic syndromes that include alterations in lipid, cholesterol, and blood glucose levels.

As with all medications prescribed to females of child-bearing age, it is important to educate patients regarding possible effects on the developing fetus if they become pregnant, or are pregnant or breast-feeding. As with any medication, clinicians try to make the best estimate of the relative risks and benefits of treatment or nontreatment and specific treatment interventions, so that the guardian and youth can make an informed decision. The education to the patient should be documented in the medical record to protect the provider in case of a negative outcome as well as document appropriate informed consent from the patient and guardian.

For treatment to succeed, the child or adolescent must come to understand that there is a problem and that it can be altered. In instances in which the patient poses an immediate danger to self or others, it is possible — and may be mandatory — to insist on hospitalization or at least to ensure that the legal guardians and any others who may be threatened are aware of the situation and its attendant risks.

PROGNOSIS

Although depression is apt to remit spontaneously over the course of 6 to 12 months, recurrences are common. In one study, 85% of depressed adolescents had a full remission within 12 months but, of those whose depression had remitted, 40% had another episode of depression within 1 year.[53]

As suggested earlier, a pivotal component to outcome is the extent to which depressive episodes interfere with other developmental tasks. Children and adolescents have much to learn about themselves and the world, and prolonged or repeated interruptions in that learning process can have serious, life-long consequences. This consideration, in addition to alleviating suffering, argues for prompt and vigorous application of effective interventions when depressed young individuals come to clinical attention.

LEGAL ISSUES

In most states, adolescents who are 14 years or older have defined rights with respect to psychiatric treatment, including the right to seek treatment even without parental consent or knowledge and the right of an independent review by a child and adolescent psychiatrist if the adolescent believes hospitalization is inappropriate. Even if that were not the case, clinicians need to remember that they have several clients when working with a depressed child or adolescent; these include the patient, the patient's parents or legal guardians, and possibly the State.

SUMMARY

Depression is now accepted as a common and significant disorder of childhood and adolescence for which effective interventions exist. Primary care physicians should be familiar with the essential features of these disorders to ensure that their patients do not suffer needlessly from their potentially devastating, even fatal, consequences. Clinical signs and symptoms of depression typically are not difficult to elicit, but patients and families may fail to volunteer them unless asked. A growing body of evidence exists to guide clinicians in their choice of treatment interventions. Treatment response to studied interventions is high, though recurrence is common. Given the paucity of child and adolescent psychiatrists, referral may have to be reserved for complicated cases or severe presentations, and consultation used to support the direct provision of care by the primary care provider.

REFERENCES

1. American Psychiatric Association. Diagnostic and statistical manual of mental disorders—3rd Edition revised. 3rd edition. Washington, DC: American Psychiatric Association; 1987.
2. American Psychiatric Association. Diagnostic and statistical manual of mental disorders—4th Edition. 4th edition. Washington, DC: American Psychiatric Association; 2000.
3. Birmaher B, Arbelaez C, Brent DA. Course and outcome of child and adolescent major depressive disorder. Child Adolesc Psychiatr Clin N Am 2002;11:619–38.
4. Costello EJ, Pine DS, Hammen C, et al. Development and natural history of mood disorders. Biol Psychiatry 2002;52:529–42.
5. Hazell P. Depression in children and adolescents. Clin Evid 2004;11:391–402.
6. Lagges AM, Dunn DW. Depression in children and adolescents. Neurol Clin 2003;21:953–60.
7. Elliott GR, Smiga S. Depression in the child and adolescent. Pediatr Clin North Am 2003;50:1093–106.
8. Costello EJ, Foley DL, Angold A. 10-year research update review: the epidemiology of child and adolescent psychiatric disorders: I. Developmental epidemiology. J Am Acad Child Adolesc Psychiatry 2006;45(1):8–25.
9. Kessler RC, Avenevoli S, Ries Merikangas K. Mood disorders in children and adolescents: an epidemiologic perspective. Biol Psychiatry 2001;49(12):1002–14.
10. Besseghini VH. Depression and suicide in children and adolescents. Ann N Y Acad Sci 1997;816:94–8.
11. Compas BE, Oppedisano G, Connor JK, et al. Gender differences in depressive symptoms in adolescence: comparison of national samples of clinically referred and nonreferred youths. J Consult Clin Psychol 1997;65:617–26.

12. Suris JC, Parera N, Puig C. Chronic illness and emotional distress in adolescence. J Adolesc Health 1996;19:153–6.
13. Stewart DE. Physical symptoms of depression: unmet needs in special populations. J Clin Psychiatry 2003;64(Suppl 7):12–6.
14. March JS, Vitiello B. Advances in paediatric neuropsychopharmacology: an overview. Int J Neuropsychopharmacol 2001;4:141–7.
15. Mann JJ, Oquendo M, Underwood MD, et al. The neurobiology of suicide risk: a review for the clinician. J Clin Psychiatry 1999;60(Suppl 2):7–11 [discussion: 18–20, 113–6].
16. Todd R, Botteron KN. Etiology and genetics of early-onset mood disorders. Child Adolesc Psychiatr Clin N Am 2002;11:499–518.
17. Bhangoo RK. Affective neuroscience and the study of normal and abnormal emotion regulation. Child Adolesc Psychiatr Clin N Am 2002;11:519–33.
18. Klein DN, Lewinsohn PM, Rohde P, et al. Psychopathology in the adolescent and young adult offspring of a community sample of mothers and fathers with major depression. Psychol Med 2005;35:353–65.
19. Klein DN, Shankman SA, Lewinsohn PM, et al. Family study of chronic depression in a community sample of young adults. Am J Psychiatry 2004;161:646–53.
20. Williams SB, O'Conor EA, Eder M, et al. Screening for child and adolescent depression in primary care settings: a systematic evidence review for the US Preventive Services Task Force. Pediatrics 2009;123:e716–35.
21. Foy JM, Kelleher KJ, Laraque D, American Academy of Pediatrics Task Force on Mental Health. Enhancing pediatric mental health care: strategies for preparing a primary care practice. Pediatrics 2010;125:S87–108.
22. Committee on Psychosocial Aspects of Child and Family Health and Task Force on Mental Health. Policy statement—the future of pediatrics: mental health competencies for pediatric primary care. Pediatrics 2009;124:410–21.
23. Rohde P, Clarke GN, Lewinsohn PM, et al. Impact of comorbidity on a cognitive-behavioral group treatment for adolescent depression. J Am Acad Child Adolesc Psychiatry 2001;40:795–802.
24. Angold A, Costello EJ, Erkanli A. Comorbidity. J Child Psychol Psychiatry 1999; 40:57–87.
25. Hughes C, Preskorn SH, Weller E, et al. The effect of concomitant disorders in childhood depression on predicting treatment response. Psychopharmacol Bull 1990;26:235–8.
26. Aseltine RH Jr, Gore S, Colten ME. The co-occurrence of depression and substance abuse in late adolescence. Dev Psychopathol 1998;10:549–70.
27. Lewinsohn PM, Pettit JW, Joiner TE Jr, et al. The symptomatic expression of major depressive disorder in adolescents and young adults. J Abnorm Psychol 2003;112:244–52.
28. Strober M, Lampert C, Schmidt S, et al. The course of major depressive disorder in adolescents: I. Recovery and risk of manic switching in a follow-up of psychotic and nonpsychotic subtypes. J Am Acad Child Adolesc Psychiatry 1993;32:34–42.
29. Kovacs M, Akiskal HS, Gatsonis C, et al. Childhood-onset dysthymic disorder. Clinical features and prospective naturalistic outcome. Arch Gen Psychiatry 1994;51:365–74.
30. Cheung AH, Zuckerbrot RA, Jensen PS, et al. Guidelines for Adolescent Depression in Primary Care (GLAD-PC): II. Treatment and ongoing management. Pediatrics 2007;120(5):e1313–26.
31. Olfson M, Gameroff MJ, Marcus SC, et al. Outpatient treatment of child and adolescent depression in the United States. Arch Gen Psychiatry 2003;60: 1236–42.

32. Emslie GJ, Mayes TL, Laptook RS, et al. Predictors of response to treatment in children and adolescents with mood disorders. Psychiatr Clin North Am 2003; 26:435–56.

33. Birhamer B, Brent D, AACAP Work Group on Quality Issues, et al. Practice parameter for the assessment and treatment of children and adolescents with depressive disorders. J Am Acad Child Adolesc Psychiatry 2007;46(11): 1503–26.

34. Hughes CW, Emslie GJ, Crimson ML, et al. Texas Children's Medication Algorithm project: update from Texas Consensus Conference Panel on medication treatment of childhood major depressive disorder. J Am Acad Child Adolesc Psychiatry 2007;46(6):667–86.

35. Zuckerbrot RA, Cheung AH, Jensen PA, et al. Guidelines for Depression in Primary Care (GLAD-PC) I. Identification, assessment, and initial management. Pediatrics 2007;120(5):e1299–312.

36. Practice parameters for the assessment and treatment of children and adolescents with depressive disorders. J Am Acad Child Adolesc Psychiatry 1998; 37(Suppl 10):63S–83S.

37. Emslie GJ, Hughes CW, Crismon ML, et al. A feasibility study of the childhood depression medication algorithm: the Texas Children's Medication Algorithm Project (CMAP). J Am Acad Child Adolesc Psychiatry 2004;43:519–27.

38. March J, Silva S, Petrycki S, et al. Fluoxetine, cognitive-behavioral therapy, and their combination for adolescents with depression: treatment for Adolescents with Depression Study (TADS) randomized controlled trial. JAMA 2004;292:807–20.

39. Brent D, Emslie G, Clarke G, et al. Switching to another SSRI or to venlafaxine with or without cognitive behavioral therapy for adolescents with SSRI-resistant depression: the TORDIA randomized controlled trial. JAMA 2008;299(8):901–13.

40. Cheung A, Emslie GJ, Mayes TL. Review of the efficacy and safety of antidepressants in youth depression. J Child Psychol Psychiatry 2005;46(7):735–54.

41. Ritvo RZ, Papilsky SB. Effectiveness of psychotherapy. Curr Opin Pediatr 1999; 11:323–7.

42. Compton SN, March JS, Brent D, et al. Cognitive-behavioral psychotherapy for anxiety and depressive disorders in children and adolescents: an evidence-based medicine review. J Am Acad Child Adolesc Psychiatry 2004;43:930–59.

43. Weisz JR, Hawley KM, Doss AJ. Empirically tested psychotherapies for youth internalizing and externalizing problems and disorders. Child Adolesc Psychiatr Clin N Am 2004;13:729–815.

44. Brent DA, Kolko DJ, Birmaher B, et al. Predictors of treatment efficacy in clinical trial of three psychosocial treatments for adolescent depression. J Am Acad Child Adolesc Psychiatry 1998;37:906–14.

45. Birmaher B, Brent DA, Kolko D, et al. Clinical outcome after short-term psychotherapy for adolescents with major depressive disorder. Arch Gen Psychiatry 2000;57:29–36.

46. Mufson L, Weissman MM, Moreau D, et al. Efficacy of interpersonal psychotherapy for depressed adolescents. Arch Gen Psychiatry 1999;56:573–9.

47. Gould MS, Greenberg T, Velting DM, et al. Youth suicide risk and preventive interventions: a review of the past 10 years. J Am Acad Child Adolesc Psychiatry 2003;42:386–405.

48. Weiss JR, McCarty CA, Valeri SM. Effects of psychotherapy for depression in children and adolescents: a meta-analysis. Psychol Bull 2006;132(1):132–49.

49. Hazell P, O'Connell D. Tricyclic drugs for depression in children and adolescents. Cochrane Database Syst Rev 2000;3:CD002317.

50. Klein RG, Mannuzza S, Koplewicz HS, et al. Adolescent depression: controlled desipramine treatment and atypical features. Depress Anxiety 1998;7:15–31.
51. Delate T, Gelenberg AJ, Simmons VA, et al. Trends in the use of antidepressants in a national sample of commercially insured pediatric patients, 1998 to 2002. Psychiatr Serv 2004;55:387–91.
52. Emslie GJ, Rush AJ, Weinberg WA, et al. A double-blind, randomized, placebo-controlled trial of fluoxetine in children and adolescents with depression. Arch Gen Psychiatry 1997;54:1031–7.
53. Emslie GJ, Rush AJ, Weinberg WA, et al. Fluoxetine in child and adolescent depression: acute and maintenance treatment. Depress Anxiety 1998;7:32–9.
54. Kastelic EA, Labellarte MJ, Riddle MA. Selective serotonin reuptake inhibitors for children and adolescents. Curr Psychiatry Rep 2000;2:117–23.
55. Baumgartner JL, Emilie GJ, Crimson ML. Citalopram in children and adolescents with depression or anxiety. Ann Pharmacother 2002;11:1692–7.
56. Vaswani M, Linda FK, Ramesh S. Role of selective serotonin reuptake inhibitors in psychiatric disorders: a comprehensive review. Prog Neuropsychopharmacol Biol Psychiatry 2003;27:85–102.
57. Ryan ND. Medication treatment for depression in children and adolescents. CNS Spectr 2003;8:283–7.
58. Wagner KD, Jonas J, Findling RL, et al. A double-blind, randomized, placebo-controlled trial with escitalopram in the treatment of pediatric depression. J Am Acad Child Adolesc Psychiatry 2006;45(3):280–8.
59. Wagner KD, Robb AS, Findling RI, et al. A randomized, placebo controlled trial of citalopram for the treatment of major depression in children and adolescents. Am J Psychiatry 2004;161(6):1079–83.
60. Emslie GJ, Croarkin P, Mayes TL. Antidepressants. In: Dulcan MK, editor. Dulcan's Textbook of Child and Adolescent Psychiatry. Washington, DC: American Psychiatric Publishing; 2009. p. 701–24.
61. Jick H, Kaye JA, Jick SS. Antidepressants and the risk of suicidal behaviors. JAMA 2004;292:338–43.
62. Whittington CJ, Kendall T, Fonagy P, et al. Selective serotonin reuptake inhibitors in childhood depression: systematic review of published versus unpublished data. Lancet 2004;363:1341–5.
63. Bridge JA, Iyengar S, Salary CB, et al. Clinical response and risk for reported suicidal ideation and suicide attempts in pediatric antidepressant treatment: a meta-analysis of randomized controlled trials. JAMA 2007;297(15):1683–96.
64. Wong IC, Besag FM, Santosh PJ, et al. Use of selective serotonin reuptake inhibitors in children and adolescents. Drug Saf 2004;27:991–1000.
65. Morrato EH, Libby AM, Orton HD, et al. Frequency of provider contact after FDA advisory on risk of pediatric suicidality with SSRIs. Am J Psychiatry 2008;165(1):42–50.
66. Gibbons RD, Brown CH, Hur K, et al. Early evidence on the effects of regulators' suicidality warnings on SSRI prescriptions and suicide in children and adolescents. Am J Psychiatry 2007;164(9):1356–63.
67. Pelkonen M, Marttunen M. Child and adolescent suicide: epidemiology, risk factors, and approaches to prevention. Paediatr Drugs 2003;5:243–65.
68. Hatcher-Kay C, King CA. Depression and suicide. Pediatr Rev 2003;24:363–71.
69. Suicide Trends among Youth and Young Adults Aged 10–24 years- United States 1990–2004. MMWR Weekly 2007;56(35):905–8. Available at: http://www.cdc.gov/mmwr/preview/mmwrhtml/mm5635a2.htm. Acceseed October 10, 2010.
70. Oxford handbook of emergency medicine. 3rd edition. p. 609.

71. Greenhill LL, Waslick B. Management of suicidal behavior in children and adolescents. Psychiatr Clin North Am 1997;20:641–66.

72. Kruesi MJ, Grossman J, Pennington JM, et al. Suicide and violence prevention: parent education in the emergency department. J Am Acad Child Adolesc Psychiatry 1999;38:250–5.

73. Biederman J, Mick E, Spencer TJ, et al. Therapeutic dilemmas in the pharmacotherapy of bipolar depression in the young. J Child Adolesc Psychopharmacol 2000;10:185–92.

74. Belpaire HA. Selective serotonin reuptake inhibitors and cytochrome P-450 mediated drug-drug interactions: an update. Curr Drug Metab 2002;3:13–37.

75. Emslie GJ, Findling RL, Yeung PP, et al. Venlafaxine ER for the treatment of pediatric subjects with depression: results from two placebo-controlled trials. J Am Acad Child Adolesc Psychiatry 2007;46(4):479–88.

76. Daviss WB, Bentivoglio P, Racusin R, et al. Bupropion sustained release in adolescent with comorbid attention-deficit/hyperactivity disorder and depression. J Am Acad Child Adolesc Psychiatry 2001;40(X):307–14.

77. Tao R, Emslie G, Mayes T, et al. Early prediction of acute antidepressant treatment response and remission in pediatric major depressive disorders. J Am Acad Child Adolesc Psychiatry 2009;48(1):71–8.

78. Heiligenstein JH, Hoog SL, Wagner KD, et al. Fluoxetine 40–60mg versus fluoxetine 20mg in the treatment of children and adolescents with a less than complete response to nine-week treatment with fluoxetine 10–20mg: a pilot study. J Child Adolesc Psychopharmacol 2006;16(1–2):207–17.

79. Emslie GJ, Kennard BD, Mayes TL, et al. Fluoxetine verses placebo in preventing relapse of major depression in children and adolescents. Am J Psychiatry 2008; 165(4):459–67.

80. Cheung A, Kusumakar V, Kutchner S, et al. Maintenance study for adolescent depression. J Child Adolesc Psychopharmacol 2008;18(4):389–94.

81. Buckley PF, Correll CU. Strategies for dosing and switching antipsychotics for optimal clinical management. J Clin Psychiatry 2008;69(Suppl 1):4–17.

82. Thase ME, Freidman ES, Biggs MM, et al. Cognitive therapy versus medication in augmentation and switch strategies as a second-step treatments: a STAR*D report. Am J Psychiatry 2007;164(5):739–52.

83. Pathak S, Johns ES, Kowatch RA. Adjunctive quetiapine for treatment-resistant adolescent major depressive disorder: a case series. J Child Adolesc Psychopharmacol 2005;15(4):696–702.

84. Carvalho AF, Machado JR, Cavalcante JL. Augmentation strategies for treatment-resistant depression. Curr Opin Psychiatry 2009;22(1):7–12.

Psychopharmacology of Pediatric Bipolar Disorders in Children and Adolescents

Tiffany Thomas, MD*, Libbie Stansifer, MD, Robert L. Findling, MD

KEYWORDS

- Pediatric bipolar disorder • Pharmacotherapy • Treatment
- Lithium • Anticonvulsants • Atypical antipsychotics

Pediatric bipolar disorder (PBD) is a chronic and disabling illness leading to serious disruption in the lives of children and adolescents with this condition.[1] Children and adolescents diagnosed with the condition experience significantly higher rates of morbidity and mortality compared with otherwise healthy children, including reduction in quality of life[2]; impairment in social, familial, and academic functioning[3]; and alarmingly high rates of suicidal ideation and behavior.[4] Recent years have shown a dramatic increase in the frequency of diagnosis of PBD, with a 40-fold increase in the number of the youth diagnosed with the disorder between 1994 and 2003, demonstrated in a national survey of office-based physicians.[5] Once considered an adult-onset illness, retrospective data indicate that most adults with bipolar disorder (BD) first showed symptoms during childhood or adolescence.[6] Pediatricians, who are likely to face the task of initial recognition and management of the youth with BD, play a crucial role in ensuring a successful outcome for youngsters with this condition.

The first step in treating children and adolescents with BD is making an accurate diagnosis. Even for the experienced child and adolescent psychiatrist, this step is often a complex clinical task for several reasons. Even as the diagnostic validity, phenomenology, and course of PBD remain active research endeavors, developmental differences in the presentation between the youth and adults have been established. Although adults exhibit distinct episodes of depression and mania, the pattern

Disclosures: Dr Findling receives or has received research support, acted as a consultant, and/or served on a speaker's bureau for Abbott, Addrenex, AstraZeneca, Biovail, Bristol-Myers Squibb, Forest, GlaxoSmithKline, Johnson & Johnson, KemPharm Lilly, Lundbeck, Neuropharm, Novartis, Organon, Otsuka, Pfizer, Sanofi-Aventis, Sepracore, Shire, Solvay, Supernus Pharmaceuticals, Validus, and Wyeth.
Division of Child and Adolescent Psychiatry, University Hospitals Case Medical Center, 10524 Euclid Avenue, Cleveland, OH 44106-5080, USA
* Corresponding author.
E-mail address: Tiffany.Thomas2@UHhospitals.org

Pediatr Clin N Am 58 (2011) 173–187
doi:10.1016/j.pcl.2010.10.001
0031-3955/11/$ – see front matter. Published by Elsevier Inc.

pediatric.theclinics.com

of illness observed in young people is often characterized by mixed or dysphoric mood states accompanied by irritability.[7] Furthermore, compared with adults, children and adolescents exhibit fewer distinct episodes, higher rates of mood switching, and fewer symptom-free intervals.[7,8] Adding to the challenge of diagnosis is the presence of additional psychiatric disorders in most patients with PBD, which is most frequently attention-deficit/hyperactivity disorder (ADHD).[9] Several symptoms of BD overlap with those of other psychiatric disorders, ADHD in particular, making it oftentimes difficult to distinguish among them. Research clarifying the expression of BD in children and adolescents is needed to facilitate early and accurate diagnosis of the condition by clinicians.

Pharmacotherapy is regarded as an essential component of treatment in PBD.[10] Historically, treatment strategies have been extrapolated from the adult literature. However, research in the treatment of psychiatric disorders has repeatedly shown that one cannot assume medications effective in treating adults are similarly effective in treating children and adolescents. Although far less is known about evidence-based treatments for pediatric versus adult BD, data to support interventions are rapidly emerging. Although PBD is considered to represent a spectrum of illness, encompassing bipolar I, bipolar II, cyclothymia, and BD not otherwise specified (NOS), the literature has largely focused on the management of acute manic and mixed states occurring in narrowly defined bipolar I. Less attention has been devoted to maintenance strategies to prevent symptom recurrence as well as to the treatment of less-classic illness phenotypes (such as BD II and BD NOS) and the depressive phase of illness. Furthermore, there is a paucity of data to guide interventions in psychiatric comorbidities of PBD and the management of the youth who are depressed and are genetically at risk for BD. The long-term safety and efficacy for agents used to treat juvenile BD is yet to be established.

Amid the challenge of recognizing and managing BD in children and adolescents, it is evident that the youth require prompt treatment to ameliorate symptoms and to prevent or reduce the psychosocial morbidity that accompanies the illness. Moreover, the probability of recovery lessens with earlier onset and longer duration of illness, further emphasizing the importance of early detection and treatment.[1] Although optimal treatment uses a comprehensive approach consisting of pharmacotherapy, psychotherapy, and psychosocial interventions,[10] this article is limited to a review of available data regarding the pharmacologic management of PBD. This article summarizes the extant literature of published studies for the treatment of manic, mixed, and depressive illness phases occurring in children and adolescents with BD as well as what is known about maintenance treatment in this population. In addition, this article reviews safety and monitoring concerns for each medication and offers practical suggestions for pediatricians initiating pharmacotherapy.

ACUTE TREATMENT OF MANIC OR MIXED STATES

Recent data suggest that children and adolescents with BD most commonly experience the manic and mixed states of the condition. Accordingly, much of the available evidence pertaining to the pharmacotherapy of PBD focuses on these illness phases.

LITHIUM

Lithium is the prototype mood stabilizer used in the treatment of mania in adults. Furthermore, lithium was the first medication approved by the United States Food and Drug Administration (FDA) for treating BD in children and adolescents who are 12 years and older. Nevertheless, this indication was based on the effectiveness of lithium among adults. Although a relatively large number of publications have considered the treatment of PBD with lithium, only a small number of studies were prospective clinical trials of methodological rigor.[11] For that reason, definitive testing of lithium treatment in the youth with BD, described later, is underway.

Multiple open-label trials have shown the favorable acute effect of lithium on symptoms occurring in the manic or mixed states of PBD. However, it has been repeatedly observed that although many patients benefit from lithium monotherapy, a substantive number of young patients do not achieve full symptom remission when lithium alone is prescribed.[12] Several clinical factors have been reported to predict poor response to lithium treatment in PBD, including prepubertal illness onset and the presence of comorbid ADHD, substance abuse, conduct disorder, and personality disorder. Furthermore, mixed manic episodes and rapid cycling, which are commonly seen in adolescents, may elicit an inadequate response to lithium treatment.[13]

A study funded by the National Institute of Mental Health (NIMH) conducted a double-blind comparison of lithium, divalproex, and placebo in the acute treatment of mixed or manic episodes occurring in the youth with bipolar I disorder. About 153 participants aged 7 to 17 years were randomized to receive lithium, divalproex, or placebo over an 8-week period. At study completion, divalproex was found to be superior to placebo on the study's primary outcome measures. In contrast, although there was a definitive trend toward efficacy, there were no differences in the results between the use of lithium and placebo.[14]

Despite a lack of methodologically stringent trials, lithium seems to be generally safe and effective in treating acute mixed and manic states in pediatric patients. Accordingly, definitive studies pertaining to the use of lithium in those with PBD (the Collaborative Lithium Trials [CoLT]) are currently in progress under the auspices of the National Institute of Child Health and Human Development funding.[15,16] The multidisciplinary CoLT trials provide data to establish evidence-based dosing strategies for lithium, describe the pharmacokinetics of lithium and biodisposition in the youth, examine the acute and long-term efficacy of lithium in pediatric bipolarity, and characterize the short- and long-term safety of lithium treatment.

ANTICONVULSANTS

Several medications originally marketed as anticonvulsants have been shown to be beneficial in treating BD in adults. As a result, it was believed that these medications may also have mood-stabilizing properties in the pediatric population. The following sections summarize what is known about this class of medications in PBD.

Carbamazepine

Although there is evidence in support of carbamazepine in the treatment of adults with mania, there are limited data regarding the safety and efficacy of this drug in younger patients. In one open-label study, participants randomized to 6 weeks of treatment with lithium, divalproex, or carbamazepine demonstrated clinically meaningful benefit in all 3 treatment groups. Furthermore, carbamazepine was reasonably well tolerated without serious adverse events.[17] A few case reports have suggested that carbamazepine may be effective in adolescents with mania who have not responded to lithium. However, on a cautionary note, there have also been case reports suggesting carbamazepine may actually worsen mania. In addition, owing to the induction of the hepatic P450 isoenzyme system by carbamazepine, there may be clinically significant drug-drug interactions that make the clinical use of this drug difficult.

Sodium Divalproex

Sodium divalproex has demonstrated efficacy in the treatment of adults with acute mania. However, much of the data pertaining to its use in PBD are from case reports. One randomized, double-blind, industry-sponsored study investigating the use of divalproex extended-release in 150 youth with BD found no statistically significant improvement in acute manic symptoms when compared with placebo.[18] However, as mentioned earlier, a randomized, double-blind, NIMH-supported trial investigating 153 youths found that divalproex was superior to placebo for treating children and adolescents with BD during a mixed or manic episode.[14] The discrepant results of these 2 studies may be explained by factors related to between-site variability. The NIMH-supported study was conducted at substantively fewer sites than the industry-supported trial. Supporting evidence for divalproex in acute mania is expanded by combination pharmacotherapy studies, suggesting that divalproex may be beneficial when coadministered with lithium, quetiapine, or risperidone.[19]

Topiramate

Preliminary data have indicated that topiramate may be effective for PBD. However, a double-blind placebo-controlled pilot investigation of topiramate for mania in PBD was discontinued prematurely when adult mania trials with topiramate failed to show efficacy. When these preliminary data were analyzed from the pediatric study, it was found that topiramate might have proven beneficial should the study have continued.[20]

Oxcarbazepine

One randomized, double-blind, placebo-controlled study investigated the use of oxcarbazepine versus placebo in 116 youths with BD. The investigators found that the results of the treatment with oxcarbazepine were not different from the results of placebo. As a result, there is no evidence to support the use of oxcarbazepine as monotherapy in the treatment of the manic phase of PBD.[21]

Gabapentin

Gabapentin has not been found to be effective for the treatment of BD in adults, and there is currently no evidence to support its use in the treatment of PBD.[22] Furthermore, gabapentin has been reported to cause behavioral disinhibition in younger children.[23]

Lamotrigine

Lamotrigine is indicated for the maintenance treatment of adults with BD to delay the time of occurrence of mood episodes (depression, mania, hypomania, mixed episodes). The effectiveness of lamotrigine in the acute management of mood episodes in adults has not been established. Open-label studies indicate that lamotrigine may be beneficial for adolescents with bipolar, manic, or mixed states,[24] although randomized controlled trials are still needed.

ANTIPSYCHOTICS

The class of medications that has the best data to support their use in the acute treatment of PBD is the atypical antipsychotics. However, as with adults, the possible metabolic complications of these drugs are important considerations, particularly over the long term. However, limited information is available about the long-term effects of these agents in children and adolescents. In addition, there are no methodologically stringent studies that have specifically compared the safety and efficacy of one atypical to another. Moreover, there are almost no data about the use of typical antipsychotics, such as haloperidol, in this patient population.

Risperidone

Risperidone, either as monotherapy or in combination with a mood stabilizer, has been reported to be effective in the treatment of PBD in case reports and open-label studies. In addition, risperidone was the first atypical antipsychotic approved by the FDA for the treatment of acute mania or mixed episodes associated with bipolar I disorder in children and adolescents in the ages of 10 to 17 years. One randomized placebo-controlled study of youth with BD found that risperidone was efficacious and relatively well tolerated at doses as low as 0.5 to 2.5 mg/d in the acute treatment of manic or mixed episodes in children and adolescents in the ages of 10 to 17 years.[25]

Olanzapine

Olanzapine is FDA approved for the acute treatment of manic or mixed episodes associated with bipolar I disorder in adolescents in the ages of 13 to 17 years. Several studies have reported the efficacy of olanzapine for the treatment of PBD. In one recent randomized placebo-controlled trial, 161 adolescents with an acute manic or mixed episode received either olanzapine (2.5–20 mg/d) or placebo in a double-blind manner. Although olanzapine demonstrated superiority over placebo, the youth treated with olanzapine had significantly greater weight gain (3.7 kg vs 0.3 kg) over the course of the 3-week trial. Furthermore, olanzapine-treated youth showed significantly greater changes in prolactin, fasting glucose, fasting total cholesterol, uric acid, and the hepatic enzymes aspartate transaminase and alanine transaminase levels.[26] Ultimately, the benefits of olanzapine for the treatment of PBD should be considered within the context of its safety profile and may lead clinicians to consider prescribing other medications first in this patient population.

Quetiapine

Quetiapine was one of the first atypical antipsychotics to be investigated in a double-blind placebo-controlled study design for the treatment of mania in adolescents. One study found that combination therapy with quetiapine and divalproex was more effective than divalproex and placebo in the acute treatment of adolescents with manic or mixed episodes.[27] An additional randomized placebo-controlled study of 277 participants, in the ages of 10 to 17 years, concluded that quetiapine, at doses of 400 and 600 mg/d, was more effective than placebo in treating acute manic symptoms in children and adolescents with BD.[28] The FDA has approved quetiapine for the acute treatment of manic episodes in pediatric patients in the ages of 10 to 17 years with bipolar I disorder.

Ziprasidone

Ziprasidone has been shown to be effective in treating mania in adults. Moreover, ziprasidone is typically associated with less weight gain than risperidone and olanzapine. One randomized, double-blind, placebo-controlled study of 238 youth with BD in the ages of 10 to 17 years found that ziprasidone at doses of 80 to 160 mg/d was effective and generally well tolerated for the treatment of mania in children and adolescents.[29] However, the United States FDA has thus far declined to approve ziprasidone for treating PBD. In April 2010, the FDA cited the drugmaker, Pfizer, for failing to properly ensure monitoring of its study investigating the use of ziprasidone in patients with PBD. The FDA reported that as a result of inadequate monitoring, widespread overdosing of patients at multiple study sites was neither detected nor corrected in a timely manner.[30]

Aripiprazole

Aripiprazole is indicated by the FDA for the acute and maintenance treatment of manic and mixed episodes associated with bipolar I disorder in pediatric patients in the ages of 10 to 17 years. One randomized, double-blind, placebo-controlled study of 296 youths in the ages of 10 to 17 years with bipolar I disorder has shown that aripiprazole, at doses of 10 and 30 mg, is superior to placebo in the acute treatment of manic and mixed episodes.[31]

Clozapine

Open trials and case reports have suggested that clozapine may be beneficial in the treatment of pediatric patients with BD who have not shown adequate response to other agents.[32] However, the side effect profile of clozapine, which may include sedation, considerable weight gain, increased salivation, seizures, myocarditis, as well as potentially lethal agranulocytosis, limits the use of this medication. For these reasons, clozapine is generally recommended only for highly treatment-resistant youth.

MAINTENANCE TREATMENT

PBD is characterized by a chronic and relapsing course, often necessitating long-term treatment. Although several evidence-based options exist for the maintenance treatment of adult BD, limited data are available to guide clinicians in optimal maintenance pharmacotherapy in younger populations.

As mentioned earlier, lithium is a mainstay in the maintenance treatment of adult BD. Kafantaris and colleagues[33] used a discontinuation study design to evaluate the efficacy of lithium in the treatment of mania in adolescents. About 40 children and adolescents in the ages of 12 to 18 years who responded to open-label treatment with lithium (mean serum lithium level 0.99 mEq/L) for up to 4 weeks were randomly assigned to continue or discontinue lithium in a 2-week, double-blind, placebo-controlled phase. Investigators found that although 57.5% of participants experienced a clinically significant symptom exacerbation during the 2-week double-blind phase, the rate of exacerbation did not differ between the 2 treatment groups. However, investigators noted that the rate of symptom relapse, which was higher and more rapid than expected, observed in subjects who continued lithium use may have been because of the relatively short stabilization period of the study; a longer period of open-label treatment may have been required to demonstrate lithium's superiority for symptom prevention during the discontinuation phase.

An 18-month trial compared divalproex and lithium as maintenance monotherapy in children and adolescents with bipolar disoprder.[34] About 60 youths in the ages of 5 to 17 years who had achieved 4 consecutive weeks of symptom remission during open-label combination therapy with divalproex and lithium were randomized to receive either drug as monotherapy in a double-blind fashion. Results demonstrated a median survival time before symptom return of 114 and 112 days for subjects randomized to lithium and divalproex, respectively, suggesting that these agents are equally effective in maintaining mood stability. The investigators also noted that concomitant treatment of comorbid ADHD with stimulant medication was not associated with earlier time to relapse.

Another study evaluated the long-term efficacy of aripiprazole in the treatment of pediatric bipolar mania. Children and adolescents in the ages of 10 to 17 years

(296 total) were randomized to receive 10 mg of aripiprazole, 30 mg of aripiprazole, or placebo in a 4-week double-blind trial. Subjects then continued their randomly assigned treatments in a 26-week extension phase. Both doses of aripiprazole were found to be superior to placebo at 4 weeks and study completion at 30 weeks.[35] Safety and tolerability data demonstrated that adverse events, which were mild to moderate in general, appeared to be dose related.[36] No clinically significant weight gain or change in serum lipids or glucose was observed in any treatment arm.

There is insufficient evidence available regarding maintenance pharmacotherapy strategies in the youth with BD. Further work is needed to identify safe and effective agents for this purpose and to determine optimal duration of therapy.

TREATMENT OF PEDIATRIC BIPOLAR DEPRESSION

Adults with BD have been shown to spend most of their symptomatic time in the depressed phase of illness[37]; however, less is known about the course and prevalence of depression in PBD. Nonetheless, it is evident that children and adolescents with BD experience depressive symptoms and episodes.[38] Unfortunately, evidence-based treatment options for the youth with depression and bipolar illness are limited.

Earlier studies have supported the use of lithium for the management of adults in the depressed phase of bipolar illness. To evaluate lithium's efficacy in treating acute depression in younger patients with BD, a 6-week open-label investigation was conducted by Patel and colleagues.[39] About 27 participants in the ages of 12 to 18 years received lithium adjusted to achieve a therapeutic serum level of 1.0 to 1.2 mEq/L. At the conclusion of the trial, lithium was associated with statistically significant improvements in response and remission based on the outcome measures of the trial. The most commonly reported adverse events were headache (74%) and nausea/vomiting (67%), and these were generally mild to moderate in severity. This study indicates that lithium may be a useful acute treatment for the youth with depression and BD, but placebo-controlled studies are needed.

Lamotrigine has emerged as a first-line agent in the long-term treatment of bipolar depression in adults. Chang and colleagues[40] evaluated the effectiveness of lamotrigine as an adjunctive or monotherapy for the treatment of pediatric bipolar depression in an 8-week open-label trial involving 20 children and adolescents in the ages of 12 to 17 years. Findings included statistically significant improvement in depressive symptoms, with 63% of participants considered to be treatment responders. No significant weight change and rash or other adverse events were reported. Controlled trials are needed to clarify the role of lamotrigine in treating bipolar depression in the pediatric population.

Quetiapine, which has strong evidence supporting its use in adult bipolar depression, was investigated by DelBello and colleagues[41] in the first published double-blind controlled study on the treatment of bipolar depression in adolescents. Around 32 subjects in the ages of 12 to 18 years were randomized to receive quetiapine (dose range 300–600 mg/d) or placebo over an 8-week period. Contrary to findings among adult patients, neither was quetiapine superior to placebo in treating depressive symptoms as defined by the trial's primary outcome measure nor did it significantly differ from placebo in overall response rate (placebo, 67%; quetiapine, 71%). However, controlled pharmacotherapy trials for pediatric unipolar depression have repeatedly shown that subjects commonly respond to placebo and that the magnitude of placebo response may contribute to a lack of demonstrated treatment effect.[42] Similarly, the high rate of placebo response observed in this study may have played a role in its failure to demonstrate the superiority of quetiapine to placebo. Furthermore, findings illustrate the importance for age-specific treatment studies in individuals with BD.

The role of antidepressants for the treatment of depressive symptoms occurring in the youth with BD has not been established. There are currently no published prospective trials on antidepressant therapy in those with PBD. Antidepressant-induced mania is a well-recognized phenomenon in adults with BD; however, the potential mood-destabilizing effects of antidepressants are less clear in children and adolescents.[43] Consequently, treatment recommendations have generally advised to avoid antidepressant monotherapy in the youth with BD.[44]

The number of studies investigating the treatment of depression in those with PBD is limited. The few open-label studies of established pharmacotherapies for adults in the depressed phase of bipolar illness show promise for treating adolescents, but more methodologically stringent studies are needed to confirm this finding. The only published double-blind study in this population failed to show quetiapine's superiority when compared with placebo. The efficacy and safety of treating pediatric bipolar depression with antidepressants has not been established. In short, evidence-based information about how best to treat the youth with BD is lacking.

TREATMENT OF PSYCHIATRIC COMORBID DISORDERS

Pediatric bipolar illness rarely occurs in the absence of comorbid psychiatric disorders. Comorbid conditions complicate the management of PBD and seem to worsen the prognosis. Of these, ADHD is the most common psychiatric comorbidity in the youth with BD. Up to 90% of prepubertal children and 30% to 50% of adolescents with BD have ADHD.[45] Other disorders occurring less frequently with pediatric BD include oppositional defiant disorder (53%), conduct disorder (19%), anxiety disorders (38%), substance use disorders (40%), and pervasive developmental disorders (11%).[9] Unfortunately, there are few controlled studies regarding the treatment of comorbid conditions occurring in young persons with BD. Clinical trials that have considered interventions in this patient population have been limited to those diagnosed with either concomitant ADHD or substance abuse.

ADHD

In one study examining the treatment of PBD with co-occuring ADHD, 40 patients (ages 6–17 years) treated with open-label divalproex were randomized to receive mixed amphetamine salts (MASs) or placebo.[46] The investigators found that treatment with MAS was superior to placebo in the reduction of ADHD symptoms. Furthermore, worsening of manic symptoms did not occur with MAS coadministration.

Another study investigated the short-term efficacy of methylphenidate in 16 youths with bipolar illness who were euthymic on at least 1 mood stabilizer but continued to experience clinically significant symptoms of comorbid ADHD. While maintaining their mood-stabilizing medication, participants received 1 week each of placebo, 5 mg methylphenidate twice daily, 10 mg methylphenidate twice daily, and 15 mg methylphenidate twice daily in a crossover design. Findings demonstrated that treatment with methylphenidate was superior to placebo in treating ADHD symptoms, and its administration was not associated with mood destabilization.[47]

These studies provide preliminary evidence to support the use of adjunctive psychostimulants for treating ADHD in the youth with bipolar illness who are already receiving mood stabilizers.

Substance Abuse

Co-occuring substance use disorders are common among the youth with bipolar illness, particularly if the onset of PBD occurs during adolescence.[9] In one study examining the treatment of BD and comorbid substance abuse, 25 teenagers were randomly assigned to lithium or placebo for up to 6 weeks.[48] Investigators found that lithium was superior to placebo with a significantly greater reduction in substance abuse and improvement in overall function.

MEDICATION ADVERSE EFFECTS AND MONITORING

Although some atypical antipsychotics and traditional mood stabilizers have emerging data supporting their efficacy in treating PBD, many are associated with side effects that require careful monitoring. In addition, long-term safety for these agents has not been established in children or adolescents.

Lithium

The same therapeutic levels of lithium used for treating adult patients (0.6–1.2 mEq/L) have been recommended for treating children and adolescents because definitive youth-specific data to guide dosing are lacking. A possible approach to reaching the target blood level of 0.6 to 1.2 mEq/L is to initiate lithium at the lesser of 20 mg/kg/d or 900 mg/d, divided into 2 or 3 daily doses, followed by gradual increases moderated by consideration of the patient's clinical response to the medication and reported side effects.[11]

Lithium's narrow therapeutic window calls for meticulous attention to safety and side-effect concerns. Early signs of lithium toxicity include ataxia, dysarthria, and reduced motor coordination. At levels substantially above the therapeutic window, severe toxicity can result in seizures, coma, or even death. Monitoring serum lithium levels is important to reduce the risk of toxicity. Frequent monitoring is recommended when dose adjustments are made. Once a therapeutic level has been achieved on a stable dose for 3 consecutive months, lithium levels should generally be checked every 3 months.[11]

The well-known side effects of lithium among adults may also occur in children and adolescents. Although it has been asserted that younger children may be more vulnerable to lithium-related side effects than older adolescents, this assertion has not been definitively confirmed.[49,50] Common side effects associated with lithium use include nausea, abdominal pain, sedation, diarrhea, polyuria, polydipsia, tremor, acne, hypothyroidism, and weight gain. Long-term treatment may also result in nephrogenic diabetes insipidus. Baseline laboratory examination should include serum electrolytes level tests, renal function tests, thyroid function tests, and complete blood cell count. In addition, because lithium may adversely affect renal tubular function secondary to a deficit in urine concentrating ability, renal function tests should be checked every 2 to 3 months during the first 6 months of treatment and every 6 months thereafter. Because of lithium's effect on the thyroid gland, thyroid function should be monitored every 6 months. A negative pregnancy test result should be verified before initiating treatment because of lithium's association with cardiac malformations, including Ebstein anomaly, in infants exposed during the first trimester.[12] Lithium is associated with cardiac side effects ranging from benign T-wave flattening to more serious conduction disturbances, such as tachycardia and/or sinoatrial block. Although serious lithium-induced cardiac side effects appear to be rare in the youth without pre-existing cardiac disease, it is generally recommended that an electrocardiogram (ECG) is obtained at baseline after a few months of treatment and yearly thereafter.[11]

Anticonvulsants

Many of the anticonvulsants have adverse effects in children and adolescents who require careful monitoring. Common side effects of divalproex in children are weight gain, nausea, sedation, and tremor. Less commonly, pancreatitis, thrombocytopenia, alopecia, weight gain, and hepatic failure may occur. In addition, there is some debate regarding the relationship between divalproex and the development of polycystic ovarian syndrome (PCOS) in girls. Therefore, it is recommended that clinicians monitor female patients treated with divalproex for signs of PCOS, including weight gain, menstrual abnormalities, hirsutism, or acne.[51] Key side effects of topiramate include anorexia, weight loss, and sedation. In addition, paresthesia, metabolic acidosis, word-finding difficulties, and glaucoma have been reported. Although there are no methodologically rigorous data on this topic, some clinicians appear to use the weight loss properties of topiramate as an adjunctive treatment in the youth with BD who have gained weight as a result of treatment with other psychotropic agents.[51] Carbamazepine has been associated with agranulocytosis, aplastic anemia, hepatotoxicity, hyponatremia, and dermatologic reactions, such as Stevens-Johnson syndrome. As mentioned earlier, induction of the hepatic P450 isoenzyme system by carbamazepine may lead to clinically significant drug-drug interactions by accelerating the metabolism of several medications, including oral contraceptives and many anticonvulsants. In addition, because carbamazepine induces its own metabolism, stable concentrations usually occur 3 to 5 weeks after achieving a fixed dose.[52] Lamotrigine carries the risk of potentially lethal cutaneous reactions such as Stevens-Johnson syndrome and toxic epidermal necrolysis. Compared with adults, this risk is greater in the youth younger than 16 years. Dosing guidelines using a more conservative dose titration may lower the risk of such serious rashes.[51] Many of the anticonvulsants may pose a risk of fetal harm if administered to pregnant women. Therefore, it is recommended that women of child-bearing age undergo pregnancy testing before treatment onset, be regularly advised of their teratogenic effects, and be referred for concurrent contraceptive use as clinically indicated.[52]

Atypical Antipsychotics

Despite their efficacy, atypical antipsychotics are commonly associated with untoward side effects. For many of these medications, weight gain has emerged as one of the most common and concerning adverse effects. As a result of weight gain, metabolic problems, including type 2 (noninsulin dependent) diabetes and elevations in serum lipids and hepatic transaminases levels, may occur. Children who experience significant weight gain should be monitored closely for these complications and should be referred for exercise and nutrition counseling.[13] In collaboration with the American Diabetes Association, the American Psychiatric Association developed a monitoring protocol for patients receiving treatment with an atypical antipsychotic medication.[53] This protocol recommends obtaining the following baseline parameters before initiating an atypical antipsychotic agent: (1) a personal and family history of obesity, diabetes, dyslipidemia, hypertension, or cardiovascular disease; (2) weight, height, and body mass index; (3) waist circumference; (4) blood pressure; (5) fasting plasma glucose; and (6) fasting lipid profile. Guidelines also recommend that weight should be reassessed at 4, 8, and 12 weeks after initiating or changing therapy with an atypical antipsychotic agent and every 3 months thereafter. If there is an increase of initial weight of more than 5%, an alternative agent should be substituted. Of note, these guidelines were not specifically designed for pediatric patients; therefore, the 5% weight gain limit may not be valid for this younger population.

In addition to weight gain and metabolic complications, atypical antipsychotics may cause hyperprolactinemia, QTc changes, extrapyramidal symptoms (EPS), and tardive dyskinesia (TD). Ziprasidone in particular has been associated with QTc prolongation in children and adolescents and should therefore be used with caution. It is recommended that an ECG be obtained at baseline and with significant increases in dosage.[54] Clozapine's side effect profile, which may include sedation, weight gain, increased salivation, seizures, myocarditis, as well as potentially lethal agranulocytosis, limits the usage of this medication. Extrapyramidal symptoms, although rare, have been reported in children and adolescents taking atypical antipsychotics and most commonly include parkinsonism and akathisia. Benztropine and diphenhydramine may be useful for managing EPS, whereas propranolol may be effective for treating akathisia. To minimize the risk of TD, the lowest effective dose of an atypical antipsychotic should be used. In addition, patients should be monitored for abnormal involuntary movements using a standardized instrument such as the Abnormal Involuntary Movement Scale.

PRACTICAL SUGGESTIONS FOR INITIATING PHARMACOTHERAPY

Drawing on recently published expert consensus guidelines and practice parameters,[10,44] the aim of this section is to summarize practical evidence-based strategies for pediatricians faced with treating bipolar illness. Although the literature has expanded since these recommendations were published, particularly for the use of atypical antipsychotics, they continue to provide a useful framework for initial treatment decisions. Key recommendations, incorporating new evidence where relevant, are summarized.

The recommended first-line treatment for bipolar I acute manic or mixed episodes without psychosis is monotherapy with lithium, divalproex, or an atypical antipsychotic that has been FDA approved for pediatric use. Patients failing to respond should receive monotherapy with a medication from a different class, whereas those exhibiting partial response should receive augmentation with a second medication from a different class. For presentations accompanied by psychosis, initial combination therapy with lithium or divalproex and an atypical antipsychotic is suggested. A minimum of 4 to 6 weeks at therapeutic blood levels and/or adequate dose for each medication trial is recommended before determining the effectiveness of each regimen.

When guidelines were written, lithium was the only medication with an FDA indication for the treatment of BD in young people. After publication, 4 additional medications, all atypical antipsychotics, have received FDA approval for the acute treatment of manic or mixed episodes occurring in pediatric bipolar I disorder. As stated earlier, aripiprazole, quetiapine, and risperidone are indicated for the youth who are 10 years and older, and olanzapine is indicated for adolescents older than 13 years. Notably, many of the atypical antipsychotic treatment trials compared 2 medication doses (or dose ranges) with placebo; in these cases, the lower doses used were as efficacious as higher doses but with fewer side effects. Although these atypical antipsychotic medications have received an FDA indication for the short-term treatment of PBD, it is worth emphasizing that the safety and effectiveness of prolonged treatment with these agents remain pressing research questions.

In cases of comorbid psychiatric disorders, it is recommended that pharmacotherapy targeting mood stabilization should take priority over treating the associated comorbidities. Once mood stabilization has been achieved, other disorders should be addressed with the best available treatment strategies. Concomitant ADHD may be cautiously treated with stimulant medication once adequate mood stabilization therapy is in place.

With limited data to inform long-term pharmacotherapy strategies for the prevention of symptom relapse, experts have generally suggested that medications helping patients to achieve symptom remission seem to be the most likely to keep them well. Although there is no body of evidence to guide pharmacotherapy duration, it is suggested that gradual medication discontinuation be considered in patients who have achieved remission for a minimum of 12 to 24 months. It is advised that medication discontinuation be undertaken with greater caution in patients with a history of suicidal behavior, severe aggression, and/or psychotic symptoms. Some youth require lifelong pharmacotherapy, necessitating an ongoing discussion of the risks and benefits of long-term treatment.

As is the case for maintenance pharmacotherapy, the evidence base for treating acute depression occurring in the youth with BD is scarce. The only controlled trial that has been conducted in this population to date failed to show a difference between quetiapine and placebo. Less-stringent open-label studies of lithium and lamotrigine, on the other hand, have shown potential. Suggested treatment options include either lithium or adjunctive treatment with an antidepressant after adequate mood stabilization. Nonetheless, the need for more methodologically stringent investigation of these agents remains.

In addition to evidence for efficacy, phase of illness, and the presence of comorbid conditions, treatment selection should be guided by several other principles. The side-effect spectrum and safety profile for each medication should be considered with regard to each patient's presentation, including medical and family history (for instance, an overweight child with a strong family history of type 2 diabetes may be most appropriately treated with an agent having evidence for a lower propensity for weight gain). Agent monitoring requirements should be reviewed with families, and potential barriers to adequate monitoring should be considered. Previous response to a given medication in patients' parents may provide valuable information, both regarding likelihood of treatment response and patient and family preferences. Developmental differences in pharmacokinetics may have important consequences on both medication dosing and side effect burden. Therefore, age-appropriate dosing strategies, with regard to both size and interval, are crucial. Ultimately, treatment selection should be a collaborative decision between the provider and the patient, tailored to the clinical situation and based on the best available evidence.

SUMMARY

PBD is a serious and debilitating illness associated with significant morbidity and mortality. Once considered a condition primarily affecting adults, it is now evident that its onset most commonly occurs during childhood or adolescence. Prompt treatment is crucial for the prevention of long-term morbidity. Historically, treatment schemes have been predicated on strategies shown to be effective in treating adults; however, developmental differences in treatment response among children and adults are now well recognized. Evidence has rapidly emerged in support of some pharmacologic interventions for the acute manic and mixed states of PBD, particularly in the case of atypical antipsychotics; however, data concerning the safety and efficacy of long-term use of these medications are critically needed. On the contrary, evidence informing the management of pediatric bipolar depression, treatment of psychiatric comorbidity, and interventions for symptomatic genetically at-risk youth is, for the most part, lacking. With research underway to investigate all aspects of treating

PBD, clinicians encountering this illness may someday have access to adequate methodologically stringent data to guide them in best caring for their patients.

REFERENCES

1. Birmaher B, Axelson D, Goldstein B. Four-year longitudinal course of children and adolescents with bipolar spectrum disorders: the Course and Outcome of Bipolar Youth (COBY) Study. Am J Psychiatry 2009;166:795–804.
2. Freeman AJ, Youngstrom EA, Michalak E, et al. Quality of life in pediatric bipolar disorder. Pediatrics 2009;123:e446–52.
3. Goldstein TR, Birmaher B, Axelson D, et al. Psychosocial functioning among bipolar youth. J Affect Disord 2009;114(1–3):174–83.
4. Goldstein TR. Suicidality in pediatric bipolar disorder. Child Adolesc Psychiatr Clin N Am 2009;18(2):339–52.
5. Moreno C, Laje G, Blanco C, et al. National trends in outpatient diagnosis and treatment of bipolar disorder in youth. Arch Gen Psychiatry 2007;64:1032–9.
6. Chang K. Adult bipolar disorder is continuous with pediatric bipolar disorder. Can J Psychiatry 2007;52:418–25.
7. Geller B, Tillman R, Craney JL, et al. Four-year prospective outcome and natural history of mania in children with a prepubertal and early adolescent bipolar disorder phenotype. Arch Gen Psychiatry 2004;61:459–67.
8. Birmaher B, Axelson D, Strober M, et al. Clinical course of children and adolescents with bipolar spectrum disorders. Arch Gen Psychiatry 2006;63:175–83.
9. Joshi G, Wilens T. Comorbidity in pediatric bipolar disorder. Child Adolesc Psychiatr Clin N Am 2009;18(2):291–319.
10. McClellan J, Kowatch R, Findling RL. Practice parameter for the assessment and treatment of children and adolescents with bipolar disorder. J Am Acad Child Adolesc Psychiatry 2007;46(1):107–25.
11. Findling RL, Pavuluri MN. Lithium. In: Geller B, DelBello M, editors. Treatment of bipolar disorder in children and adolescents. New York: The Guilford Press; 2008. p. 43–68.
12. Madaan V, Chang KD. Pharmacotherapeutic strategies for pediatric bipolar disorder. Expert Opin Pharmacother 2007;8(12):1801–19.
13. Kowatch RA, DelBello MP. Pharmacotherapy of children and adolescents with bipolar disorder. Psychiatr Clin North Am 2005;28(2):385–97.
14. Kowatch RA, Findling RL, Scheffer RE, et al. Pediatric bipolar collaborative mood stabilizer trial. Poster presentation at the Annual Meeting of the American Academy of Child and Adolescent Psychiatry. Boston, October 23–28, 2007.
15. Findling RL. Treatment of childhood-onset bipolar disorder. In: Zarate CA, Manji HK, editors. Bipolar depression: molecular neurobiology, clinical diagnosis and pharmacotherapy. Verlag (Switzerland): Birkhauser; 2009. p. 241–52.
16. Findling RL, Frazier JA, Karantaris V, et al. The Collaborative Lithium Trials (CoLT): specific aims, methods, and implementation. Child Adolesc Psychiatry Ment Health 2008;2(1):21.
17. Kowatch RA, Suppes T, Carmody TJ, et al. Effect size of lithium, divalproex sodium, and carbamazepine in children and adolescents with bipolar disorder. J Am Acad Child Adolesc Psychiatry 2000;39(6):713–20.
18. Wagner KD, Redden L, Kowatch RA, et al. A double-blind, randomized, placebo-controlled trial of divalproex extended-release in the treatment of bipolar disorder in children and adolescents. J Am Acad Child Adolesc Psychiatry 2009;48(5): 519–32.

19. Findling RL, Kuich K. Bipolar disorders. In: Findling RL, editor. Clinical manual of child and adolescent psychopharmacology. New York: Guilford Press; 2008. p. 229–63.
20. DelBello MP, Findling RL, Kushner S, et al. A pilot controlled trial of topiramate for mania in children and adolescents with bipolar disorder. J Am Acad Child Adolesc Psychiatry 2005;44(6):539–47.
21. Wagner KD, Kowatch RA, Emslie GJ, et al. A double-blind, randomized, placebo-controlled trial of oxcarbazepine in the treatment of bipolar disorder in children and adolescents. Am J Psychiatry 2006;163(7):1179–86.
22. Smarty S, Findling RL. Psychopharmacology of pediatric bipolar disorder: a review. Psychopharmacology 2007;191(1):39–54.
23. Kowatch RA. Pharmacotherapy 1: mood stabilizers. In: Kowatch RA, Fristad MA, editors. Clinical manual for management of bipolar disorder in children and adolescents. Arlington (VA): American Psychiatric Publishing, Inc; 2009. p. 133–56.
24. Pavuluri MN, Henry DB, Moss M, et al. Effectiveness of lamotrigine in maintaining symptom control in pediatric bipolar disorder. J Child Adolesc Psychopharmacol 2009;19(1):75–82.
25. Haas M, DelBello MP, Pandina G, et al. Risperidone for the treatment of acute mania in children and adolescents with bipolar disorder: a randomized, double-blind, placebo-controlled study. Bipolar Disord 2009;11:687–700.
26. Tohen M, Kryzhanovskaya L, Carlson G, et al. Olanzapine versus placebo in the treatment of adolescents with bipolar mania. Am J Psychiatry 2007;164:1547–56.
27. DelBello MP, Kowatch RA, Adler CM, et al. A double-blind randomized pilot study comparing quetiapine and divalproex for adolescent mania. J Am Acad Child Adolesc Psychiatry 2006;45(3):305–13.
28. DelBello MP, Findling RL, Earley WR, et al. Efficacy of quetiapine in children and adolescents with bipolar mania: a 3-week, double-blind, randomized, placebo-controlled trial. Poster presentation at the Annual Meeting of the American Academy of Child and Adolescent Psychiatry. Boston, October 23–28, 2007.
29. DelBello MP, Findling RL, Wang PP, et al. Efficacy and safety of ziprasidone in pediatric bipolar disorder. Poster presentation at the Annual Meeting of American Psychiatric Association. Washington, DC, May 3–8, 2008.
30. Geodon and Pediatric Bipolar Disorder. U.S. Food and Drug Administration website. Available at: http://www.fda.gov/ICECI/EnforcementActions/WarningLetters/ucm208976.htm. Accessed August 11, 2010.
31. Findling RL, Nyilas M, Forbes RA, et al. Acute treatment of pediatric bipolar I disorder, manic or mixed episode, with aripiprazole: a randomized, double-blind, placebo-controlled study. J Clin Psychiatry 2009;70(10):1441–51.
32. Masi G, Mucci M, Millepiedi S. Clozapine in adolescent inpatient mania. J Child Adolesc Psychopharmacol 2002;12(2):93–9.
33. Kafantaris V, Coletti DJ, Dicker R, et al. Lithium treatment of acute mania in adolescents: a placebo-controlled discontinuation study. J Am Acad Child Adolesc Psychiatry 2004;43(8):984–93.
34. Findling RL, McNamara NK, Youngstrom EA, et al. Double-blind 18-month trial of lithium versus divalproex maintenance treatment in pediatric bipolar disorder. J Am Acad Child Adolesc Psychiatry 2005;44(5):409–17.
35. Wagner KD, Nyilas M, Johnson B, et al. Long-term efficacy of aripiprazole in children (10–17 years old) with mania. Poster presentation at the Annual Meeting of the American Academy of Child and Adolescent Psychiatry. Boston, October 23–28, 2007.
36. Correll CU, Nyilas M, Aurang C, et al. Safety and tolerability of aripiprazole in children (10–17) with mania. Poster presentation at the Annual Meeting of the American Academy of Child and Adolescent Psychiatry. Boston, October 23–28, 2007.

37. Judd LL, Akiskal HS, Schettler PJ, et al. The long-term natural history of the weekly symptomatic status of bipolar I disorder. Arch Gen Psychiatry 2002;59:530–7.

38. Chang K. Challenges in the diagnosis and treatment of pediatric bipolar depression. Dialogues Clin Neurosci 2009;11(1):73–80.

39. Patel NC, DelBello MP, Bryan HS, et al. Open-label lithium for the treatment of adolescents with bipolar depression. J Am Acad Child Adolesc Psychiatry 2006;45(3):289–97.

40. Chang K, Saxena K, Howe M. An open-label study of lamotrigine adjunct or monotherapy for the treatment of adolescents with bipolar depression. J Am Acad Child Adolesc Psychiatry 2006;45(3):298–304.

41. DelBello MP, Chang K, Welge JA, et al. A double-blind, placebo-controlled pilot study of quetiapine for depressed adolescents with bipolar disorder. Bipolar Disord 2009;11:483–93.

42. Bridge JA, Birmaher B, Iyengar S, et al. Placebo response in randomized controlled trials of antidepressants for pediatric major depressive disorder. Am J Psychiatry 2009;166:42–9.

43. Joseph M, Youngstrom EA, Soares JC. Antidepressant-coincident mania in children and adolescents treated with selective serotonin reuptake inhibitors. Future Neurol 2009;4(1):87–102.

44. Kowatch RA, Fristad M, Birmaher B, et al. Treatment guidelines for children and adolescents with bipolar disorder. J Am Acad Child Adolesc Psychiatry 2005; 44(3):213–35.

45. Biederman J, Faraone SV, Mick E, et al. Attention deficit hyperactivity disorder and juvenile mania: an overlooked comorbidity? J Am Acad Child Adolesc Psychiatry 1996;35(8):997–1008.

46. Scheffer RE, Kowatch RA, Carmody T, et al. Randomized, placebo controlled trial of mixed amphetamine salts for symptoms of comorbid ADHD in pediatric bipolar disorder after mood stabilization with divalproex sodium. Am J Psychiatry 2005; 162:58–64.

47. Findling RL, Short EJ, McNamara NK, et al. Methylphenidate in the treatment of children and adolescents with bipolar disorder and attention-deficit/hyperactivity disorder. J Am Acad Child Adolesc Psychiatry 2007;46:1445–53.

48. Geller B, Cooper TB, Sun K, et al. Double-blind and placebo-controlled study of lithium for adolescent bipolar disorders with secondary substance dependency. J Am Acad Child Adolesc Psychiatry 1998;37:171–8.

49. Campbell M, Silva RR, Kafantaris V, et al. Predictors of side effects associated with lithium administration in children. Psychopharmacol Bull 1991;27(3):373–80.

50. Hagino OR, Weller EB, Weller RA, et al. Untoward effects of lithium treatment in children aged four through six years. J Am Acad Child Adolesc Psychiatry 1995;34(12):1584–90.

51. Kowatch RA, DelBello MP. Pediatric bipolar disorder: emerging diagnostic and treatment approaches. Child Adolesc Psychiatr Clin N Am 2006;15(1):73–108.

52. Kowatch RA. Mood stabilizers. In: Geller B, DelBello M, editors. Treatment of bipolar disorder in children and adolescents. New York: The Guilford Press; 2008. p. 109–25.

53. American Diabetes Association. American Psychiatric Association. Consensus development conference on antipsychotic drugs and obesity and diabetes. Diabetes Care 2004;27(2):596–601.

54. Blair J, Scahill L, State M, et al. Electrocardiographic changes in children and adolescents treated with ziprasidone: a prospective study. J Am Acad Child Adolesc Psychiatry 2005;44(1):73–9.

Cognitive-Adaptive Disabilities

Joseph L. Calles Jr, MD[a,b,*]

KEYWORDS

- Cognitive-adaptive disabilities • Developmental disorders
- Pharmacologic treatment • Epidemiology

The term "cognitive-adaptive disabilities" (CADs) denotes a group of disorders associated with significant impairments in mental abilities and in functional capabilities. Subsumed under CAD are other terms that similarly denote global or specific dysfunctions (**Box 1**). As in other areas of medical practice, the early identification of and interventions for CADs is extremely important, the goals being prevention of mortality, reduction of morbidity, and improvement of functional status. To that end the American Academy of Neurology has developed a practice parameter for the evaluation of children with global developmental delays.[1] The work-up should include thorough personal and family histories, complete physical, neurologic and dysmorphology examinations, and screening for visual and auditory disorders. If not already done as part of universal newborn screening, metabolic testing and evaluations for autistic and communication disorders should be considered.

EPIDEMIOLOGY

The determination of prevalence of CADs has been fraught with methodologic problems, and has therefore yielded variable results. A relatively recent review on the epidemiology of mental retardation has reasonably estimated that the prevalence of severe mental retardation (intelligence quotient <35) is 1.4 per 1000, and the prevalence of mild mental retardation (IQ 50–70) is 10.6 per 1000.[2] The US Centers for Disease Control and Prevention reported that for 8 year olds surveyed in 2006, the overall average prevalence of autism spectrum disorders (ASDs) was 9 per 1000.[3] This means that, on average, approximately 1 child in every 110 was classified as having an ASD, an increase of 57% from the 2002 surveillance year. Epidemiologic

[a] Department of Psychiatry, College of Human Medicine, Michigan State University, A236 East Fee Hall, East Lansing, MI 48824, USA
[b] Child and Adolescent Psychiatry, Psychiatry Residency Training Program, Michigan State University/Kalamazoo Center for Medical Studies, 1722 ShafferRoad, Suite 3, Kalamazoo, MI 49048, USA
* Psychiatry Residency Training Program, Michigan State University/Kalamazoo Center for Medical Studies, 1722 Shaffer Road, Suite 3, Kalamazoo, MI 49048.
E-mail address: calles@kcms.msu.edu

Pediatr Clin N Am 58 (2011) 189–203
doi:10.1016/j.pcl.2010.10.003
0031-3955/11/$ – see front matter © 2011 Elsevier Inc. All rights reserved.

> **Box 1**
> **Cognitive-adaptive disabilities**
>
> Intellectual disabilities (formerly known as mental retardation)
>
> • Implies below normal performance on standardized intellectual testing and a functional level below that expected for chronologic age or the individual requires varying levels of environmental support.
>
> Autism spectrum disorders (pervasive developmental disorders); includes autistic disorder, Asperger disorder, Rett syndrome, childhood disintegrative disorder, and pervasive developmental disorder not otherwise specified
>
> • Implies a variable combination of impaired socialization, communication, and interests, often accompanied by some level of intellectual disabilities.
>
> Specific learning disorders
>
> • Unlike intellectual disabilities and autism spectrum disorders, these are specific, not global, in their effects; more likely to affect academic performance in the areas of reading, writing, and mathematics.
>
> Communication disorders
>
> • May be seen in the absence of other disabilities; can affect the reception or expression of language, or the articulation of speech.

studies have also found that intellectual disabilities (IDs) and ASDs are highly comorbid, because 50% to 70% of those with an ASD also have an ID, whereas 28% to 40% of individuals with an ID have an ASD.[4]

Studies that have looked at the presence of psychopathology in youth with CADs have also found variable results, although they are consistent in reporting more emotional and behavioral problems in those with versus those without CADs. A survey from the United Kingdom examined 10,438 children, between the ages of 5 and 15 years, for psychiatric disorders.[5] Compared with children with no ID, those with IDs were seven times more likely to have received any psychiatric diagnosis. In addition, rates for conduct disorders, anxiety disorders, attention-deficit/hyperactivity disorder (ADHD), and pervasive developmental disorders were statistically higher among the children with ID than among their peers without ID. The emotional and behavioral problems in children with IDs do not seem to substantially resolve as they transition into adulthood. For example, an Australian study evaluated a cohort of youth with ID (5–19.5 years of age at study entry) at four points in time, the last occurring 10 years after the end of the initial evaluation period.[6] The prevalence of subjects meeting criteria for obvious psychopathology, or a definite psychiatric disorder, had only decreased from 41% to 31% between the first and last assessments. One possible explanation is that only 10% of those with diagnosed psychopathology received any mental health treatment during the study period. A Dutch study similarly evaluated two cohorts of youth (ages 6–18 years at study entry) with and without IDs at three points in time over 6 years.[7] The results revealed that children with IDs continued to have a greater risk for psychopathology compared with children with no ID, although the risk for aggression was less pronounced at age 18 years than it was at age 6 years.

To better evaluate and treat child and adolescent patients with CADs, specific, relatively common developmental syndromes are discussed here in terms of epidemiology, comorbid psychiatric disorders, and psychopharmacologic treatments.

DEVELOPMENTAL DISORDERS
Down Syndrome

Down syndrome (DS) is the most common chromosomal disorder associated with ID. In the United States, a cross-sectional study found a DS prevalence rate of 10.3 per 10,000 children and adolescents (0–19 years old).[8] Individuals with DS are at risk for developing certain psychiatric and behavioral problems.

Mood disorders

Depression in children and adolescents with DS seems to be uncommon; however, the vulnerability increases as those individuals age into adulthood.[9] This has implications for the care provided by pediatricians, who are often the default clinicians for patients with DS even after they reach legal adulthood. Bipolar disorder is rare in the DS population, occurring at a lower rate than that seen in either the general population or in CAD patients without DS.[10] Symptoms that could be interpreted as bipolar-like (eg, motor hyperactivity) are much more likely to be secondary to other psychiatric disorders (see later).

Obsessive-compulsive disorder

Adults with DS seem to have rates of obsessive-compulsive disorder (OCD) that are higher than reported in the non-DS ID and general populations.[11] In a study comparing children with DS with typically developing children (mean age ~5 years) there were no differences between them in terms of the number of compulsive-like behaviors they engaged in, although subjects with DS did engage in repetitive behaviors more frequently and intensely.[12] This is consistent with reports that, in individuals with DS, the onset of OCD symptoms is typically in adolescence or young adulthood.[11]

Attention-deficit/hyperactivity disorder

Similar to rates seen in the general population, ADHD in DS is more common in those under 20 years of age (6.1%) than in those over age 20 (2.4%).[9]

Psychosis

Studies are mixed regarding the occurrence of delusions and hallucinations in individuals with DS. Given the limitations in communication associated with CADs, patients may not report psychotic symptoms, or clinicians may not specifically inquire about them. In a retrospective chart review of adults with IDs, there was no significant difference between the group with DS and the group without DS in terms of psychotic symptomatology.[13] The subjects with DS were less likely to display aggressive or self-injurious behaviors, which could have lowered the index of suspicion of an underlying psychotic process.

Dementia

Contrary to popular belief, the rate of Alzheimer dementia in DS may be only slightly higher than in the general population; however, the average age of onset is much younger.[14] Given that the presence of dementia greatly complicates the care of individuals with DS, early identification and possible treatment are very important. The recommendation has, therefore, been made that a baseline assessment of functioning should be performed by age 35 years, and that follow-up should occur yearly thereafter.

Treatments

Evidence-based treatments for the underlying pathology in DS are lacking; treatments are aimed at correcting presumed neurotransmitter abnormalities.[15] For depression, the selective serotonin reuptake inhibitor (SSRI) antidepressants are a good choice; they have demonstrated some reversal of functional decline associated with either depression or early dementia in adults with DS.[15] A small case series of adults with DS with OCD yielded positive responses to SSRIs, either alone or in combination with risperidone.[16] The SSRIs can presumably be used for other anxiety disorders. Because there are no specific guidelines for the treatment of ADHD symptoms in DS, general approaches to treatment should be followed (ie, beginning with standard stimulant medications).[17] Psychotic symptoms in young people with developmental disorders can respond to risperidone or olanzapine.[18] Patients should be monitored for dyskinesias, especially in females, and for other side effects. Although research into treatments for Alzheimer disease in the ID population is limited, the use of donepezil for dementia in patients with DS may be a reasonable choice.[19]

Fragile X Syndrome

Fragile X syndrome (FXS) is the most common form of inherited ID, involving excessive repeats of the CGG trinucleotide. The screening of newborn boys for full-mutation FXS, using a highly accurate assay of methylated *FMR1* gene DNA, yielded an incidence of 1 in 5161.[20]

Mood disorders

A study examined 119 males and 446 females (ages 18–50 years) selected from either the general population or from families with a history of FXS.[21] Subjects were categorized into three groups: (1) noncarriers (≤40 CGG repeats); (2) intermediate allele carriers (41–60 repeats); and (3) premutation allele carriers (61–199 repeats). Results demonstrated a linear association between CGG repeat length and negative affect in both males and females, and with depression only in males. In a study of females (ages 4–27 years) with FXS versus those without FXS, those with FXS had higher rates of mood disorders (47% vs 6%), with one-half of those meeting criteria for major depressive disorder (MDD).[22] In another study that compared males and females with FXS, there was no statistical difference in either "anxious-depressed" or "withdrawn" scores between the two genders.[23]

Anxiety disorders

In the previously cited premutation study,[21] the results did not find any association between CGG repeat length and anxiety (state or trait), social phobia, or agoraphobia. Given that cognitive and language impairments are common in children with FXS, the detection of anxiety in that population may have to be through observation rather than direct inquiry. When asked to identify anxiety symptoms by the presence of specific behaviors in a group of children with FXS, the parents rated 26% as having "clinically significant anxiety problems," whereas the teachers rated 42% of the children as having high levels of anxiety.[24]

Attention-deficit/hyperactivity disorder

The symptoms of ADHD are common in FXS. When compared with same-age peers, parental ratings were consistent with ADHD in 53.7% of children with FXS; similarly, teachers rated 59.2% as meeting ADHD criteria, but with higher scores for hyperactivity-impulsivity than were reported by the parents.[25]

Aggression

Using a standardized behavioral rating form, parents of 49 boys (mean age 8.5 years) with FXS reported that 40.8% of their children scored in the borderline and clinical ranges for aggressive behaviors (compared with only 5% of the normative population that scored in those ranges).[26]

Treatments

The SSRI antidepressants can be used to treat both depression and anxiety in patients with FXS.[27] Alternative medications for depression include the serotonin-norepinephrine reuptake inhibitor antidepressants (eg, venlafaxine or duloxetine) or bupropion; the latter should be used with caution, given its potential for lowering the seizure threshold. Alternative medications for anxiety include buspirone or the α_2-agonists clonidine or guanfacine. The symptoms of ADHD in FXS respond to the usual stimulant medications, such as methylphenidate or mixed amphetamine salts. If the stimulants are ineffective, intolerable, or exacerbate other symptoms (eg, irritability), the α_2-agonists can be very useful, particularly guanfacine,[28] the long-acting form of which is now approved for the treatment of ADHD. The treatment of aggression should start with the α_2-agonists, especially if ADHD is also present. Other medications to consider for treating aggressive behaviors in youth with FXS are the atypical antipsychotics (AAs) risperidone and aripiprazole (low doses, because agitation occurs at higher doses).[28]

Fetal Alcohol Syndrome

Fetal alcohol syndrome (FAS) and fetal alcohol spectrum disorders (FASD) are the most common preventable causes of ID. Prevalence estimates of FAS and FASD have varied widely, but extrapolating from school populations (where rates of FAS-FASD are higher) to the general population has yielded a prevalence of greater than or equal to 2 to 7 per 1000 for FAS and a prevalence of 2 to 5 per 100 for FASD in younger school children.[29]

Mood disorders

One study looked at a group of children who had been exposed prenatally to high levels of alcohol, but who did not have ID.[30] They were classified into three groups: (1) full FAS, (2) partial FAS, and (3) alcohol-related neurodevelopmental deficits (ARND). There were no cases of MDD in the full FAS and partial FAS groups; however, 33% were diagnosed with bipolar disorder. In the ARND group, 18% were diagnosed with MDD and 35% with bipolar disorder. Based on these data, children with FAS and FASD may be at more risk of developing bipolar disorder than of developing depression.

Attention-deficit/hyperactivity disorder

A chart review of 2231 children (mean age 8.7 years) referred for FASD divided the patients into four risk categories based on prenatal alcohol exposure: (1) confirmed high exposure, (2) confirmed low exposure, (3) unknown exposure, and (4) confirmed lack of exposure.[31] Using a standardized diagnostic system, rates of ADHD varied by level of exposure risk, with 49.4% of those in the highest risk group meeting criteria for ADHD, whereas only 0.8% of the no-risk group met criteria.

Psychosis

Children with prenatal exposure to alcohol (PEA) were compared with nonexposed children on a personality inventory completed by caregivers.[32] The PEA group (which included children with FAS) scored statistically higher on the "psychosis" subscale (which discriminates children with psychotic symptomatology from normal, behaviorally disturbed nonpsychotic, and children with ID). There was no statistical difference in psychotic symptoms between children with FAS and those with PEA without FAS.

Aggression

The connection between FAS and aggressive behavior is somewhat puzzling and counterintuitive. Children and adolescents with a history of PEA, versus those without prenatal exposure, show higher rates of delinquent behaviors, including fighting.[33]

However, in those with PEA, but without FAS, one-half met probable conduct disorder criteria, compared with none of the patients with FAS. Similarly, another study[34] found that patients with partial FAS had significantly higher anger scores (a risk factor for aggression) than did those with full FAS.

Treatments

There are no specific guidelines available for the treatment of bipolar disorder in youth with FAS or FASD. It is reasonable to follow the recommendations for treatment of bipolar disorder proposed for children and adolescents without PEA. A recent, comprehensive literature review of the psychopharmacology of pediatric bipolar disorder[35] found that AAs and mood stabilizers are equally effective in their treatment of manic symptoms, but that the AAs achieve mood stabilization more quickly. Risperidone and aripiprazole are both approved for the treatment of bipolar disorder I in children greater than or equal to 10 years of age. As with the other CADs, the treatment of depression in FAS should begin with the SSRIs. The symptoms of ADHD in FASD respond to psychostimulants; dextroamphetamine or mixed amphetamine salts may be preferable to methylphenidate as first-line agents.[36] The stimulants may be more effective in ameliorating hyperactivity-impulsivity than in improving attention span.[37] For the treatment of psychosis in FAS, either risperidone or aripiprazole can be used (both are approved for the treatment of schizophrenia in adolescents ≥13 years of age). Risperidone (and possibly other AAs) can be used to treat aggression in children with FAS that has not responded to an SSRI or a stimulant.[36]

Autism Spectrum Disorders

As previously noted, the Centers for Disease Control and Prevention estimated the overall average prevalence of ASDs to be 9 per 1000, or 1 out of every 110 children in the general population.[3] The etiology of ASDs is unknown, but evidence suggests an interaction between genetic vulnerability and environmental factors.[38]

Mood disorders

Children (9–14 years old) with Asperger syndrome or high-functioning autism (higher IQs, better communication skills) were evaluated for psychiatric problems approximately 6 years after the ASD diagnoses were made.[39] Of the children with ASDs, 16.9% scored at least two standard deviations above the population mean on a measure of depression (P<.001). Prevalence numbers for depression in individuals with ASDs are not necessarily reliable, and may be underreported, because subjective reporting of depression can be inhibited by deficient language skills, and caretaker reporting may be inaccurate, because depressive symptoms could be attributed to the core features of the ASDs, such as social withdrawal.[40] Bipolar disorder can also be identified in youth with ASDs. A Japanese sample of outpatients (≥12 years of age) with ASDs (excluding autistic disorder) and IQs greater than or equal to 70 were evaluated for mood disorders.[41] Of the 44 subjects, 16 (36.4%) were diagnosed with a mood disorder, and of those 4 were diagnosed with MDD, the rest (75%) with a bipolar spectrum disorder. The authors make the statement that the "major comorbid mood disorder" in the ASDs is bipolar disorder, rather than MDD.

Anxiety disorders

In the previously cited follow-up study,[39] the investigators also identified significant numbers of the children with ASD as having anxiety; specifically, 13.6% were "overanxious" (ie, with generalized anxiety) and 8.5% had separation anxiety. In another study, parents of 171 medication-free children (5–17 years) used a standardized symptom inventory to rate anxiety symptoms.[42] Of the total sample, 43% met screening cut-off criteria for at least one anxiety disorder. Compared with children with IQs less than 70, those with higher IQs were significantly more likely to have generalized anxiety disorder, somatization disorder, and separation anxiety disorder.

Attention-deficit/hyperactivity disorder
Identical to the rate of depression in children with ASDs, 16.9% of a follow-up sample of children with Asperger syndrome and high-functioning autism scored high on a measure of ADHD.[39] There is bidirectional comorbidity between ASDs and ADHD: 20% to 50% of children with ADHD meet criteria for an ASD, whereas 30% to 80% of ASD children meet criteria for ADHD.[43] This may indicate some shared genetic factors.

Aggression
A study of 160 children with ASDs reported that 32% displayed aggressive behaviors, either toward themselves or toward others.[44] A school-based study compared teacher and parent ratings of students (mean age 9.6 years) with identified pervasive developmental disorders.[45] The combined moderate and severe behavioral scores from parents and teachers, respectively, were 9.6% and 14.9% for cruelty/meanness; 11.3% and 11.5% for property destruction; 5.3% (both raters) for physical fights; 9.9% and 14.8% for attacking people; and 4.5% and 7.6% for threatening people. The students with lower adaptive skills scored higher on the conduct problems and hyperactivity subscales. In another study of children and adolescents with ASDs, recruited from clinical and community settings, behavioral ratings were made by the parents or other caregivers.[46] Aggression toward others was reported in 50% (severe in 10.2%); yelling or shouting at others in 44.3% (10.8%); property destruction in 42.6% (13.6%); throwing objects at others in 36.9% (7.4%); kicking objects in 35.8% (10.2%); and pulling others' hair in 14.8% (4.5%).

Treatments
The treatment of depression in youth with ASDs usually begins with an SSRI, although there are no controlled studies to justify that practice.[47] Nonetheless, if one chooses to use an antidepressant, fluoxetine is considered to be the safest first choice. Treatment studies are also lacking in the area of comorbid ASDs and bipolar disorder, although expert recommendations include the use of mood stabilizers or AAs.[48] The approach to the pharmacotherapy of anxiety in the ASDs is the same as that proposed for the treatment of depression (ie, the use of SSRIs based on clinical indication) but without the backing of good studies.[47] For the treatment of ADHD symptoms in children with ASDs, either methylphenidate or atomoxetine can be used, although treatment responses are lower and adverse events are greater than seen in children with ADHD without ASDs.[49] A better choice may be an α_2-agonist, especially the long-acting preparation of guanfacine. The most commonly prescribed agents for treating aggression in individuals with ASDs are the AAs. Two of them (risperidone and aripiprazole) have received Food and Drug Administration approval to treat the irritability (including aggressive symptoms) associated with autistic disorder. It is reasonable to extend their use to treat aggression in all of the ASDs. If the AAs are ineffective or intolerable, mood stabilizers may be tried.[48]

Neurofibromatosis Type 1

Neurofibromatosis 1 (NF1) is an autosomal-dominant disorder with an estimated prevalence of 1 in 2000 to 1 in 5000, although it may be more common, because detection of milder forms can be missed.[50]

Mood and anxiety disorders

Parent ratings of children with NF1 yielded significantly higher scores of anxious-depressed symptoms compared with a normative sample and with unaffected siblings.[51] A different study did not identify any significant problems for most children with NF1 regarding anxiety-depression, with one exception: an interaction between NF1 and age (ie, older children with NF1were viewed by their mothers as having more symptoms of depression and anxiety).[52] The authors speculate that social problems may contribute to the development of anxious and depressive symptomatology.

Attention-deficit/hyperactivity disorder

In the previously cited study, parent ratings of children with NF1 also yielded significantly higher scores on an attention problems scale.[51] Teacher ratings were also significantly higher than the normal for attention problems. An outpatient study of 93 consecutive children with NF1 found that 46 (49.5%) met diagnostic criteria for ADHD.[53]

Aggression

Parents of children with NF1 rated them significantly higher on aggressive behaviors compared with a normative sample, but not compared with unaffected siblings.[51] Children with NF1 rate even higher on aggression scores when they have comorbid ADHD.[53]

Treatments

The treatment study that used methylphenidate to treat ADHD in patients with NF1 found that not only did the medication improve attention scores, but it also significantly reduced scores on the anxiety-depression and aggression scales.[53] What is encouraging is that the methylphenidate dose (given twice daily) averaged only 7.4 mg, thus avoiding high-dose treatment and its associated adverse effects.

Velocardiofacial Syndrome

Technically known as the 22q11.2 deletion syndrome, but traditionally called the velocardiofacial syndrome (VCFS), this CAD is fairly common, with a prevalence of 1 in 5950 total births; between 1 in 6000 and 1 in 6500 white, black, and Asian births; and 1 in 3800 Hispanic births.[54]

Mood disorders

A study compared 84 children with VCFS (mean age 11.75 years; 55% male) with matched sibling and community controls.[55] In the VCFS group, 10 subjects (12%) were diagnosed with MDD, which was significantly higher than in either control group. The VCFS group was also the only group in which children were diagnosed with dysthymic disorder and bipolar disorder (neither was significant). Regarding bipolar disorder in VCFS, a group of 26 patients (ages 5–34 years) with molecularly confirmed VCFS were evaluated for psychiatric disorders.[56] Considering the diagnoses in the bipolar disorder spectrum (ie, bipolar I, bipolar II, cyclothymia, and schizoaffective-manic), 12 of 19 patients under age 18 years and 6 of 7 of those over age 18 years met diagnostic criteria for a bipolar spectrum diagnosis.

Anxiety disorders

In addition to mood disorders, the previous study found significant numbers of children with VCFS with simple phobias (22.6%) and generalized anxiety disorder (16.7%).[55] The rate of OCD was not elevated in this study. However, in another study of 43 subjects with VCFS (mean age 18.3 years), 14 (32.6%) met diagnostic criteria for OCD.[57] What is interesting is that, for those subjects, the onset was early for both obsessive-compulsive symptoms (mean 10.7 years of age) and for actual OCD (mean 13.1 years of age).

Attention-deficit/hyperactivity disorder

The subjects in two of the previously noted studies[55,57] were diagnosed with ADHD at high rates (42.8% and 37.2%, respectively), which makes it one of the most common psychiatric comorbidities in VCFS.

Psychosis

The rate of psychosis (mostly schizophrenia) in individuals with VCFS is about 30%.[58] Although psychotic symptoms tend to develop beyond childhood, structured interviews of adolescents with VCFS have found that 45% have positive psychotic symptoms (eg, auditory hallucinations), whereas most (85%) have negative psychotic symptoms (eg, anhedonia).[59]

Treatment

Over the last decade, not much progress has been made in the pharmacotherapy of psychiatric disorders in VCFS.[36] For the treatment of depression and anxiety, caution must be used if choosing SSRIs, because they could precipitate mania in these patients at high risk for bipolar disorder. However, fluoxetine has been used successfully to treat OCD without destabilizing mood.[57] Similarly, the theoretical potential that methylphenidate has to precipitate mania in vulnerable individuals was not seen in a small, open-label trial in patients with VCFS and ADHD.[60] Treating the psychosis associated with VCFS can proceed using any of the AAs, except perhaps clozapine, which has the greatest potential of lowering the seizure threshold (7% of children with VCFS can have unprovoked seizures[61]).

Tuberous Sclerosis Complex

The tuberous sclerosis complex (TSC) is a multisystem disorder with autosomal-dominant genetics. In whites it has a prevalence of 1 in 25,000.[62]

Mood disorders

In a United Kingdom mail survey of children with TSC, parents reported that 23% of the children (all under age 18 years; over half under age 10 years) had "depressed mood."[63] There were no statistical differences in rates of depression whether or not ID was present, nor between males and females. A retrospective chart review of 241 patients with TSC (average age 20 years) found that 27% had a history of mood disorder symptoms, and of 43 evaluated by a psychiatrist, 11 (26%) received a formal mood disorder diagnosis.[64]

Anxiety disorders

Parents in the United Kingdom mail survey also reported that 40% of their children with TSC had anxiety.[63] Similar to the results related to depression, the rates of anxiety did not differ based on gender or IQ level. The chart review study also found that 27% of subjects with TSC had a history of anxiety disorder symptoms, and of 43 evaluated by a psychiatrist, 12 (28%) received a formal anxiety disorder diagnosis, over half of which were for generalized anxiety disorder.[64]

Attention-deficit/hyperactivity disorder

The United Kingdom survey also asked the parents of children with TSC about "disruptive behaviors and attention deficit symptoms." Overactivity, restlessness, and impulsive behavior were seen in 56%, 54%, and 52%, respectively, of the children.[63] The chart review study identified 30% of those with TSC as having a history

Table 1
Cognitive-adaptive disabilities, comorbid psychiatric disorders, and recommended psychopharmacologic treatment options

CAD	Depr	BD	Anxiety	ADHD	Aggr	Psych	Dem
DS	SSRIs	—	SSRIs; may add RISP for OCD	MPH or MAS; ATX; α_2-agonists	—	RISP or OLZ	Donepezil
FXS	SSRIs; SNRIs; BUP	—	SSRIs; buspirone; α_2-agonists	MPH or MAS; α_2-agonists	α_2-agonists; RISP or ARI	—	—
FAS	SSRIs	RISP/ARI or AEDs	—	DEX or MAS; MPH	First treat depression or ADHD; RISP	RISP or ARI	—
ASD	FLU; other SSRIs	RISP/ARI or AEDs	SSRIs	MPH/ATX or α_2-agonists	RISP or ARI	—	—
NF1	MPH	—	MPH	MPH	MPH	—	—
VCFS	SSRIs	—	SSRIs (FLU for OCD)	MPH	—	AAs[a]	—
TSC	SSRIs	—	SSRIs	MPH; MAS or ATX; α_2-agonists or RISP/ other AAs	First treat depression, anxiety or ADHD; RISP or other AAs	—	—

Abbreviations: AAs, atypical antipsychotics; ADHD, attention-deficit/hyperactivity disorder; AEDs, antiepileptic drugs/mood stabilizers; Aggr, aggression; ARI, aripiprazole; ASDs, autism spectrum disorder; ATX, atomoxetine; BD, bipolar disorder; BUP, bupropion; CAD, cognitive-adaptive disability; Dem, dementia; Depr, depression; DEX, dextroamphetamine; DS, Down syndrome; FAS, fetal alcohol syndrome; FLU, fluoxetine; FXS, fragile X syndrome; MAS, mixed amphetamine salts; MPH, methylphenidate; NF1, neurofibromatosis 1; OCD, obsessive-compulsive disorder; OLZ, olanzapine; Psych, psychosis; RISP, risperidone; SNRIs, serotonin-norepinephrine reuptake inhibitors; SSRIs, selective serotonin reuptake inhibitors; TSC, tuberous sclerosis complex; VCFS, velocardiofacial syndrome.

[a] Except clozapine.

of ADHD symptoms; of 43 evaluated by a psychiatrist, 9 (21%) received a formal ADHD diagnosis, all but 1 of which were of the combined type.[64] The lower rates of ADHD symptoms in this study (vs the United Kingdom study) are likely caused by the older average age of the participants.

Aggression

More than half of the children with TSC in the United Kingdom survey were reported to have aggressive outbursts (58%) and temper tantrums (57%).[63] In the chart review study, 28% of patients with TSC had a history of aggressive-disruptive behavior disorder symptoms.[64] Although there were no formal diagnoses made specifically related to aggression, those in the aggressive group had high degrees of overlap with other diagnostic groups: 43% in the group with mood disorders, 29% in the group with anxiety disorders, and 49% in the group with ADHD.[64]

Treatments

The pharmacotherapy of psychiatric disorders in TSC is complicated, as in many other CADs, by the high rates of comorbid epilepsy, ID, and autism.[65] There has also been very little research on the use of psychotropic agents to treat specific psychopathologies in individuals with TSC. Despite the limited database, pharmacotherapies can be used. The treatment of depression and anxiety should start with the SSRIs[65]; citalopram was shown to be effective in the treatment of both.[64] The use of bupropion should be avoided, given its well-known ability to lower the seizure threshold. For children with ADHD and TSC, the usual ADHD medications (stimulants and atomoxetine) can be used, provided that a seizure disorder is absent or, if present, well-controlled; methylphenidate may be the safest and most efficacious agent to use in this population.[66] If the stimulants or atomoxetine are ineffective or intolerable, the α_2-agonists or AAs (especially risperidone) may be used to treat ADHD.[65,66] Finally, the treatment of aggression in TSC should begin with identifying and treating underlying psychiatric disorders, such as ADHD, depression, or anxiety. Refractory aggression may respond to risperidone[64–66] or other AAs.

SUMMARY

Children and adolescents with CADs make up small percentages of the general and clinical pediatric populations; however, they may require an inordinate amount of providers' time and resources, given the high rates of comorbidity that they experience. Psychiatric disorders are common in the CADs, and may be some of the more demanding and difficult conditions that pediatricians and other primary care clinicians are asked to treat. This article reviews a select number of the more common CADs and the rates of psychopathology seen in them, and presents best-evidence approaches to their psychopharmacologic treatments (which are summarized in **Table 1**).

REFERENCES

1. Shevell M, Ashwal S, Donley D, et al. Practice parameter: evaluation of the child with global developmental delay: report of the Quality Standards Subcommittee of the American Academy of Neurology and The Practice Committee of the Child Neurology Society. Neurology 2003;60:367–80.
2. Leonard H, Wen X. The epidemiology of mental retardation: challenges and opportunities in the new millennium. Ment Retard Dev Disabil Res Rev 2002; 8(3):117–34.

3. Centers for Disease Control and Prevention. Prevalence of autism spectrum disorders. Autism and Developmental Disabilities Monitoring Network, United States, 2006. MMWR Surveill Summ 2009;58(No. SS-10):1–20.

4. Matson JL, Shoemaker M. Intellectual disability and its relationship to autism spectrum disorders. Res Dev Disabil 2009;30(6):1107–14.

5. Emerson E. Prevalence of psychiatric disorders in children and adolescents with and without intellectual disability. J Intellect Disabil Res 2003;47(Pt 1):51–8.

6. Einfeld SL, Piccinin AM, Mackinnon A, et al. Psychopathology in young people with intellectual disability. JAMA 2006;296(16):1981–9.

7. de Ruiter KP, Dekker MC, Verhulst FC, et al. Developmental course of psychopathology in youths with and without intellectual disabilities. J Child Psychol Psychiatry 2007;48(5):498–507.

8. Shin M, Besser LM, Kucik JE, et al. Prevalence of Down syndrome among children and adolescents in 10 regions of the United States. Pediatrics 2009; 124(6):1565–71.

9. Myers BA, Pueschel SM. Psychiatric disorders in persons with Down syndrome. J Nerv Ment Dis 1991;179(10):609–13.

10. Craddock N, Owen M. Is there an inverse relationship between Down's syndrome and bipolar affective disorder? Literature review and genetic implications. J Intellect Disabil Res 1994;38(6):613–20.

11. Prasher VP, Day S. Brief report: obsessive-compulsive disorder in adults with Down's syndrome. J Autism Dev Disord 1995;25:453–8.

12. Evans DW, Gray FL. Compulsive-like behavior in individuals with Down syndrome: its relation to mental age level, adaptive and maladaptive behavior. Child Dev 2000;71(2):288–300.

13. Hurley AD. Delusions and hallucinations in Down syndrome: literature review and comparison with non-down syndrome patients. Ment Health Aspect Dev Disabil 2003;6(4):135–46.

14. Nieuwenhuis-Mark RE. Diagnosing Alzheimer's dementia in Down syndrome: problems and possible solutions. Res Dev Disabil 2009;30(5):827–38.

15. Dierssen M, Ortiz-Abalia J, Arque G, et al. Pitfalls and hopes in Down syndrome therapeutic approaches: in the search for evidence-based treatments. Behav Genet 2006;36(3):454–68.

16. Sutor B, Hansen MR, Black JL. Obsessive compulsive disorder treatment in patients with Down syndrome: a case series. Downs Syndr Res Pract 2006; 10(1):1–3.

17. Huang H, Ruedrich S. Recent advances in the diagnosis and treatment of attention-deficit/hyperactivity disorder in individuals with intellectual disability. Ment Health Aspect Dev Disabil 2007;10(4):121–8.

18. Friedlander R, Lazar S, Klancnik J. Atypical antipsychotic use in treating adolescents and young adults with developmental disabilities. Can J Psychiatry 2001; 46:741–5.

19. Prasher VP. Review of donepezil, rivastigmine, galantamine and memantine for the treatment of dementia in Alzheimer's disease in adults with Down syndrome: implications for the intellectual disability population. Int J Geriatr Psychiatry 2004; 19(6):509–15.

20. Coffee B, Keith K, Albizua I, et al. Incidence of fragile X syndrome by newborn screening for methylated FMR1 DNA. Am J Hum Genet 2009;85(4):503–14.

21. Hunter JE, Allen EG, Abramowitz A, et al. Investigation of phenotypes associated with mood and anxiety among male and female fragile X premutation carriers. Behav Genet 2008;38(5):493–502.

22. Freund LS, Reiss AL, Abrams MT. Psychiatric disorders associated with fragile X in the young female. Pediatrics 1993;91(2):321–9.
23. Hessl D, Dyer-Friedman J, Glaser B, et al. The influence of environmental and genetic factors on behavior problems and autistic symptoms in boys and girls with fragile X syndrome. Pediatrics 2001;108(5):E88.
24. Sullivan K, Hooper S, Hatton D. Behavioural equivalents of anxiety in children with fragile X syndrome: parent and teacher report. J Intellect Disabil Res 2007;51(1): 54–65.
25. Sullivan K, Hatton D, Hammer J, et al. ADHD symptoms in children with FXS. Am J Med Genet A 2006;140(21):2275–88.
26. Backes M, Genç B, Schreck J, et al. Cognitive and behavioral profile of fragile X boys: correlations to molecular data. Am J Med Genet 2000;95(2):150–6.
27. Berry-Kravis E, Potanos K. Psychopharmacology in fragile X syndrome: present and future. Ment Retard Dev Disabil Res Rev 2004;10(1):42–8.
28. Hagerman RJ, Berry-Kravis E, Kaufmann WE, et al. Advances in the treatment of fragile X syndrome. Pediatrics 2009;123(1):378–90.
29. May PA, Gossage JP, Kalberg WO, et al. Prevalence and epidemiologic characteristics of FASD from various research methods with an emphasis on recent in-school studies. Dev Disabil Res Rev 2009;15(3):176–92.
30. O'Connor MJ, Shah B, Whaley S, et al. Psychiatric illness in a clinical sample of children with prenatal alcohol exposure. Am J Drug Alcohol Abuse 2002;28(4): 743–54.
31. Bhatara V, Loudenberg R, Ellis R. Association of attention deficit hyperactivity disorder and gestational alcohol exposure: an exploratory study. J Atten Disord 2006;9(3):515–22.
32. Roebuck TM, Mattson SN, Riley EP. Behavioral and psychosocial profiles of alcohol-exposed children. Alcohol Clin Exp Res 1999;23(6):1070–6.
33. Schonfeld AM, Mattson SN, Riley EP. Moral maturity and delinquency after prenatal alcohol exposure. J Stud Alcohol 2005;66(4):545–54.
34. Burd L, Klug MG, Martsolf JT, et al. Fetal alcohol syndrome: neuropsychiatric phenomics. Neurotoxicol Teratol 2003;25(6):697–705.
35. Hamrin V, Iennaco JD. Psychopharmacology of pediatric bipolar disorder. Expert Rev Neurother 2010;10(7):1053–88.
36. Hagerman RJ. Psychopharmacological interventions in fragile X syndrome, fetal alcohol syndrome, Prader-Willi syndrome, Angelman syndrome, Smith-Magenis syndrome, and velocardiofacial syndrome. Ment Retard Dev Disabil Res Rev 1999;5:305–13.
37. Doig J, McLennan JD, Gibbard WB. Medication effects on symptoms of attention-deficit/hyperactivity disorder in children with fetal alcohol spectrum disorder. J Child Adolesc Psychopharmacol 2008;18(4):365–71.
38. Herbert MR. Contributions of the environment and environmentally vulnerable physiology to autism spectrum disorders. Curr Opin Neurol 2010;23(2):103–10.
39. Kim JA, Szatmari P, Bryson SE, et al. The prevalence of anxiety and mood problems among children with autism and Asperger syndrome. Autism 2000;4(2): 117–32.
40. Stewart ME, Barnard L, Pearson J, et al. Presentation of depression in autism and Asperger syndrome: a review. Autism 2006;10(1):103–16.
41. Munesue T, Ono Y, Mutoh K, et al. High prevalence of bipolar disorder comorbidity in adolescents and young adults with high-functioning autism spectrum disorder: a preliminary study of 44 outpatients. J Affect Disord 2008;111(2–3): 170–5.

42. Sukhodolsky DG, Scahill L, Gadow KD, et al. Parent-rated anxiety symptoms in children with pervasive developmental disorders: frequency and association with core autism symptoms and cognitive functioning. J Abnorm Child Psychol 2008;36(1):117–28.

43. Rommelse NN, Franke B, Geurts HM, et al. Shared heritability of attention-deficit/hyperactivity disorder and autism spectrum disorder. Eur Child Adolesc Psychiatry 2010;19(3):281–95.

44. Xue M, Brimacombe M, Chaaban J, et al. Autism spectrum disorders: concurrent clinical disorders. J Child Neurol 2008;23(1):6–13.

45. Lecavalier L. Behavior and emotional problems in young people with pervasive developmental disorders: relative prevalence, effects of subject characteristics, and empirical classification. J Autism Dev Disord 2006;36(8):1101–14.

46. Matson JL, Wilkins J, Macken J. The relationship of challenging behaviors to severity and symptoms of autism spectrum disorders. J Ment Health Res Intellect Disabil 2009;2(1):29–44.

47. Williams K, Wheeler DM, Silove N, et al. Selective serotonin reuptake inhibitors (SSRIs) for autism spectrum disorders (ASD). Cochrane Database Syst Rev 2010;8:CD004677.

48. Hamrin V, McDonnell MA, Moffett J, et al. Psychopharmacological treatment of non-comorbid and comorbid pervasive developmental disorder and pediatric bipolar disorder. Minerva Pediatr 2008;60(1):87–101.

49. Blankenship K, Erickson CA, McDougle CJ. Pharmacotherapy of autism and related disorders. Psychiatr Ann 2010;40(4):203–9.

50. Rasmussen SA, Friedman JM. NF1 gene and neurofibromatosis 1. Am J Epidemiol 2000;151(1):33–40.

51. Johnson NS, Saal HM, Lovell AM, et al. Social and emotional problems in children with neurofibromatosis type 1: evidence and proposed interventions. J Pediatr 1999;134(6):767–72.

52. Noll RB, Reiter-Purtill J, Moore BD, et al. Social, emotional, and behavioral functioning of children with NF1. Am J Med Genet A 2007;143(19):2261–73.

53. Mautner VF, Kluwe L, Thakker SD, et al. Treatment of ADHD in neurofibromatosis type 1. Dev Med Child Neurol 2002;44(3):164–70.

54. Botto LD, May K, Fernhoff PM, et al. A population-based study of the 22q11.2 deletion: phenotype, incidence, and contribution to major birth defects in the population. Pediatrics 2003;112(1):101–17.

55. Antshel KM, Fremont W, Roizen NJ, et al. ADHD, major depressive disorder, and simple phobias are prevalent psychiatric conditions in youth with velocardiofacial syndrome. J Am Acad Child Adolesc Psychiatry 2006;45(5):596–603.

56. Carlson C, Papolos D, Pandita RK, et al. Molecular analysis of velo-cardio-facial syndrome patients with psychiatric disorders. Am J Hum Genet 1997;60(4):851–9.

57. Gothelf D, Presburger G, Zohar AH, et al. Obsessive-compulsive disorder in patients with velocardiofacial (22q11 deletion) syndrome. Am J Med Genet B Neuropsychiatr Genet 2004;126(1):99–105.

58. Murphy KC. Annotation: velo-cardio-facial syndrome. J Child Psychol Psychiatry 2005;46(6):563–71.

59. Stoddard J, Niendam T, Hendren R, et al. Attenuated positive symptoms of psychosis in adolescents with chromosome 22q11.2 deletion syndrome. Schizophr Res 2010;118(1–3):118–21.

60. Gothelf D, Gruber R, Presburger G, et al. Methylphenidate treatment for attention-deficit/hyperactivity disorder in children and adolescents with velocardiofacial syndrome: an open-label study. J Clin Psychiatry 2003;64(10):1163–9.

61. Kao A, Mariani J, McDonald-McGinn DM, et al. Increased prevalence of unprovoked seizures in patients with a 22q11.2 deletion. Am J Med Genet 2004;129: 29–34.
62. Morrison PJ. Tuberous sclerosis: epidemiology, genetics and progress towards treatment. Neuroepidemiology 2009;33(4):342–3.
63. de Vries PJ, Hunt A, Bolton PF. The psychopathologies of children and adolescents with tuberous sclerosis complex (TSC): a postal survey of UK families. Eur Child Adolesc Psychiatry 2007;16(1):16–24.
64. Muzykewicz DA, Newberry P, Danforth N, et al. Psychiatric comorbid conditions in a clinic population of 241 patients with tuberous sclerosis complex. Epilepsy Behav 2007;11(4):506–13.
65. Asato MR, Hardan AY. Neuropsychiatric problems in tuberous sclerosis complex. J Child Neurol 2004;19(4):241–9.
66. D'Agati E, Moavero R, Cerminara C, et al. Attention-deficit hyperactivity disorder (ADHD) and tuberous sclerosis complex. J Child Neurol 2009;24(10):1282–7.

Psychopharmacology of Schizophrenia in Children and Adolescents

L. Lee Carlisle, MD*, Jon McClellan, MD

KEYWORDS

- Schizophrenia • Psychopharmacology • Child • Adolescent
- Psychiatry • Pharmacology

The past 5 years have seen major advances in the diagnosis and treatment of schizophrenia in children and adolescents. This article reviews the clinical and diagnostic characteristics of schizophrenia in youth with an eye toward recent findings. This article also provides a more extensive review and update of the psychopharmacology of early-onset schizophrenia (EOS).

DEFINITIONS
Schizophrenia

Schizophrenia is a chronic debilitating disorder associated with deficits in affect, cognition, and the ability to relate socially with others. Symptoms are traditionally described as positive, which include delusions, hallucinations, disorganized speech, and disorganized behavior (including catatonia) or negative, which include flattened affect, paucity of thought, and diminished and/or slowed speech.

EOS

EOS is defined as schizophrenia with onset of psychotic symptoms before 18 years of age. It is typically a chronic condition associated with elevated rates of premorbid abnormalities, significant long-term morbidity, and poor outcome.

Childhood-Onset Schizophrenia

Childhood-onset schizophrenia (COS) is defined as schizophrenia that develops before 13 years of age.

The authors have nothing to disclose.
Division of Child and Adolescent Psychiatry, Department of Psychiatry and Behavioral Sciences, University of Washington School of Medicine, PO Box 356560, Seattle, WA 98195, USA
* Corresponding author. Child Study and Treatment Center, 8805 Steilacoom Boulevard SW, W27-25, Lakewood, WA 98498-4771.
E-mail address: carlill@dshs.wa.gov

Pediatr Clin N Am 58 (2011) 205–218
doi:10.1016/j.pcl.2010.11.006

HISTORICAL PERSPECTIVE

Kraepelin[1] viewed COS as a rare form of the more typical adult-onset disorder. Over time, however, COS was characterized as part of a general category of childhood developmental syndromes that included infantile autism.[2] When the American Psychiatric Association's *Diagnostic and Statistical Manual of Mental Disorders* (DSM), Second Edition was published in 1968, this opinion still held. Thus, research from this time reflects a broad rubric of pervasive developmental problems.

EOS was eventually recognized as distinct from autism and continuous with the adult-onset disorder.[3–5] The DSM Third Edition[6] modified the diagnostic criteria for schizophrenia in childhood, using the same criteria as adults regardless of the age of onset. This convention has been maintained with subsequent revisions of both the DSM current edition DSM Fourth Edition (IV) Text Revision (TR)[7] and the *International Classification of Diseases* (ICD).[8] The evidence to date suggests that results from research on adult-onset schizophrenia can be reasonably extrapolated to children and adolescents, provided developmental differences are taken into account.

EPIDEMIOLOGY

The prevalence of EOS is not known. COS is extremely rare, with an estimated prevalence of 1 in 10000.[9] The rate of onset increases during adolescence, with the prime ages of onset for schizophrenia ranging from 15 to 30 years.[7] EOS, particularly COS, presents more often in males. As the age increases, the gender ratio tends to even out.

CLINICAL FEATURES

The diagnostic criteria for schizophrenia as delineated in DSM-IV-TR[7] are age-independent. These criteria are briefly summarized. To make a diagnosis of EOS, the DSM-IV-TR or ICD criteria should be followed. It is important to stress that, despite the historical ambiguity, a consensus has emerged that schizophrenia does develop in childhood, albeit rarely, and can be diagnosed using the DSM criteria.[10]

Overview of Diagnostic Criteria and Characteristic Symptoms

Schizophrenia characteristically presents with positive and negative symptoms. The former include hallucinations, especially auditory, delusions, and disordered behavior and/or speech. Negative symptoms include a generalized loss of energy, apathy, and flattening of affect. At least 2 positive symptoms or 1 positive and 1 negative symptom must be present for a 1 month in order to diagnose EOS, unless the symptoms are treated successfully within that time. An exception to this rule exists wherein this portion of the criteria can be fulfilled by hallucinations or delusions that are particularly florid and/or continuous. The remaining criteria essentially involve evidence of at least 6 months of deterioration in some area of social functioning and exclusion of other disorders (see discussion later).

Diagnostic Challenges and Differential Diagnosis

Although the criteria for diagnosing EOS in children are identical to those for adults, the younger age group presents some specific diagnostic challenges, which is especially true for COS. The main issues are with differentiating psychotic mood disorders, posttraumatic phenomena, and symptom reports suggestive of psychosis when taken out of developmental context. Immature responses of normal children can occasionally be confused with psychotic symptoms; it has been reported that 10% of children from the community may report experiences suggestive of hallucinations or delusions, yet do not have a true psychotic illness.[11]

CLINICAL COURSE OF EOS

Before the onset of schizophrenia, most patients experience prodromal symptoms associated with deteriorating social and intellectual functioning. During this time, children may appear depressed and anxious, while also developing unusual or bizarre behaviors. In teenagers, substance abuse is common, which confounds the diagnostic presentation. In addition, patients who develop EOS, particularly COS, have high rates of premorbid conditions, including early language abnormalities, cognitive disabilities, social withdrawal, and delayed motor development.[11] Patients diagnosed with COS generally have an insidious onset, whereas some adolescents experience an acute onset of the illness.[12]

The onset of positive symptoms (ie, hallucinations, delusions, and disorganized speech and behavior) marks the acute phase of the illness. This phase generally lasts anywhere from 1 to 6 months.[13] Once the acute symptoms are controlled, the patient typically remains impaired, with a predominance of negative symptoms (eg, flat affect, loss of energy, social withdrawal). Patients may also develop a postschizophrenic depression and flat affect. Acute symptoms may recur at varying intervals, and long-term impairment from the negative symptoms is, unfortunately, common.

PROGNOSIS

Follow-up studies of EOS suggest moderate to severe impairment across the lifespan.[14] Poor long-term outcome is predicted by low premorbid functioning, insidious onset, higher rates of negative symptoms, childhood onset, and low intellectual functioning.[15–20] When followed up into adulthood, youth with EOS demonstrated greater social deficits, lower levels of employment, and a lesser likelihood of living independently relative to those with other psychiatric disorders.[20,21]

Suicidal behavior is higher in adolescents with first-episode psychosis.[22] In follow-up studies, at least 5% of individuals with EOS die by completed suicide or by accidental death directly because of behaviors influenced by psychotic thinking.[23,24] Individuals with schizophrenia are also at a higher risk of other morbidities, such as heart disease, obesity, human immunodeficiency virus infection, hepatitis, and diabetes.[25]

ASSESSMENT OF EOS

The effective treatment of EOS relies on an accurate diagnosis and a thorough assessment to identify any other contributing medical or psychiatric condition and/or psychosocial stressors. **Fig. 1** lists the differential diagnosis for EOS.

Psychiatric Assessment

To screen for psychosis, the clinician can ask the child age-appropriate questions, such as "Do you hear voices talking to you when you are alone?" or "You know how you have dreams at night, do you sometimes feel like you have dreams when you are awake in the day?" Youth are sometimes responsive to direct questions about having "trouble thinking" or having their "thoughts now being more confused." When interviewing intellectually disabled children and children younger than 12 years, the clinicians must ensure that the child truly understands the question. Parents are important sources of information when trying to determine whether a child has

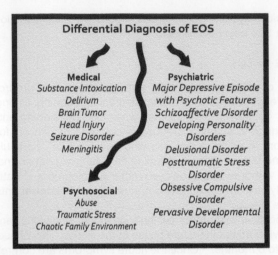

Differential Diagnosis of EOS

Medical
Substance Intoxication
Delirium
Brain Tumor
Head Injury
Seizure Disorder
Meningitis

Psychiatric
Major Depressive Episode
with Psychotic Features
Schizoaffective Disorder
Developing Personality
Disorders
Delusional Disorder
Posttraumatic Stress
Disorder
Obsessive Compulsive
Disorder
Pervasive Developmental
Disorder

Psychosocial
Abuse
Traumatic Stress
Chaotic Family Environment

Fig. 1. Differential diagnosis of EOS.

difficulty with thinking or perceptions. Changes in behavior and signs of responding to internal stimuli are most easily described by those who know the child best.

Children who do not have true psychotic illnesses sometimes report symptoms suggestive of psychosis. This reporting is particularly true for youth with trauma histories and for those with other types of emotional and conduct problems. Schizophrenia is defined by overt psychotic symptoms and observable mental status changes rather than solely by positive responses to a checklist of questions. Atypical psychotic symptom reports differ qualitatively from those associated with true psychosis. Reports of hallucinations are often much more detailed and organized, with content related to traumatic experiences, anxiety, or demonstrative imaginations. Atypical psychotic symptoms are also more likely to be situationally specific, for example, children who describe hallucinations only when adults are setting limits or telling them "no."

The diagnosis of schizophrenia should be reassessed as the symptoms evolve over the natural course of the disorder. It is not uncommon that the clinical presentation will change over time.[26] Reevaluation and/or a second opinion becomes more critical when the clinical presentation is atypical and/or the symptoms appear treatment refractory. Structured diagnostic interviews developed for use in pediatric populations with modules specific to psychotic disorders, such as Kiddie-Schedule for Affective Disorders and Schizophrenia for School-Aged Children (K-SADS),[27] may help improve the diagnostic accuracy.[28]

PHARMACOLOGIC MANAGEMENT OF EOS
Introduction

This section focuses on the medication management of EOS. It is important to recognize that effective management of EOS requires both psychosocial interventions and medication. Because EOS encompasses a pediatric population, psychosocial interventions should include developmentally appropriate treatment strategies and address family issues.

Antipsychotic medications are the foundation of treatment of EOS (**Table 1**). Because of a paucity of controlled clinical studies in children and adolescents, medication treatment of EOS has been guided primarily by extrapolation from adult literature and clinical experience.

Table 1
Antipsychotic indications for schizophrenia

	FDA Indication for Adults	FDA Indication for Adolescents 13–17 Years	Positive-Controlled Trials in Pediatric Population
First-Generation Antipsychotics			
Haloperidol	✔	✔	✔
Perphenazine	✔	—	—
Chlorpromazine	✔	✔	—
Molindone[a]	✔	✔	✔
Loxapine	✔	—	✔
Thioridazine	✔	✔	✔
Thiothixene	✔	✔	✔
Second-Generation Antipsychotics			
Risperidone	✔	✔	✔
Olanzapine	✔	✔	✔
Quetiapine	✔	✔	✔
Aripiprazole	✔	✔	✔
Ziprasidone	✔	—	—
Asenapine	✔	—	—
Paliperidone	✔	—	—
Clozapine	✔	—	✔
Iloperidone	✔	—	—

Abbreviation: FDA, Food and Drug Administration.
[a] Molindone is no longer available for sale as of June 2010.

Second-generation antipsychotic agents (SGAs) (with the exception of clozapine) have generally been considered the first-line treatment of EOS, and until recently were widely thought to be safer and more effective than first-generation agents. However, several large adult trials, including the Clinical Antipsychotic Trials of Intervention Effectiveness (CATIE) study,[29] the Cost Utility of the Latest Antipsychotic Drugs in Schizophrenia (CutLASS) study,[30] and the European First Episode Schizophrenia Trial (EUFEST) study[31] failed to demonstrate the superiority of SGAs over first-generation (typical) antipsychotics. Furthermore, regardless of the medication choice, many patients discontinue their treatment because of lack of efficacy, side effects, or noncompliance.

Efficacy of Antipsychotics in Children and Adolescents

There have been 11 published randomized controlled trials of antipsychotics in children and adolescents (**Table 2**). Positive findings are noted for several agents, including both first-generation medications (loxapine, haloperidol, thiothixene, thioridazine, and molindone) and second-generation medications (risperidone, olanzapine, and clozapine). Although molindone would seem to be a useful agent for EOS, it has been taken off the market and is no longer available.

As presented in **Table 2**, the number needed to treat (NNT) is a measure of the treatment effectiveness. NNT represents the number of patients who would need to be treated with a specified intervention in order to obtain one additional positive outcome that would not have occurred had the patient received the comparison treatment. Alternatively, it is the number of patients who would need to be treated in order to

Table 2
Efficacy of antipsychotics for EOS: evidence from randomized controlled trials in children and adolescents

Study	Design				Age (y)			Drug	Mean Dose (mg/d)	NNT	Outcome	
	Weeks	DB-RPCT	DB-RCT	SB-RCT	N	Ave Mean	Range				Measure	Findings
Pool et al,[32] 1976	4	✓	—	—	75	15.5	13–18	LOX HAL PBO	87.5 9.8 —	—	BPRS CGI-S	Both medications superior to PBO; ns between LOX and HAL; EPS & sedation problematic
Realmuto et al,[33] 1984	4–6	—	—	✓	21	15.6	11–18	THIX THIO	0.26 2.57	—	BPRS	Both medications significantly reduced symptoms
Spencer et al,[34] 1992	8	✓	—	—	12	8.8	5–12	HAL PBO	2.02 —	—	CGI-S CGI-I	HAL superior PBO; sedation problematic
Kumra et al,[35] 1996	6	—	✓	—	21	14.0	—	CLO HAL	176 16	—	BPRS-C	CLO superior to all measures; however, neutropenia and seizures lead to one-third of the patients discontinuing on CLO
Sikich et al,[36] 2004	8	—	✓	—	50	14.8	8–19	RIS OLA HAL	4.0 12.3 5.0	5 3 —	BPRS-C	Significant improvement with RIS, OLA, HAL; ns between medications; EPS and weight gain higher in youth compared with reports in adults
Shaw et al,[37] 2006	8	—	✓	—	25	12.2	7–16	CLO OLA	403.1 26.2	6 —	CGI-S/SANS SAPS	Significant improvement with CLO & OLA; ns between medications; marked weight gain in both groups
Haas et al,[38] 2007	6	✓	—	—	160	15.6	13–17	RIS RIS PBO	2.6 5.3 —	6 5 —	PANSS	RIS 1–3 mg & RIS 4–6 mg superior to PBO; higher dose had greater incidence of EPS

Findling et al,[39] 2008	6	✓	—	—	302	15.5	—	ARI ARI PBO	9.5 27.8 —	8 6 —	PANSS	ARI 10 mg & ARI 30 mg superior to PBO
Kumra et al,[40] 2008	12	—	✓	—	39	15.6	10–18	CLO OLA	403.1 26.2	3 —	BPRS-C	CLO & OLA caused significant improvement; ns between medications; 13% (3 patients on CLO, 2 patients on OLA) gained more than 7% of baseline body weight
Sikich et al,[41] 2008	8	—	✓	—	119	—	8–19	OLA RIS MOL[a]	11.4 2.8 59.9	— —	CGI-I PANSS	OLA, RIS, & MOL significant improvement; ns between medications; OLA & RIS greater weight gain; OLA greatest risk of weight gain and increased levels of cholesterol; MOL[a] most reports of akathisia
Kryzhanovskaya et al,[42] 2009	6	✓	—	—	107	16.2	13–17	OLA PBO	11.1 —	6 —	BPRS-C PANSS/CGI-S	OLA superior to PBO; 46% vs 15% PBO; patients on OLA gained ≥7% of body weight (higher and more severe in youth compared with reports in adults)

Abbreviations: ARI, aripiprazole; BPRS, Brief Psychiatric Rating Scale; BPRS-C, Brief Psychiatric Rating Scale for Children; CGI-I, Clinical Global Impressions Improvement Scale; CGI-S, Clinical Global Impressions Severity of Symptoms Scale; CLO, clozapine; DB, double-blind; HAL, haloperidol; LOX, loxapine; MOL, molindone; NNT, number needed to treat; ns, no significant difference/not significant; OLA, olanzapine; PANSS, Positive and Negative Syndrome Scale; PBO, placebo; RCT, randomized controlled trial; RIS, risperidone; RPCT, randomized, placebo-controlled trial; SANS, Schedule for the Assessment of Negative Symptoms; SAPS, Schedule for the Assessment of Positive Symptoms; SB, single-blind; THIO, thioridazine; THIX, thiothixene.

[a] No longer available as of June 2010.

prevent one negative outcome that would have occurred had the patient received the comparison treatment.[43] With an NNT of 3 as compared with a range of 5–8 for the other medications, clozapine has the best-documented effectiveness. Clozapine's use, however, is limited because of its side effects.

There is one large publicly-funded comparative trial for EOS, the Treatment of Early Onset Schizophrenia Spectrum Disorders Study (TEOSS).[41] TEOSS compared the effectiveness and safety of olanzapine, risperidone, and molindone for youth with EOS spectrum disorders. Less than 50% of the participants (n = 119) responded over 8 weeks of short-term treatment. Only 12% remained on their original treatment after 12 months.[44] The treatment groups did not differ significantly in the response rates or the magnitude of symptom reduction. Patients receiving olanzapine gained significantly more weight than those in the other 2 treatment arms to a degree that the data safety monitoring board discontinued the olanzapine arm midway through the study. These results of TEOSS replicate those of the large comparative adult trials and further challenge the presumed superiority of second-generation agents.

Side Effects of Antipsychotics in Children and Adolescents

Side effect profiles for first- and second-generation antipsychotic medications are outlined in **Table 3**. While the side effects reported in pediatric samples are similar to those seen in the adult population, some studies report different degrees of risk. Children and adolescents seem to be more vulnerable to prolactin abnormalities and extrapyramidal side effects (EPS), especially akathisia (involuntary movement disorder characterized by motor restlessness) and withdrawal dyskinesia (involuntary movement disorder [usually] occurring after the abrupt withdrawal of antipsychotics, which include chorea, athetosis, spasmodic torticollis, tongue protrusions, and other dystonic reactions). Children also typically experience more difficulty with weight gain and metabolic abnormalities than reported in adults. However, this observation may be attributable to the higher proportion of youth in antipsychotic trials who are treatment naive.[45]

First-generation antipsychotics generally produce higher rates of EPS, whereas the second-generation drugs are more often associated with metabolic abnormalities, including diabetes mellitus and weight gain. The degree of metabolic problems associated with olanzapine raises concerns regarding its use as a first-line agent.[41] Clozapine is associated with neutropenia and seizures and thus is reserved for refractive cases.[46] In addition, use of clozapine is difficult because it requires weekly blood draws, which can be especially problematic in younger patients.

Monitoring

Long-term safety monitoring is critical for children taking antipsychotic medications. Baseline blood pressure, weight, and body mass index should be recorded, electrocardiogram obtained, and metabolic studies including levels of fasting glucose and lipids should be performed before treatment. Blood pressure and weight should be recorded routinely at each visit. Recording levels of fasting glucose and lipids and electrocardiogram should be repeated at 3 months and annually thereafter, or more frequently, depending on the clinical situation. Given the risk of metabolic problems, preventative dietary education and/ or consultation with a nutritionist or dietitian may be useful before and during the treatment. Family education is critical as well.

TREATMENT GUIDELINES

Before discussing specific guidelines for the treatment of EOS, it is important to review the general principles regarding the pharmacologic management of children and

Table 3
Side effects of antipsychotic medications

Side Effects	First-Generation Antipsychotics			Second-Generation Antipsychotics						
	Haloperidol	Perphenazine	Molindone[a]	Risperidone	Olanzapine	Quetiapine	Aripiprazole	Ziprasidone	Paliperidone	Clozapine
Acute Parkinson Syndrome	++++++	++++	++++	++++	++	-	++	++	++++	-
Akathisia	++++++	++++	++++	++	++	++	++++	+++	++	++
Diabetes Mellitus	++	++	+	++	++++++	++++	+	+	++	+++++
Diabetes Insipidus	-	-	-	-	-	-	-	-	-	+
⇑ Lipid Levels	+	++	+	++	++++	+++	+	+	++	+++
Neutropenia	+	+	+	+	+	+	+	+	+	++++
Orthostatic hypotension	+	++	++	++	++++	++++	+	-	++	++++++
⇑ Prolactin level	++++	++++	++++	++++++	+++	-	-	++	+++++	-
⇓ Prolactin level	-	-	-	-	-	-	++++	-	-	-
⇑ QT interval	+	++	++	++	+	++	+	++++	++	++
Sedation	+	++	++	++	++++	++++	+	+	++	++++++
Seizures	+	+	+	+	+	+	+	+	+	++++
Tardive Dyskinesia	++++	++++	+++	+	+	+	+	+	+	-
Withdrawal Dyskinesia	++++	+++	+++	++	+	+	++++	++	++	++
Weight Gain	++	++++	+	++++	++++++	++++	++	++	+++	++++++

Abbreviations: ⇓, decreased; ⇑, increased; -, none; + to ++++, mild to severe.
[a] No longer available as of June 2010.
Data from Refs.[48–50]

adolescents with mental illness. Whenever possible, medication options are based on the efficacy and safety data from pediatric populations, while also considering patient and family preferences and costs. Before initiating treatment, it is important to review the target symptoms, anticipated outcomes, and potential risks with the patient and family. Rating scales are often useful for monitoring the symptom response. Potential side effects need to be systematically monitored, with laboratory assessments and physical examinations conducted at set defined intervals as clinically indicated. If symptoms do not improve or intolerable side effects develop, a different course of treatment should be implemented following the same guidelines. Although some youth may require more than one medication, as a general rule polypharmacy is best avoided.

In **Fig. 2** the authors offer an algorithm for treating EOS, with the caveat that this guideline is only a suggestion based on data available at present. The authors suggest risperidone as the first choice because (1) it has the most empirical data in youth, (2) it is

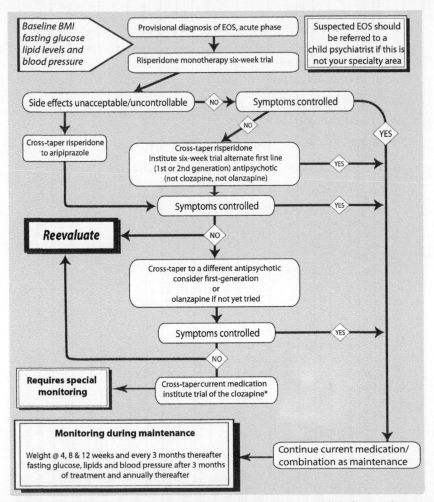

Fig. 2. Suggested algorithm for the treatment of EOS. The asterisk indicates that use of clozapine requires coordination between physician, laboratory and pharmacy. BMI, body mass index.

available as a generic drug and is therefore less expensive, and (3) it is approved by the Food and Drug Administration for EOS. If risperidone is not tolerated, aripiprazole is suggested as the next choice because of safety issues (lower metabolic side effects).

Results from the TOESS indicate that the first-generation antipsychotic could also be used as the first choice. Consideration should be given to perphenazine at this point, given the results of the CATIE trial,[29] the higher incidence of EPS with haloperidol, and the fact that molindone is no longer available. Olanzapine is only recommended after the failure of another agent, given its association with substantial weight gain and risk for long-term metabolic problems. Ziprasidone is not currently considered an option for EOS because of an industry-sponsored, double-blind, placebo-controlled trial in which it was discontinued because of a lack of efficacy.[47] For the treatment of refractory cases, clozapine should be considered.

Some providers prefer to try a combination of 2 antipsychotics for patients with refractory EOS. Although this option may be beneficial for some patients, empirical data are not available to support this practice at present. If multiple medications are deemed necessary, each agent should be initiated and monitored systematically to allow an accurate assessment of effectiveness and safety. Otherwise, patients end up on multiple agents with no clear understanding of how each medication affects the illness and side effect profile.

Antipsychotic medications can provide substantial benefit for EOS, which when left untreated is a devastating illness. However, none of the available agents are associated with substantial rates of illness remission, and all are linked with significant side effects.

New treatments are needed, with mechanisms based on advances in research unraveling the genetic and neurobiological pathways underlying schizophrenia (see **Fig. 2**).

REFERENCES

1. Kraepelin E. In: Dementia praecox and paraphrenia. [Barclay RM, Trans. 8th German edition of the Textbook of Psychiatry, Vol. III, Part 2, on "Endogenous Dementias" 1913.] Edinburgh (UK): E. & S. Livingstone; 1919.
2. Fish B, Ritvo E. Psychoses of childhood. In: Noshpitz JD, Berlin I, editors. Basic handbook of child psychiatry. New York: Basic Books; 1979. p. 249–304.
3. Kolvin I. Studies in the childhood psychoses. Br J Psychiatry 1971;6:209–34.
4. Rutter M. Childhood schizophrenia reconsidered. J Autism Child Schizophr 1972; 2:315–37.
5. Werry JS. Psychoses. In: Quay HC, Werry JS, editors. Psychopathological disorders of childhood. Second edition. New York: Wiley; 1979. p. 43–89.
6. American Psychiatric Association. In: Diagnostic and Statistical Manual of Mental Disorders. (DSM-III). Third edition. Washington, DC: American Psychiatric Association; 1980.
7. American Psychiatric Association. In: Diagnostic and Statistical Manual of Mental Disorders. Text Revision. Fourth Edition. Washington, DC: American Psychiatric Association; 2000.
8. World Health Organization. In: ICD-10: the ICD-10 classification of mental and behavioral disorders: clinical descriptions and diagnostic guidelines. Geneva (Switzerland): World Health Organization; 1992.
9. American Academy of Child and Adolescent Psychiatry. Practice parameter for the assessment and treatment of children and adolescents with schizophrenia. J Am Acad Child Adolesc Psychiatry 2001;40:4S–23S.

10. Asarnow J, Tompson M, McGrath E. Annotation: childhood-onset schizophrenia: clinical and treatment issues. J Child Psychol Psychiatry 2004;45(2):180–94.

11. Masi G, Mucci M, Cinzia P, et al. Children with schizophrenia clinical picture and pharmacological treatment. CNS Drugs 2006;20(10):841–66.

12. Khurana A, Aminzadeh A, Bostic JQ, et al. Childhood-onset schizophrenia: diagnostic and treatment challenges. SPECIAL REPORT SCHIZOPHRENIA. Psychiatr Times 2007;XXIV(2):33.

13. Werry JS, Taylor E. Schizophrenia and allied disorders. In: Rutter M, Hersov L, Taylor E, editors. Child and adolescent psychiatry: modern approaches. Third edition. Oxford (UK): Blackwell Scientific; 1994. p. 594–615.

14. McClellan J. Early onset schizophrenia. In: Kaplan HI, Kaplan, editors. Sadock's comprehensive textbook of psychiatry/VIII. Baltimore (MD): Lippincott Williams and Wilkins; 2005. p. 2782–9.

15. McClellan J, McCurry C, Snell J, et al. Early onset psychotic disorders: course and outcome over a two year period. J Am Acad Child Adolesc Psychiatry 1999;38:1380–9.

16. Vyas NS, Hadjulis M, Vourdas A, et al. The Maudsley early onset schizophrenia study: predictors of psychosocial outcome at 4-year follow-up. Eur Child Adolesc Psychiatry 2007;16(7):465–70.

17. Werry JS, McClellan J. Predicting outcome in child and adolescent (early onset) schizophrenia and bipolar disorder. J Am Acad Child Adolesc Psychiatry 1992; 31:147–50.

18. Röpcke B, Eggers C. Early-onset schizophrenia: a 15-year follow-up. Eur Child Adolesc Psychiatry 2005;14(6):341–50.

19. Maziade M, Bouchard S, Gingras N, et al. Long-term stability of diagnosis and symptom dimensions in a systematic sample of patients with onset of schizophrenia in childhood and early adolescence. II: postnegative distinction and childhood predictors of adult outcome. Br J Psychiatry 1996;169(3): 371–8.

20. Jarbin H, Ott Y, Von Knorring AL. Adult outcome of social function in adolescent-onset schizophrenia and affective psychosis. J Am Acad Child Adolesc Psychiatry 2003;42(2):176–83.

21. Hollis C. Adult outcomes of child- and adolescent-onset schizophrenia: diagnostic stability and predictive validity. Am J Psychiatry 2000;157(10):1652–9.

22. Falcone T, Mishra L, Carlton E, et al. Suicidal behavior in adolescents with first-episode psychosis. Clin Schizophr Relat Psychoses 2010;4(2):34–40.

23. Werry JS, McClellan J, Chard L. Early-onset schizophrenia, bipolar and schizoaffective disorders: a clinical follow-up study. J Am Acad Child Adolesc Psychiatry 1991;30:457–65.

24. Eggers C. Course and prognosis in childhood schizophrenia. J Autism Child Schizophr 1978;8:21–36.

25. Goff DC, Sullivan LM, McEvoy JP, et al. A comparison of ten-year cardiac risk estimates in schizophrenia patients from the CATIE study and matched controls. Schizophr Res 2005;80(1):45–53.

26. Schwartz JE, Fennig S, Tanenberg-Karant M, et al. Congruence of diagnoses 2 years after a first-admission diagnosis of psychosis. Arch Gen Psychiatry 2000; 57:593–600.

27. Kaufman J. Kiddie-Sads-Present and Lifetime version (K-SADS-PL). University of Pittsburgh Department of Psychiatry; 2010. Available at: http://www.wpic.pitt.edu/ksads/default.htm. Modified Thursday, 9:16:12 AM. Accessed September 8, 2010.

28. Carlisle L, McClellan J. Diagnostic interviews. In: Dulcan M, editor. Dulcan's texbook of child and adolescent psychiatry. Chicago: American Psychiatric Publishing; 2010. p. 79–88.
29. Lieberman JA, Stroup TS, McEvoy JP, et al. Effectiveness of antipsychotic drugs in patients with chronic schizophrenia. N Engl J Med 2005;353(12):1209–23.
30. Jones PB, Barnes TR, Davies L, et al. Randomized controlled trial of the effect on Quality of Life of second- vs first-generation antipsychotic drugs in schizophrenia: Cost Utility of the Latest Antipsychotic Drugs in Schizophrenia Study (CUtLASS 1). Arch Gen Psychiatry 2006;63(10):1079–87.
31. Kahn RS, Fleischhacker WW, Boter H, et al. EUFEST study group. Effectiveness of antipsychotic drugs in first-episode schizophrenia and schizophreniform disorder: an open randomized clinical trial. Lancet 2008;371(9618):1085–97.
32. Pool D, Bloom W, Mielke DH, et al. A controlled evaluation of loxitane in seventy-five adolescent schizophrenic patients. Curr Ther Res Clin Exp 1976;19:99–104.
33. Realmuto G, Erickson W, Yellin A, et al. Clinical comparison of thiothixene and thioridazine in schizophrenic adolescents. Am J Psychiatry 1984;141:440–2.
34. Spencer E, Kafantaris V, Padron-Gayol M, et al. Haloperidol in schizophrenic children: early findings from a study in progress. Psychopharmacol Bull 1992;28: 183–6.
35. Kumra S, Frazier J, Jacobsen, et al. Childhood-onset schizophrenia: a double-blind clozapine-haloperidol comparison. Arch Gen Psychiatry 1996;53:1090–7.
36. Sikich L, Hamer R, Bashford R, et al. A pilot study of risperidone, olanzapine, and haloperidol in psychotic youth: a double-blind, randomized, 8-week trial. Neuropsychopharmacology 2004;29(1):133–45.
37. Shaw P, Sporn A, Gogtay N, et al. Childhood-onset schizophrenia: a double-blind, randomized clozapine-olanzapine comparison. Arch Gen Psychiatry 2006;63:721–30.
38. Haas M, Unis A, Copenhaver M, et al. Efficacy and safety of risperidone in adolescents with schizophrenia [abstract]. In: Programs and Abstracts of the Annual Meeting of the American Psychiatric Association. San Diego (CA), May 2007.
39. Findling RL, Robb A, Nyilas M, et al. A multiple-center, randomized, double-blind, placebo-controlled study of oral aripiprazole for treatment of adolescents with schizophrenia. Am J Psychiatry 2008;165(11):1432–41.
40. Kumra S, Oberstar JV, Sikich L, et al. Efficacy and tolerability of second generation antipsychotics in children and adolescents with schizophrenia. Schizophr Bull 2008;34:60–71.
41. Sikich L, Frazier JA, McClellan J, et al. Double-blind comparison of first- and second-generation antipsychotics in early onset schizophrenia and schizoaffective disorder: findings from the treatment of early onset schizophrenia spectrum disorders (TEOSS) study. Am J Psychiatry 2008;165:1420–31.
42. Kryzhanovskaya L, Schulz C, McDougle C, et al. Olanzapine versus placebo in adolescents with schizophrenia: a 6-week, randomized, double-blind, placebo-controlled trial. J Am Acad Child Adolesc Psychiatry 2009;48(1):60–70.
43. Pinson L, Gray GM. Psychopharmacology: number needed to treat: an underused measure of treatment effect. Psychiatr Serv 2003;54(2):145–54.
44. Findling RL, Johnson JL, McClellan J, et al. Double-blind maintenance safety and effectiveness findings from the Treatment of Early-Onset Schizophrenia Spectrum (TEOSS) study. J Am Acad Child Adolesc Psychiatry 2010;49(6):583–94.
45. Correll CU, Manu P, Olshanskiy V, et al. Cardiometabolic risk of second-generation antipsychotic medications during first-time use in children and adolescents. JAMA 2009;302(16):1765–73.

46. Toren P, Rainer S, Laor N, et al. Benefit-risk assessment of atypical antipsychotics in the treatment of schizophrenia and comorbid disorders in children and adolescents. Drug Saf 2004;27(14):1135–56.

47. Safety and efficacy of ziprasidone in adolescents with schizophrenia. U.S. Department of Health & Human Services; 2010. Available at: http://www.clinicaltrials.gov/ct2/show/NCT00257192?term=NCT00257192&rank=1. Modified Wednesday, 4:14:24 PM. Accessed September 8, 2010.

48. Haddad PM, Sharma SG. Adverse effects of atypical antipsychotics differential risk and clinical implications. CNS Drugs 2007;21(11):911–36.

49. Conley R, Kelly D. A review of current drug targets and pharmacology of antipsychotic treatment. Med Chem Rev Online 2005;2(3):177–82.

50. Ananth J, Parameswaran S, Hara B. Drug therapy in schizophrenia. Curr Pharm Des 2004;10:2205–17.

Management of Nonpsychiatric Medical Conditions Presenting with Psychiatric Manifestations

Manmohan K. Kamboj, MD[a], Ruqiya Shama Tareen, MD[b,c],*

KEYWORDS

• Medical conditions • Psychiatric conditions • Management

One of the most significant dilemmas arise when there is an underlying medical disorder presenting as a psychiatric presentation. It is important to identify the medical condition because treatment and management strategies need to be directed not only to the presenting symptoms but also to the underlying medical condition for appropriate success in the treatment of the patient. Some systemic disorders are known to present with psychiatric manifestations more often than others. The pattern of psychiatric disturbance seen may be specific for a particular medical disorder but also may be varied. Many drug formulations and medications also may produce well-recognized psychiatric presentations. The spectrum of medical disorders that may present with psychiatric clinical presentations is listed in **Box 1**. Many endocrine system disorders may present with a wide range of psychiatric symptoms. This article discusses the overlapping of psychiatric clinical features in these endocrine disorders and addresses appropriate management strategies in these scenarios.

THYROID DISORDERS

Hypothyroidism and hyperthyroidism may present with signs and symptoms that closely overlap a variety of psychiatric features. The presence of coexistent

---

The authors have no disclosures.

[a] Section of Endocrinology, Metabolism and Diabetes, Nationwide Children's Hospital, 700 Children's Drive (ED425), Columbus, OH 43205, USA

[b] Department of Psychiatry, Michigan State University College of Human Medicine, East Lansing, MI, USA

[c] Psychiatry Residency Program, Kalamazoo Center for Medical Studies, 1722 Shaffer Road, Suite 3, Kalamazoo, MI 49048, USA

* Corresponding author. Psychiatry Residency Program, Kalamazoo Center for Medical Studies, 1722 Shaffer Road, Suite 3, Kalamazoo, MI 49048.

E-mail address: tareen@kcms.msu.edu

Pediatr Clin N Am 58 (2011) 219–241

doi:10.1016/j.pcl.2010.10.008

Box 1
Spectrum of medical disorders that may present with psychiatric symptoms

Endocrine disorders[a]

- Thyroid

  Hypothyroidism

  Hyperthyroidism

- Parathyroid disorders

  Hypoparathyroidism

  Hyperparathyroidism

- Adrenal disorders

  Hypoadrenocorticism/adrenal insufficiency

  Hypercorticism/Cushing syndrome

  Pheochromocytoma

- Disorders of glycemic control

  Hyperglycemia/diabetes mellitus

  Hypoglycemia

- Genetic syndromes

  Klinefelter syndrome

  Turner syndrome

Metabolic disorders

- Porphyrias

- Vitamin deficiencies

  B_1 deficiency

- Hepatic disorders

  Hepatic encephalopathy

  Wilson disease

Immunologic disorders

- Systemic lupus erythematosus

- Multiple sclerosis

- Fibromyalgia

Central nervous system disorders

Infectious diseases

- Rheumatic fever

- Human immunodeficiency virus infections

- Syphilis

- Malaria

- Typhoid

[a] These disorders are discussed in this article.

neuropsychiatric manifestations may cause a more serious and insidious functional decline. At times, psychiatric symptoms may be the only, or the most prominent, presenting symptoms of thyroid disequilibrium and these are the patients who may be misdiagnosed with a primary psychiatric illness.[1] Cognitive dysfunction with slowing of the mental processes, difficulties in short-term memory, decreased concentration, inattention, and attention deficit hyperactivity disorder (ADHD), are some of the clinical features that may mislead the diagnosis. **Table 1** lists some of the common psychiatric presentations seen in various thyroid disorders.

Hypothyroidism

Clinical features

Clinical presentation varies greatly based on severity of hypothyroidism and on whether the hypothyroidism develops acutely or is more chronic in onset. The chronic, slow-developing hypothyroidism presents with vague, nonspecific features and has the potential for a delayed diagnosis. Children and adolescents may be asymptomatic but, on routine physical examination, may be noted to show evidence of suboptimal growth. They may complain of being lethargic with low energy levels, fatigue, loss of appetite, weight gain, sallow complexion, memory loss, menstrual disturbances generally with increased and prolonged bleeding, dry skin, temperature intolerance, and hair loss.

Psychiatric features

Depression as the hallmark of hypothyroidism has been well documented in literature. However, manic presentation is uncommon, even in patients with established bipolar disorder, but there are reports of mania induced by thyroxine treatment in hypothyroid patients.[2,3] Myxedema madness was once a common initial presentation of hypothyroidism but now accounts for only about 5% to 15% of cases.[4,5] A wide variety of symptoms have been reported with myxedema madness, including depression and restlessness, perceptual disturbances in the form of auditory and visual hallucinations, delusions of a persecutory nature, paranoia, and loosening of associations. The presence of psychosis usually signifies chronic hypothyroidism. The severity of illness does not always correlate with the occurrence of psychotic symptoms and therefore cannot be used as a predicting factor.[6] Two types of encephalopathy have been reported in hypothyroidism. Hashimoto encephalopathy in children and adolescents 9 to 17 years of age is reported to present with dysphoric mood, hallucinations, decreased alertness, decline in cognition, anxiety, hyperactivity, and various neurologic symptoms including myoclonus, hemiperesis/hemiplegia, and focal and generalized seizure activity.[7] Acute exhaustion psychosis or delirium has been reported in older studies citing mortality rate as high as 70%.[8] The incidence of hypothyroidism in patients being treated with lithium is reported to be around 2% to 10%.[9] Clinicians

---

Table 1
Frequency of occurrence of various psychiatric disorders in thyroid disorders

Thyroid Disorders	Depression	Mania	Anxiety Spectrum	Psychosis	ADHD	Delirium	Cognitive Dysfunction
Hypothyroidism	+++	+	++	++	+	+	+++
Hyperthyroidisms	++	++	+++	++	+	+	++
Subclinical hypothyroidism	+	+	+	±	+	±	+

must counsel their patients regarding the possibility of hypothyroidism when starting on this treatment. It is also prudent to do baseline thyroid function tests, including antithyroid antibodies, before initiation of lithium therapy.[9] The risk of rapid-cycling bipolar disorder (4 or more manic, hypomanic, or depressive episodes occurring in 1 year) is seen in 10% to 12% of patients with bipolar disorder. Bauer and colleagues[10] reported that grade 1 hypothyroidism in bipolar patients is a risk factor for development of rapid cycling.

Medical work-up

Thyroid function tests, including free thyroxine (FT_4) and thyroid stimulating hormone (TSH) levels, are the main diagnostic laboratory studies used to diagnose thyroid disorders (**Table 2**). If thyroid dysfunction is noted, further testing, including antithyroperoxidase and antithyroglobulin antibodies, may be done to establish any underlying autoimmune cause. Imaging studies, including thyroid ultrasound, may be done only if needed. This further work-up is best addressed in coordination with a pediatric endocrinologist.

Psychiatric work-up

Diagnosis of depression poses a diagnostic dilemma in the presence of hypothyroidism because many of the clinical features of hypothyroidism mimic the neurovegetative symptoms of depression. The high association of the 2 disorders should alert any clinician to do a mandatory screen for depression. Use of psychiatric testing measures for the identification of psychiatric illness and for the ongoing monitoring of these disorders is gaining some popularity in primary care settings.

Medical treatment

It is recommended that overt hypothyroidism be treated adequately; however, the consensus about treatment of subclinical or compensated hypothyroidism is not as clear.[11] Initial presentation with borderline, mild, or subclinical hypothyroidism should be followed with a repeat of FT_4 and TSH testing in several weeks for confirmation and to watch for a trend. Treatment decisions need to be individualized and may depend on multiple factors including growth pattern, symptoms, thyroid enlargement, antibody status, and the laboratory values.[12,13] Thyroid hormone preparations recommended for use are the recombinant levothyroxine (LT_4) preparations. FT_4 and TSH levels are repeated in 4 weeks after initiating treatment to make appropriate dose titrations.

Psychiatric treatment

Selective serotonin reuptake inhibitors (SSRIs) have now become the first-line treatment of depression and anxiety in adults because of their efficacy. The relative safety of SSRIs versus their predecessors, the tricyclic antidepressants (TCAs), has revolutionized the way patients with medical comorbidities can be treated for their

Table 2		
Laboratory findings in hypothyroidism		
	Free Thyroxine	**Thyroid Stimulating Hormone**
Subclinical/compensated hypothyroidism	Normal	Increased
Overt hypothyroidism	Low	Increased
Central hypothyroidism	Low	Low/normal

psychiatric illness. The SSRIs have equal clinical efficacy but only few are approved for use in pediatric populations (**Table 3**). The selection of a particular agent depends on multiple factors including age, previous response to any particular SSRI, any contra-indications, side effects, possible drug interactions, and previous good response to a particular SSRI in the patient or in another family member. The other factors affecting the choice of SSRI include ease of dosing (eg, availability of different formulations, ie, suspensions and tablets) and daily dosing options (ie, once daily vs 2 to 3 times a day). The most important factor can be the cost of the particular SSRI, insurance coverage, and the availability of generic versus brand name formulations. Hashimoto encepha-lopathy is a steroid-responsive encephalopathy associated with Hashimoto thyroiditis and usually responds well to high-dose glucocorticoid therapy. Treatment usually starts with intravenous therapy followed by prednisone 1 to 2 mg/kg/d for 6 to 8 weeks. Relapses have been reported in spite of initial good response.[7] Cognitive defi-cits may persist even after successful treatment.

Hyperthyroidism

Clinical features

Patients with hyperthyroidism may present with a wide spectrum of symptoms depending on severity and acuity of onset, including weight loss with increased appe-tite, heat intolerance, menstrual disturbances generally with menorrhagia/metorrha-gia, palpitations, warm and flushed skin, diaphoresis, exophthalmos, proptosis, and lid lag.

Table 3			
Psychotropics approved by the US Food and Drug Administration for the pediatric population			
	Psychotropic	**Indication**	**Age (y)**
SSRIs	Fluoxetine	Depression	≥ 8
		OCD	≥ 7
	Fluvoxamine	OCD	≥ 8
	Sertraline	OCD	≥ 6
	Escitalopram	Depression	≥ 12
Tricyclic antidepressants	Imipramine	Depression	≥ 12
	Clomipramine	OCD	≥ 10
	Doxepin	Depression	≥ 12
Mood stabilizers	Carbamazepine	Epilepsy monotherapy/adjunctive	All ages
	Oxcarbazepine	Epilepsy monotherapy	≥ 4
	Lamotrigine	Epilepsy monotherapy	≥ 16
	Gabapentin	Epilepsy adjunctive therapy	≥ 3
	Topiramate	Epilepsy monotherapy	≥ 10
Typical antipsychotics	Chlorpromazine	Severe behavior problems	0.5–12
	Haloperidol	Severe behavior problems	≥ 3
	Pimozide	Tourette disorder	≥ 12
Atypical antipsychotics	Risperidone	Schizophrenia	≥ 13
		Bipolar disorder type I	≥ 10
		Irritability in autistic disorder	5–16
	Apiprazole	Schizophrenia	≥ 13
		Bipolar disorder type I	≥ 10
		Irritability in autistic disorder	6–17

Abbreviation: OCD, obsessive-compulsive disorder.

Psychiatric features

The debate about the role of thyroid dysfunction in children and adolescents with ADHD continues, with strong arguments on both sides without any clear conclusion. Children with hyperthyroidism may display deterioration in school performance, hyperactivity, and inattention. The onset of neuropsychological symptoms generally precedes the diagnosis of abnormality of thyroid function. The spectrum of anxiety disorders has a strong correlation with hyperthyroidism. Neuropsychiatric symptoms, including anxious dysphoria and irritability, may predate the diagnosis of thyrotoxicosis by up to a year.[14] Studies have also found a strong correlation between depression and anxiety among hyperthyroid patients. A survey of 137 patients with Graves disease found irritability in 78%, shakiness in 77%, and anxiety in 72% of patients.[15] Specific phobias have also been reported as a presenting symptom in hyperthyroidism.[16] Panic disorder with agoraphobia (fear of having a panic attack in a situation from which escape is difficult, which can make the patient housebound) is a debilitating disorder and at times is the presenting symptom of hyperthyroidism. Psychotic symptoms with mania and hypomania have been associated with more morbidity and loss of functioning than a hyperthyroid state without mania, and are associated with a higher lifetime risk of hospitalization for psychiatric reasons.[17]

Medical work-up

FT_4 and TSH are primary laboratory tests for diagnosis of hyperthyroidism. Further testing if needed may include free T_3 levels, antithyroperoxidase and antithyroglobulin antibodies, and thyroid-stimulating immunoglobulin levels (**Table 4**).

Psychiatric work-up

It is prudent to complete a thorough initial psychiatric evaluation. The focus should be on developmental psychology to differentiate between the concerns and fears normally associated with a given developmental stage versus an anxiety disorder. Separation anxiety, situational anxiety related to school, gender and sexual identity, and so forth are age-appropriate developmental responses with features of anxiety but usually are transient and resolve on their own. Several screening tests can be used in children more than 8 years of age for the diagnosis of anxiety disorders, for example the Multidimensional Anxiety Scale for Children or the Screen for Child Anxiety-related Emotional Disorders (**Table 5**).

Medical treatment

Hyperthyroidism may be treated with medications, surgery, or radioactive iodine (RAI). Medical therapy includes 2 main groups of medications: methimazole/tapazole or thionamides such as propyl thiouracil. RAI therapy for Graves disease is becoming increasingly popular in the adolescent age group, whereas it is the treatment of choice in adults. Total or partial thyroidectomy may have to be undertaken in younger children in situations in which RAI may be contraindicated, or if the thyroid gland is very large.

Table 4
Laboratory findings in hyperthyroidism

Thyroid Disorder	FT$_4$	TSH	Free Triiodothyronine
Overt hyperthyroidism	Increased high	Low	Not needed
Subclinical hyperthyroidism	Normal	Low	Not needed
Triiodothyronine toxicosis	Normal	Low	High

Table 5
Psychological screening tests for psychiatric disorder in children and adolescents

Presentation	Psychological Tests	Ages (y)	Time (min)
Depression	Weinberg Depression Scale for Children and Adolescents	5–17	3–5
	Children's Depression Rating Scale-Revised	6–12 and adolescent	15–20
	Beck Depression Inventory for Youth	7–14	3–5
	Reynolds Child/Adolescent Depression Scales:		
	Child	8–12	10
	Adolescent	11–20	10
	Center for Epidemiologic Studies	6–17	5
	Depression Scale for Children		
	Children Depression Inventory	7–17	10–15
Bipolar disorder	Young Mania Rating Scale	5–17	15–30
	Parent version of the Young Mania Rating Scale	5–17	5
	Mood Disorder Questionnaire	≥12	5–10
	Weinberg Affective Scale	7–17	5
Suicide risk assessment	Suicidal Ideation Questionnaire	13–18	10
Anxiety spectrum disorders	Depression and Anxiety in Youth Scale	6–19	15–20
	Beck Anxiety Inventory for Youth	7–14	10
	Self-report for Childhood Anxiety-related Emotional Disorders	≥8	5
	How I Feel Questionnaire	7–17	5–10
	Children's Yale-Brown Obsessive Compulsive Scale	6–14	40
ADHD	Conners Rating Scale Scales Revised short form	3–17	5–10
	Vanderbilt ADHD Diagnostic Parent Rating Scale	6–12	10
	Conners-Wells Self-report	12–17	5–10
Psychotic disorders	Kiddie Schedule for Affective Disorders and Schizophrenia	6–18	90–120
Delirium/encephalopathy	Pediatric Anesthesia Emergence Scale	19 mo to 6 y	1
	Delirium Rating Scale in Children and Adolescents	6 mo to 19 y	
Achievement/development/ learning	Wide Range Assessment of Visual Motor Abilities	3–17	4–10 per subset
	Test of language Development-Primary, 4th edition	4–8	60
	Test of Visual Perceptual Skills, 3rd edition	4–18	30–40
	Test of Nonverbal Intelligence 4th edition	6–11 onward	20

Data from School Psychiatry Program & MADI Resource Center http://www2.massgeneral.org/schoolpsychiatry/screeningtools_table.asp.

Propranolol or atenolol may be used initially to control some of the sympathomimetic effects of hyperthyroidism.

Psychiatric treatment
The ADHD-like symptoms respond well to antithyroid treatment if the treatment is initiated early. However, a delay in diagnosis and treatment may result in persistence of the neuropsychiatric and cognitive issues.[13] The anxiety symptoms of hyperparathyroidism generally respond well to medical treatment. However, if a comorbid anxiety disorder is present, psychiatric intervention may be indicated. The initial treatment of anxiety spectrum disorders is psychotherapy, with some data to support the efficacy of psychodynamic therapy, cognitive behavioral therapy (CBT), and parent-child and family therapy.[18] SSRIs offer efficacious therapeutic options in anxiety disorders if psychotherapy alone is unsuccessful.[18,19] Other anxiolytics approved for adults, but not clearly approved in the pediatric population, such as benzodiazepines, buspar, venlafaxine, bupropion, and TCAs, have also been used alone or in combination for treatment of childhood anxiety disorders.[18] Psychotic symptoms usually resolve spontaneously when TSH levels normalize. However, atypical antipsychotics may be useful in the short-term.[20]

PARATHYROID DISORDERS

Disturbances in parathyroid hormone metabolism comprise mainly hypoparathyroidism and hyperparathyroidism. The main clinical presentation is caused by features of hypocalcemia or hypercalcemia respectively.

Hypoparathyroidism

Clinical features
Children and adolescents with hypoparathyroidism may present with generalized weakness, fatigue, and listlessness; signs of muscle irritability, twitching, tetany, or frank seizures; and slow cognition or severe cognitive impairment. Chevostek and Trousseau signs may be present. Abnormalities of cardiac rhythm may be present. These patients may also present for attention with psychiatric symptoms even before the physical features described.

Psychiatric features
Psychiatric symptoms are usually associated with long-standing hypoparathyroidism.[21] Velasco and colleagues[22] studied the frequency of occurrence of psychiatric symptoms and noted that cognitive impairment (39%) is the commonest followed by nonspecific psychiatric symptoms (21%), neurotic symptoms (12%), and psychosis (11%). Electrolyte studies should be done in these patients before the start of therapy because hypocalcaemia and hypomagnesemia may cause treatment resistance to psychotropics.

Medical work-up
Laboratory findings for hypoparathyroidism are noted in **Table 6**. Serum magnesium levels may also be low.

Psychiatric work-up
Screening questions and suspicion of psychiatric comorbidity guide further work-up. In children and adolescents, a decline in school performance may be the first indication of cognitive dysfunction. A pediatric version of Confusion Assessment Method for the Intensive Care Unit (CAM-ICU) has been proposed as an algorithm for evaluation of pediatric delirium and is considered suitable for children more than 5 years of age.[23]

Table 6			
Laboratory findings in parathyroid disorders			
Parathyroid Disorder	Ca	P	Parathyroid Hormone
Hypoparathyroidism	Decreased	Increased	Decreased
Hyperparathyroidism	Increased	Decreased	Increased
Pseudohypoparathyroidism	Decreased	Increased	Increased

CAM consist of only 4 questions establishing acute onset, fluctuating course, inattention, disorganized speech, and altered level of consciousness. The Pediatric Anesthesia Emergence Delirium Scale (PAED) is another simple tool that can be easily adopted for assessment of delirium in pediatric populations.[19]

Medical treatment

The severity of the presentation dictates selection of treatment modalities. Acute presentations of severe hypocalcemia presenting with tetany or seizures require pediatric intensive care management including intravenous calcium given most commonly with intravenous calcium gluconate or lactate either by a continuous drip or in 4- to 6-hourly doses. It is important to treat hypomagnesemia if present. Vitamin D levels, even if drawn at admission, may not be available for evaluation for a few days. Vitamin D replacement may even be needed intravenously until the patient is ready to tolerate it orally. Once oral intake is safe, oral calcium as well as vitamin D supplementation may be instituted for optimal absorption and use. After the acute phase, short- and longer-term follow-up is important for further treatment and for maintaining adequacy of calcium and vitamin D levels.

Psychiatric treatment

Most of the psychiatric symptoms respond well to appropriate medical treatment, but residual issues may remain in some patients even after adequate medical treatment. The first and foremost treatment of delirium is to identify and treat the parathyroid disorder promptly, which usually results in resolution of delirium. There are no specific guidelines available to treat delirium in children and adolescent populations. A literature review from 1980 to 2009 concluded that delirium was underdiagnosed in the pediatric population and is treated based on "slim empirical evidence."[24] Antipsychotic agents are the mainstay of the treatment of delirium. Gold standard treatment of delirium in adults is haloperidol; a typical high-potency neuroleptic. Because of the strong dopamine 2 antagonism of haloperidol, it can cause extrapyramidal side effects including acute muscle dystonias, occulogyric crisis, akathisia, and other disturbing dystonias. Chlorpromazine is another atypical antipsychotic agent that can be used. Atypical antipsychotic agents such as risperidone should be used when typical agents are not indicated. Agitated patients with hyperactive delirium may benefit from valproic acid, or benzodiazepines such as diazepam or clonazepam. Close monitoring for excessive sedation or respiratory depression is prudent.

HYPERPARATHYROIDISM

Hyperparathyroidism has a low prevalence: 0.1% in the general population, but it is more common in patients suffering from psychiatric illness, especially if they are being treated with lithium.[22]

Clinical Features

The well-known mnemonic, bones, stones, groans, and psychic moans, sums up features of hyperparathyroidism/hypercalcemia. Nonspecific symptoms such as weakness, tiredness, lethargy, nausea, vomiting, loss of appetite, polyuria, depression, and lack of concentration and focus are common. Mobilization of calcium from the bones leads to osteoporosis causing bone and joint pains or fractures that may be pathologic or caused by minimal trauma. Kidney stones and nephrocalcinosis may also be seen.

Psychiatric Features

A wide range of psychiatric features, including mild to psychotic depression, confusion, lethargy, fatigue, disorientation, encephalopathy, and catatonia, may be noted.[22,25] Lithium is known to cause dysregulation of calcium metabolism and hyperparathyroidism, with a reported incidence of 10% to 40%.[25] Successful response in mania to calcium channel blockers also indicates that there may exist a more direct role of calcium in the causation of this disorder than was initially believed.[26] The severity of neuropsychiatric symptoms was also shown to be in correlation with level of hypercalcemia.[27]

Medical Work-up

Laboratory values are listed in **Table 6**. Urinary calcium excretion may be increased, and imaging may reveal nephrocalcinosis and/or renal calculi. Parathyroid glands may be imaged by ultrasonography or more specifically using the Sestamibi scan.

Psychiatric Work-up

A brief but specific psychiatric screening test may be used to establish a diagnosis when there is suspicion of a psychiatric disorder coexisting with hyperparathyroidism (see **Table 5**).

Medical Treatment

The medical treatment of hypercalcemia depends on the severity of hypercalcemia and also on the underlying cause. For mild hypercalcemia, no immediate treatment may be needed, but further testing and close follow-up may be warranted to detect any underlying cause. For severe hypercalcemia (serum calcium of >14 mg/dL) or if the child/adolescent has systemic symptoms, including cardiac arrhythmias and neurologic or gastrointestinal concerns, more emergent treatment is indicated with hospital admission, intravenous hydration with isotonic fluids, and loop diuretics (furosemide) to promote calciuresis. Hemodialysis may be used in extremely sick patients to lower the serum calcium levels. Additional measures, including the use of calcitonin and bisphosphonates, may be indicated in cases in which bone resorption is the primary underlying disorder.[28] However, tachyphylaxis (decreased efficiency with continued use) limits the use of calcitonin; and there is still limited experience with the use of bisphosphonates in the pediatric population.[29,30] Glucocorticoids offer additional treatment options to lower gastrointestinal tract absorption of calcium, as well as to inhibit activity of the 1α hydroxylase enzyme, thereby minimizing conversion of 25-hydroxyvitamin D to 1,25-dihydroxyvitamin D. Glucocorticoids are especially useful in vitamin D toxicity. Newer options, including calcimimetics, are useful in hyperparathyroidism secondary to renal failure or caused by parathyroid concerns. However, these agents are not yet approved for the pediatric population. Surgical options, including removal of affected parathyroid gland to total parathyroidectomy with autotransplantation of some parathyroid tissue, generally in the forearm, may be done depending on underlying pathophysiology. Postoperative monitoring is needed in all these patients to evaluate and treat for hypocalcaemia and/or hypercalcemia (in the case of autotransplanted parathyroid tissue).

Psychiatric Treatment

When used appropriately, SSRIs are a very effective treatment of not only depressive disorders but also for generalized anxiety disorder, anxiety disorders of childhood, social phobia, specific phobias, and other symptoms such as irritability and anger associated with general medical conditions. The altered prescribing pattern by pediatricians and primary care physicians resulting from the US Food and Drug Administration (FDA) black box warning regarding emergence of suicidal ideation has paradoxically resulted in an increased rate of suicides in teenagers.[31] The landmark study Sequenced Treatment Alternatives to Relieve Depression (STAR*D), concluded that, if depression is properly treated, remission can be achieved equally effectively in a primary care setting or in a psychiatrist's office.[32]

ADRENAL DISORDERS

Disorders of adrenal function result in hypercortisolemia or hypocortisolemia. Psychiatric features may be seen in both situations but are more common in hypercortisolemia.

Adrenal Insufficiency

Adrenal insufficiency (AI) with resultant hypocortisolemia may be primary, with the disorder in the adrenal cortex itself, whereas secondary AI is caused by an underlying disorder in the pituitary or hypothalamus. AI may be congenital or acquired, but nevertheless presents with some common clinical features that are caused by the hypocortisolemia. Additional clinical features may be noted because of the specific underlying disorder.

Clinical features

The main features of glucocorticoid deficiency include fatigue, lethargy, hypoglycemia, loss of appetite, nausea, vomiting, and abdominal pain. Additional features caused by concomitant mineralocorticoid deficiency, including muscle weakness, weight loss, hypotension, hyponatremia, hyperkalemia, and salt craving, may also be noted. Hyperpigmentation is usually seen with primary AI.

Psychiatric features

Popkin and Mackenzie reported that 60% to 90% of patients with Addison disease experienced some psychiatric symptoms such as low drive, lack of interest and enjoyment, easy fatigue, social withdrawal, negativism, and apathy.[21(p97)] Other studies have reported presence of depression, mood disturbances, cognitive impairment, behavioral problems, lethargy, and anorexia in this population.[33] The most severe psychiatric symptoms are seen in Addisonian crisis in the form of confusion, delirium, and psychosis.[21] Patients with adrenoleukodystrophy present with mania, psychosis, and cognitive impairment.[34]

Medical work-up

Hypocortisolemia is shown by documenting low serum cortisol levels, preferably 8 AM levels. Serum cortisol levels exhibit diurnal variation, therefore it is important to consider the time of blood draw and to compare with appropriate reference ranges. In primary hypoadrenocorticism, adrenocorticotropic hormone (ACTH) levels are significantly increased; whereas they are low in secondary hypoadrenocorticism. ACTH stimulation test may be undertaken for more definitive diagnosis, especially in the early stages of AI, when no increase in cortisol is noted after ACTH stimulation. Different protocols and reference ranges are needed with low-dose and high-dose ACTH stimulation tests. Further diagnostic testing is directed toward delineating underlying disorders.

Psychiatric work-up

The diagnosis of depression can be challenging in the presence of comorbid AI. Symptoms of AI closely resemble the neurovegetative symptoms of the major depressive disorder, and this may mislead the clinician to make a primary psychiatry diagnosis. Several simple screening questionnaires specifically asking for depressive symptoms may be used (see **Table 5**).

Medical treatment

Glucocorticoids are used for treatment of hypocortisolemia. The glucocorticoid replacement is done by using hydrocortisone or, less commonly, prednisone. The normal physiologic replacement dose of hydrocortisone is variable and needs to be individualized in the range of 8 to 15 mg/m^2/d divided into 3 daily doses. For concomitant mineralocorticoid deficiency, replacement is done with fludrocortisone. It is important to educate the patient and families about the need for stress dosing of glucocorticoids for covering stress periods of illness, trauma, surgery, and so forth. Families are taught to administer injectable hydrocortisone intramuscularly in situations in which oral stress dosing may not be tolerated.

Psychiatric treatment

The psychosocial interventions are the first-line and, in some cases, the most needed treatment. Supportive therapy with an emphasis on counseling for the patient and family may be important in devising a successful treatment plan in these cases. If symptoms fail to respond to treatment with glucocorticoids, further options to treat depression are explored including SSRIs. Because of inherent risk of the syndrome of inappropriate antidiuretic hormone and risk of hyponatremia with SSRIs, caution must be exercised to closely monitor electrolytes in a patient with AI.

Hyperadrenocorticism

Patients who have hypercortisolemia are at a higher risk of not only developing a comorbid psychiatric illness but also one with a higher risk of disability. A statistically significant correlation between the psychiatric disability scores and the level of cortisol and ACTH has been shown.[35] Hyperadrenocorticism may be characterized by increased cortisol, increased aldosterone levels, or, depending on the underlying cause, conditions with increased androgen levels. Only issues related to hypercortisolemia are discussed in this article. Hypercortisolemia may be primary (Cushing syndrome) or secondary, caused by disorders in pituitary/hypothalamus (Cushing disease).

Clinical features

Hypercortisolemia may affect body metabolism at multiple levels and result in significant physiologic disturbances. Disturbances in lipid, protein, and carbohydrate metabolism results in hyperlipidemia, hypercholesterolemia, hyperglycemia, and even frank diabetes. The typical physical appearance, cushingoid features, is characterized by generalized obesity, body fat redistribution causing truncal obesity, moon facies, temporal fat pads, and buffalo hump, in contrast with limb muscle wasting;

and skin changes including thinning, purple striae, and easy bruising. Patients with chronic hypercortisolemia exhibit stunting of growth presenting with short stature. These children are short and obese-looking, to be differentiated from children with exogenous obesity who are tall and obese. Electrolyte imbalance includes hypernatremia resulting in hypertension and hypokalemia with severe muscle weakness.

Psychiatric features

Mild increase of cortisol is seen in depression, anxiety, and alcoholism, putting these conditions in the group of pseudo-Cushing syndromes.[36] Low-dose dexamethasone suppression test was used in the past as a biologic marker of the depressed state. The depressive state most commonly seen in Cushing syndrome is of the agitated restless type. Kelly and colleagues[37] reported depression as the main psychiatric diagnosis comorbid in these patients. In a study of 209 patients with Cushing syndrome, 65% of patients were found to be suffering from a psychiatric illness of some kind.[38] Not only was depression the predominant psychiatric disorder, it was also found to be linked to the higher probability of having adverse life events. Other psychiatric illnesses were anxiety (12%), active psychosis (8%), mania or hypomania (3%), and confusion was found in 1% of these patients.[38] Cushing disease was associated with 79% of severe mental illness, whereas adrenal adenoma and adrenal carcinoma were found to be less likely, at 8.6% and 4.7% respectively.[38] Starkman and colleagues found irritability to be the commonest at 86%, and also the earliest symptoms to develop in patients with Cushing disease, anxiety and impaired concentration, were found in 66% of cases. Less-common symptoms reported were elated mood, perceptual disturbances, and mental slowing at 11% each. Paranoia and hyperactivity were seen in 9% of these patients.[21]

Pheochromocytoma

These catecholamine-secreting tumors are notorious for causing debilitating anxiety and panic attacks. Some of the clinical features of pheochromocytoma, such as palpitation, diaphoresis, tremors, weakness, and nausea, are also common features of anxiety and panic attacks. Both disorders are episodic in nature and can pose a diagnostic dilemma initially; however, plasma metanephrine level is the best and most specific marker for pheochromocytoma.

Medical work-up

The medical treatment and subsequent prognosis of hypercortisolemia depend on the underlying cause. If the hypercortisolemia is caused by excessive exogenous glucocorticoids given to treat other conditions, these need to be lowered, stopped, or changed to alternative therapy if possible.

Psychiatric work-up

Anxiety in children is a common developmentally appropriate response to the environment. Fears and worries are part of growing up unless they become excessive and begin to affect a child's ability to function at the age-appropriate level.[18] Diagnosing anxiety in children and adolescent patients is not easy because they do not present with the typical symptoms that meet the criteria of generalized anxiety disorder (GAD) according to the Diagnostic and Statistical Manual of Mental Disorders, Fourth Edition (DSM-IV). There are several screening tests that can be used in children more than 8 years old, for example the Multidimensional Anxiety Scale for Children or Screen for Child Anxiety-related Emotional Disorders. It is prudent to take time and do a thorough clinical evaluation to differentiate between the concerns and fears normally associated with developmental stages of early life. Overanxious disorders of childhood share many characteristics with GAD.

Medical treatment

The treatment of hypercortisolemia caused by Cushing disease or an adrenal gluco-corticoid-producing tumor is primarily surgical removal. Cushing disease results in bilateral adrenal hyperplasia, and therefore bilateral adrenalectomy was done to cure the hypercortisolemia. However, significant morbidity secondary to total adrenal insufficiency was noted and other options have come up more recently. Targeting the primary source of a pituitary ACTH-producing adenoma is seen as a more direct option but, again, is accompanied by other possible morbidity. Surgical removal using transphenoidal surgery; radiation therapy, with options including radiation of the sella turcia and fractionated radiation therapy; and γ knife radiosurgery techniques are available.[39–45] A high level of surgical expertise is required for these procedures. Deficiency of other pituitary hormones may be a cause of significant side effects. Treatment to suppress ACTH secretion, such as cyproheptadine, or to suppress adrenal cortex secretion, such as metyrapone and aminoglutethimide, may be used in the short-term but do not offer effective treatment.

Psychiatric treatment

Anxiety symptoms caused by underlying endocrine disorders generally respond well to the medical treatment of these disorders. However, the co-occurring anxiety disorders in association with endocrine abnormality require specific treatment. All SSRIs are found to be equally efficacious in the treatment of anxiety spectrum disorders in adults, but only fluoxetine, sertraline and fluvoxamine are approved for use in children. Some of the anxiety spectrum disorders, especially posttraumatic stress disorder and obsessive-compulsive disorder, may require much higher doses than are recommended for depression or generalized anxiety. A study found that sertraline is a safe and effective treatment of anxiety at dose of 50 mg/d.[46] There is some evidence of efficacy of serotonin-norepinephrine reuptake inhibitors like extended-release venlafaxine for short-term treatment of GAD.[18]

Diabetes Mellitus

A broad spectrum of psychiatric and behavioral clinical features may be seen in patients with diabetes mellitus (DM). Manifestations of behavioral disturbances seen with acute episodes of hypoglycemia include sweating, irritability, confusion, delirium, combativeness, lack of attention, emotional outbursts, and anxiety. These episodes need to be recognized by the patient and/or the caretaker for these children. Patients recognize their own symptoms and often learn to say "I feel low." There may be a phase of hyperglycemia for many months before the diagnosis of DM is made. Generalized symptoms of weakness, weight loss, fatigue, low energy, lack of attention, polyuria, polydipsia, nausea, and abdominal pain may often be mistaken for depression, behavioral concerns, and mood disorders before a diagnosis of DM is made. On a more long-term basis, children and adolescents with DM exhibit significant psychiatric and behavioral issues including depression, anxiety, and anger that accompany the awareness and frustration of the diagnosis of a chronic illness that they have to deal with every moment of their lives. The realization of their limitations and the demands of intensive diabetes management often lead to frustration in individuals and families. Earlier in the diagnosis, there is a disconnect about how well these patients may feel even with poor diabetes care and risk of long-term chronic complications promoting the belief that the intensive diabetes care expected of them may be unnecessary.

Psychiatric features

Depression in DM occurs at 2 to 3 times the prevalence in the general population.[47] When DM and depression coexist, there is a frequent association with poor compliance with diabetes care, resulting in poor glycemic control and hence increased risk of long-term complications. There is a bimodal relationship between diabetes and depression, and, by virtue of the inherent characteristics of both these conditions, there is a cause and effect relationship in both directions. Depression is known to cause anhedonia, resulting in lack of involvement in physical activity, lack of interest in a healthy lifestyle, and a lack of motivation to comply with treatment recommendation. A longitudinal cohort study of 4623 patients in primary care with coexistent type 2 DM (T2DM) and major depressive disorder (MDD) had a higher risk of developing macrovascular complications independent of variables such as prior complications, type of treatment, and diabetes self care.[48] Adolescents with recent onset of T2DM are 30% more likely to have a previous diagnosis of depression than their age-matched controls, and depression also increased the risk of developing T2DM in young adults by as much as 23%.[49] Patients with DM have a 20% lifetime risk of developing an anxiety disorder, and MDD was found to be present in between 11.4% and 31% of DM patients according to different studies.[49,50] Eating disorders have been reported in association with diabetes, especially in late adolescence and in young women with type 1 DM (T1DM). Jones and colleagues[51] conducted a study in adolescent girls aged 12 to 19 years with DM of at least 1 year duration. Ten percent of girls with T1DM versus 4% of age-matched control met the DSM-IV diagnostic criteria of an eating disorder. An additional 14% of subjects and 8% of controls displayed some symptoms but did not meet the full criteria of an eating disorder ($P = .001$). In girls with T1DM, deliberate omission or manipulation of the insulin dose was the second commonest way of controlling weight after dieting. Girls with T1DM comorbid with eating disorders had higher mean hemoglobin A1c levels then girls with DM who did not have a comorbid eating disorder.[51] Another study followed the young girls with T1DM and disorderly eating behaviors and, after 4- to 5-year follow-up, concluded that eating disorders tend to persist in these women and that they are highly associated with development of microvascular complications of T1DM.[52]

Neurocognitive difficulties of T1DM in children and adolescents have been reported by various investigators, mostly agreeing that earlier onset of diabetes and the effects of recurrent hypoglycemia and hyperglycemia on the developing brain predisposes for long-term neurocognitive deficits like reduced memory and learning capacity. Northam and colleagues[53] studied 116 subjects between the ages of 3 to 14 years with T1DM, soon after the diagnosis and after 2 years, and they found a negative influence of T1DM on performance intelligence quotient. A meta-analysis of 24 studies on this topic confirmed that children and adolescents with T1DM develop mild cognitive deficits and have subtle changes in overall intellectual functioning.[54]

Psychiatric work-up

Timely diagnosis and treatment of psychiatric concerns in DM have been shown to improve measurable treatment outcomes such as glycated hemoglobin levels.[55] DM in children and adolescents affects psychological development profoundly, resulting in faulty coping mechanisms including aggressiveness, lower use of active coping skills, behavioral disengagement, and disease-focused worries.[56] The presence of all these behaviors makes the diagnosis of depression and anxiety challenging. The Hospital Anxiety and Depression Scale (HADS) is a self-report scale used to measure the severity of depression and anxiety in patients with comorbid medical conditions. It has been validated in adolescents and takes only 3 to 5 minutes to complete.

Psychiatric treatment

Comprehensive management strategies for diabetes care have promoted the concept of multidisciplinary team approach, including follow-up diabetes clinic visits in which the children/adolescents and their families interact with not only their pediatric endocrinologist but also with their diabetes nurse, a diabetes educator, a nutritionist, social worker, and, preferably, a psychologist/psychiatrist. It has been shown in adults that use of health care services increases many fold when DM is complicated with depression, reflecting a 4.5-times increased burden on the health care system, translating to a monetary difference of $247 million versus $55 million. These patients also tend to use more prescriptions (43 vs 21, P<.0001) than controls.[57] A comprehensive care approach is vital for these patients and families to optimize the success of treatment. The emphasis should be on establishing long-term relationships with their professional care team to promote communication, care, and follow-ups. Patients noted to have behavioral/psychiatric issues are referred for more frequent and comprehensive counseling sessions and/or medications as needed. The importance of prompt recognition, treatment, and follow-up cannot be overemphasized. If left unaddressed, these issues greatly affect the medical management of their diabetes care. There is growing literature on the role of atypical antipsychotic medication and development of diabetes in adult populations, and there have been case reports of new onset DM in children after treatment with apiprazole, an atypical antipsychotic medication.[58]

Hypoglycemia

Hypoglycemia is the commonest diabetes-related emergency encountered by emergency response teams, although most of these situations are resolved on-site and do not result in a visit to the emergency room or hospitalization. Hypoglycemic episodes can present a serious threat to the health of the child or adolescent, worsened by many children having hypoglycemic unawareness. Younger children are at the greatest risk. T1DM is associated with a 10% to 30% possibility of having a serious hypoglycemic event annually, which decreases to less than 5% annually for T2DM treated with insulin, and to 1% for T2DM. Depression, mood lability, cognitive difficulties, confusion, disorientation, anxiety, and fear of having another attack are some of the common symptoms associated with hypoglycemia. Fear of having a hypoglycemic episode can reach a phobic proportion, not only in the patient but even more so in the parents of younger children, affecting the quality of life of the children and adolescents significantly.[59] The standard of diabetes care may also be compromised by fear of hypoglycemia.

GENETIC SYNDROMES
Klinefelter Syndrome

Klinefelter syndrome (KS) is a genetic syndrome with an incidence of about 1:1000 that is seen in males and results from the presence of more than 1 X chromosome in their karyotype.[60] The commonest presentation is the 47XXY karyotype, but some rare variants with additional X chromosomes, such as 48 XXXY and 46XY/46XXY mosaicism, can occur.[61]

Clinical features

Boys with KS present with tall stature and eunuchoid body proportions, abnormal anatomic body proportions characterized by long arms and legs compared with the truncal length, and thus a low upper segment/lower segment ratio; hypogonadism with delayed puberty or incomplete puberty; and gynecomastia.

Psychiatric features

There are multiple psychiatric and behavioral features that are characteristic of KS. These features include mild mental retardation and various cognitive and learning disabilities. The commonest are language-based difficulties, affecting up to 80% of children with KS.[62] About 50% of children with KS were identified to be reading at 1 or more grade levels lower then their age level. Deficits in executive functioning, short-term auditory memory, and auditory processing are also noted. In contrast, the visual spatial processing is preserved and may be enhanced in some cases.[62] Children with KS have difficulties in regulation of emotions and behavior, resulting in social maladjustment. Another study in 51 boys (ages 6–19 years) found that 65% had language disorders, 63% had attention deficit disorder, and 27% were identified to have an autistic spectrum disorders (ASD). Six of these children had a primary psychotic disorder and also ASD, resulting in significant behavioral dysregulation.[63] Approximately 0.81% of all adult men hospitalized for schizophrenia have a XXY karyotype, a four- to five fold increase in comparison with the general population.[64]

Medical work-up

Suspicion of KS is clinical, with tall stature, increased arm span, small testes, and gynecomastia. From clinical suspicion, blood karyotype establishes the diagnosis of KS. Chromosomal analysis reveals 47 XXY, 48 XXXY, or other aneuploid karyotypes with more than 1 X chromosome.

Psychiatric work-up

The psychiatric assessment of the children with KS should be broad based and comprehensive, including assessment of cognitive functioning, speech and language assessment, assessing the social and family systems, and a careful and thoughtful assessment of psychiatric disorders. Given the strong correlation of many psychiatric disorders in these patients, a more structured or semistructured interview approach can be taken, such as Kiddie Schedule for Affective Disorders and Schizophrenia Present and Lifetime Version (K-SADS-PL), which is a useful tool to investigate current or past episodes of psychopathology in pediatric populations. K-SADS-PL screens for a wide variety of psychiatric disorders including, but not limited to, affective, anxiety, ADHD, and psychotic disorders. It also inquires about the school and social adaptation as well as peer and family relations. Diagnosis of psychotic disorder can be challenging in children because it can be difficult to distinguish between vivid imagination, idiosyncratic thinking, and perceptions, especially when accompanied by developmental delays and exposure to traumatic events. The diagnosis can be challenging in very young children as well because the symptoms can be fluid. Isolated auditory hallucinations can be a manifestation of acute anxiety in preschool children.[65]

Medical treatment

The main medical intervention is aimed toward androgen replacement therapy because of hypogonadism and low testosterone level both for pubertal development as well as for sexual functioning in later adolescent and adult life.

Psychiatric treatment

A comprehensive team approach should be used when managing children and adolescents with KS in the presence of widely ranging and challenging psychiatric issues. If a diagnosis of childhood schizophrenia is made with certainty, the treatment plan should take into account the child's capabilities and family functioning, teaching of problem-solving skills, educating and implementing better communication skills, and relapse prevention techniques.[65] Atypical antipsychotic medications are now considered the first-line treatment of psychosis because of their favorable side effect profile. Risperidone and apiprazole are the 2 medications from this group that are approved for the treatment of schizophrenia in children and adolescents and are also useful for the irritability and behavioral issues associated with autistic spectrum disorders. Typical antipsychotics, like chlorpromazine and haloperidol, can be used with caution for short term treatment of psychosis, irritability, and behavior problems, but long term use is discouraged as it is associated with extrapyramidal symptoms like akathisia, rigidity, and muscle dystonia.

Turner Syndrome

Turner syndrome (TS) is the most common genetic syndrome in females characterized by complete or partial absence of 1 X chromosome, with an incidence of about 1:2000.[66,67] The features of TS are now known to be haploinsufficiency of the SHOX gene.[68–70]

Clinical features

A wide range of clinical features may be seen at different ages. Presentation may vary greatly depending on the karyotype, whether there is X monosomy or different mosaic presentations. Lymphedema and nuchal cystic hygromas may be seen in utero. Short stature and ovarian dysgenesis are 2 almost constant features seen in TS. Short stature presents in childhood, and girls with TS are about 20 cm shorter than their genetic potential. Delayed puberty, failure of pubertal progression, or delayed menarche may be the features of ovarian dysgenesis.[71] Multiple other dysmorphic features and congenital anomalies may be seen and are listed in **Box 2**.

Box 2
Main clinical features of TS

Skeletal feature

- Short stature
- Short neck
- Cubitus valgus
- Short fourth metacarpal
- Modeling deformity
- Micrognathia
- High arched palate

Gonadal dysgenesis

Others

- Cardiovascular abnormalities
- Renovascular abnormalities
- Cystic hygroma
- Webbed neck
- Nail dysplasia
- Edema of hands and feet
- Strabismus
- Multiple pigmented nevi

Psychiatric features

Girls with TS in general possess a normal range of intelligence and global intellectual functioning, but their other cognitive abilities are affected. Most girls with TS tend to have a higher verbal than nonverbal functioning, including a higher level of comprehension, vocabulary, and reading levels than their age-matched controls.[72] However, the visuospatial perception and visual constructional abilities tend to lag behind.[72] Problems with executive functioning, such as deficits in working memory, speed of processing information, behavioral dyscontrol, and lesser use of goal-directed strategies, have been reported. An 18-fold increase in the prevalence of ADHD has been reported in girls with TS. A higher incidence of autistic spectrum disorder has been reported but the data are inconsistent in this regard.[72]

Puberty is an especially difficult time for girls with TS because they become self-conscious about the delay in linear growth and pubertal development.[73] They have a lower self-concept and negative body image, higher risk of social isolation because of poor social coping skills, immaturity, difficulty in relating to others, and impulsivity in social interactions.[71,73] The data on the association of specific psychiatric disorders with TS are limited. The presence of shyness, social anxiety, and anxiety in general has been reported in young girls with TS. The association with depression has been reported in adult women with TS, but this has not been well established in children and adolescents with TS.[73] There have been several case reports of co-occurrence of anorexia nervosa with TS.[74]

Medical work-up

Diagnosis of TS may be made on a karyotype on amniocentesis, or on a peripheral blood karyotype after birth. Follicle-stimulating hormone levels are high in infancy and then in the pubertal period. However, specific diagnosis is based on a karyotype. Cardiology and renal work-up are essential, including consultation and a echocardiogram and renal ultrasound.[71]

Psychiatric work-up

Children with TS generally do well on intelligence quotient and in verbal skills, thus at times may not be recognized to have a subtle nonverbal learning disorder that in turn will cause functional impairment. The prepubertal and pubertal period is a crucial time for girls with TS because of the heightened anxiety regarding their psychosexual development. The anxiety and mood disorder may surface for the first time in this period. There should be a high index of suspicion, and inquiry about this should be done during regular pediatric care visits. Brief but targeted psychological testing can be done in an office setting to identify nonverbal cognitive difficulties. Psychological test batteries specifically assessing the nonverbal cognitive difficulties and visual spatial problems to detect any significant areas of cognitive deficits can be used on individual case basis to pinpoint the areas of deficit.

Medical treatment

Treatment in girls with TS is intended to address the clinical findings. Any congenital anomalies and their management are addressed as indicated. The use of growth hormone is FDA approved for short stature in TS. Although these girls are not deficient in growth hormone, timely and adequate treatment with growth hormone results in significant improvement, or even normalization, of their final adult height, and is now standard of care.[75] Estrogen therapy is generally required in gradually increasing increments to mimic normal pubertal development and then menstrual cycling. Cardiology and nephrology are other important subspecialty follow-ups that are essential because of a high incidence of cardiovascular and renal anomalies.

Psychiatric treatment

The treatment plan for the girls with TS should be dynamic and flexible enough to evolve with their growth. In young patients, psychosocial intervention may be required in identifying and treating academic and developmental problems; at puberty, the focus should be on psychosexual development and strategies to address it. Psychological education and supportive psychotherapy is the mainstay of any treatment plan not only for these children but also for parents and families. Low self-esteem and social phobia should be treated with CBT. Anxiety and mood disorders can also be effectively treated with structured CBT. Use of medications like SSRIs is indicated in cases in which response to psychosocial intervention and CBT is suboptimal.

REFERENCES

1. Heinrich TW, Graham G. Hypothyroidism presenting as psychosis: myxedema madness revisited. Prim Care Companion J Clin Psychiatry 2003;5(6):260–6.
2. Josephson AM, Mackenzie TB. Thyroid-induced mania in hypothyroid patients. Br J Psychiatry 1980;137:222–8.
3. Levitte SS. Coexistent hypomania and severe hypothyroidism. Psychosomatics 1993;34(1):96–7.
4. Dugbartey AT. Neurocognitive aspects of hypothyroidism. Arch Intern Med 1998; 158(13):1413–8.
5. Asher R. Myxoedematous madness. Br Med J 1949;2(4627):555–62.
6. Libow LS, Durell J. Clinical studies on the relationship between psychosis and the regulation of thyroid gland activity. I. Periodic psychosis with coupled change in thyroid function: report of a case. Psychosom Med 1965;27:369–76.
7. Mahmud FH, Lteif AN, Renaud DL, et al. Steroid-responsive encephalopathy associated with Hashimoto's thyroiditis in an adolescent with chronic hallucinations and depression: case report and review. Pediatrics 2003;112(3 Pt 1):686–90.
8. Dunlap HF, Moersch FP. Psychic manifestations associated with hyperthyroidism. Am J Psychiatry 1935;91:1215–38.
9. Johnston AM, Eagles JM. Lithium-associated clinical hypothyroidism. Prevalence and risk factors. Br J Psychiatry 1999;175:336–9.
10. Bauer MS, Whybrow PC, Winokur A. Rapid cycling bipolar affective disorder. I. Association with grade I hypothyroidism. Arch Gen Psychiatry 1990;47(5): 427–32.
11. Jones DD, May KE, Geraci SA. Subclinical thyroid disease. Am J Med 2010; 123(6):502–4.
12. Kaplowitz PB. Subclinical hypothyroidism in children: normal variation or sign of a failing thyroid gland? Int J Pediatr Endocrinol 2010;2010:281453.
13. Fatourechi V. Subclinical thyroid disease. Mayo Clin Proc 2001;76(4):413–6.
14. Bhatara VS, Sankar R. Neuropsychiatric aspects of pediatric thyrotoxicosis. Indian J Pediatr 1999;66(2):277–84.
15. Stern RA, Robinson B, Thorner AR, et al. A survey study of neuropsychiatric complaints in patients with Graves' disease. J Neuropsychiatry Clin Neurosci 1996;8(2):181–5.
16. Ficarra BJ, Nelson RA. Phobia as a symptom in hyperthyroidism. Am J Psychiatry 1947;103(5):831.
17. Thomsen AF, Kvist TK, Andersen PK, et al. Increased risk of affective disorder following hospitalisation with hyperthyroidism – a register-based study. Eur J Endocrinol 2005;152(4):535–43.

18. Connolly SD, Bernstein GA. Work Group on Quality Issues. Practice parameter for the assessment and treatment of children and adolescents with anxiety disorders. J Am Acad Child Adolesc Psychiatry 2007;46(2):267–83.

19. Rynn MA, Riddle MA, Yeung PP, et al. Efficacy and safety of extended-release venlafaxine in the treatment of generalized anxiety disorder in children and adolescents: two placebo-controlled trials. Am J Psychiatry 2007;164(2): 290–300.

20. Lehrmann JA, Jain S. Myxedema psychosis with grade II hypothyroidism. Gen Hosp Psychiatry 2002;24(4):275–7.

21. Levenson JL. Essential of psychosomatic medicine. Arlington (VA): American Psychiatric Publishing Inc; 2007. p. 97, 504.

22. Velasco PJ, Manshadi M, Breen K, et al. Psychiatric aspects of parathyroid disease. Psychosomatics 1999;40(6):486–90.

23. Schieveld JN, van der Valk JA, Smeets I, et al. Diagnostic considerations regarding pediatric delirium: a review and a proposal for an algorithm for pediatric intensive care units. Intensive Care Med 2009;35(11):1843–9.

24. Hatherill S, Flisher AJ. Delirium in children and adolescents: a systematic review of the literature. J Psychosom Res 2010;68(4):337–44.

25. Gatewood JW, Organ CH Jr, Mead BT. Mental changes associated with hyperparathyroidism. Am J Psychiatry 1975;132(2):129–32.

26. Brown SW, Vyas BV, Spiegel DR. Mania in a case of hyperparathyroidism. Psychosomatics 2007;48(3):265–8.

27. Brown GG, Preisman RC, Kleerekoper M. Neurobehavioral symptoms in mild primary hyperparathyroidism: related to hypercalcemia but not improved by parathyroidectomy. Henry Ford Hosp Med J 1987;35(4):211–5.

28. Diaz R. Calcium disorders in children and adolescents. In: Lifshiftz F, editor. Pediatric endocrinology. 5th edition. New York: Informa Healthcare; 2007. p. 475–95.

29. Lteif AN, Zimmerman D. Bisphosphonates for treatment of childhood hypercalcemia. Pediatrics 1998;102(4 Pt 1):990–3.

30. Pecherstorfer M, Brenner K, Zojer N. Current management strategies for hypercalcemia. Treat Endocrinol 2003;2(4):273–92.

31. American Academy of Child and Adolescent Psychiatry. Practice parameter on the use of psychotropic medication in children and adolescents. J Am Acad Child Adolesc Psychiatry 2009;48(9):961–73.

32. Trivedi MH, Rush AJ, Wisniewski SR, et al. Evaluation of outcomes with citalopram for depression using measurement-based care in STAR*D: implications for clinical practice. Am J Psychiatry 2006;163(1):28–40.

33. Anglin RE, Rosebush PI, Mazurek MF. The neuropsychiatric profile of Addison's disease: revisiting a forgotten phenomenon. J Neuropsychiatry Clin Neurosci 2006;18(4):450–9.

34. Rosebush PI, Garside S, Levinson AJ, et al. The neuropsychiatry of adult-onset adrenoleukodystrophy. J Neuropsychiatry Clin Neurosci 1999;11(3):315–27.

35. Starkman MN, Schteingart DE, Schork MA. Depressed mood and other psychiatric manifestations of Cushing's syndrome: relationship to hormone levels. Psychosom Med 1981;43(1):3–18.

36. Newell-Price J, Trainer P, Besser M, et al. The diagnosis and differential diagnosis of Cushing's syndrome and pseudo-Cushing's states. Endocr Rev 1998;19(5): 647–72.

37. Kelly WF, Checkley SA, Bender DA. Cushing's syndrome, tryptophan and depression. Br J Psychiatry 1980;136:125–32.

38. Kelly WF. Psychiatric aspects of Cushing's syndrome. QJM 1996;89(7):543–51.

39. Laws ER, Sheehan JP, Sheehan JM, et al. Stereotactic radiosurgery for pituitary adenomas: a review of the literature. J Neurooncol 2004;69(1–3):257–72.
40. Jennings AS, Liddle GW, Orth DN. Results of treating childhood Cushing's disease with pituitary irradiation. N Engl J Med 1977;297(18):957–62.
41. Styne DM, Grumbach MM, Kaplan SL, et al. Treatment of Cushing's disease in childhood and adolescence by transsphenoidal microadenomectomy. N Engl J Med 1984;310(14):889–93.
42. Mampalam TJ, Tyrrell JB, Wilson CB. Transsphenoidal microsurgery for Cushing disease: a report of 216 cases. Ann Intern Med 1988;109(6):487–93.
43. Tyrrell JB, Brooks RM, Fitzgerald PA, et al. Cushing's disease: selective transsphenoidal resection of pituitary microadenomas. N Engl J Med 1978;298(14): 753–8.
44. Tindall GT, Herring CJ, Clark RV, et al. Cushing's disease: results of transsphenoidal microsurgery with emphasis on surgical failures. J Neurosurg 1990;72(3): 363–9.
45. Brada M, Ajithkumar TV, Minniti G. Radiosurgery for pituitary adenomas. Clin Endocrinol (Oxf) 2004;61(5):531–43.
46. Rynn MA, Siqueland L, Rickels K. Placebo-controlled trial of sertraline in the treatment of children with generalized anxiety disorder. Am J Psychiatry 2001;158(12): 2008–14.
47. Levenson JL. Psychiatric issues in endocrinology: updates in psychosomatic medicine and consultation-liaison psychiatry. Prim Psychiatry 2006;13(4):27–30.
48. Lin EH, Rutter CM, Katon W, et al. Depression and advanced complications of diabetes: a prospective cohort study. Diabetes Care 2010;33(2):264–9.
49. Brown LC, Majumdar SR, Newman SC, et al. History of depression increases risk of type 2 diabetes in younger adults. Diabetes Care 2005;28(5):1063–7.
50. Li C, Barker L, Ford ES, et al. Diabetes and anxiety in US adults: findings from the 2006 Behavioral Risk Factor Surveillance System. Diabet Med 2008;25(7): 878–81.
51. Jones JM, Lawon ML, Daneman D, et al. Eating disorders in adolescent females with and without type 1 diabetes: cross sectional study. BMJ 2000;320(7249): 1563–6.
52. Rydall AC, Rodin GM, Olmsted MP, et al. Disordered eating behavior and microvascular complications in young women with insulin-dependent diabetes mellitus. N Engl J Med 1997;336(26):1849–54.
53. Northam EA, Anderson PJ, Werther GA, et al. Predictors of change in the neuropsychological profiles of children with type 1 diabetes 2 years after disease onset. Diabetes Care 1999;22(9):1438–44.
54. Naguib JM, Kulinskaya E, Lomax CL, et al. Neuro-cognitive performance in children with type 1 diabetes–a meta-analysis. J Pediatr Psychol 2009;34(3):271–82.
55. Aina Y, Susman J. Understanding comorbidity with depression and anxiety disorders. J Am Osteopath Assoc 2006;106(5 Suppl 2):S9–14.
56. Graue M, Wentzel-Larsen T, Bru E, et al. The coping styles of adolescents with type 1 diabetes are associated with degree of metabolic control. Diabetes Care 2004;27(6):1313–7.
57. Egede LE, Zheng D, Simpson K. Comorbid depression is associated with increased health care use and expenditures in individuals with diabetes. Diabetes Care 2002;25(3):464–70.
58. Dhamjia R, Verma R. Diabetic ketoacidosis induced by aripiprazole in a 12-year-old boy. Diabetes Care 2008;31(6):e50.

59. Bailey CJ, Day C. Hypoglycaemia: a limiting factor. Br J Diabetes Vasc Dis 2010; 10:2.
60. Bojesen A, Juul S, Gravholt CH. Prenatal and postnatal prevalence of Klinefelter syndrome: a national registry study. J Clin Endocrinol Metab 2003;88(2):622-6.
61. Paulsen CA, Gordon DL, Carpenter RW, et al. Klinefelter's syndrome and its variants: a hormonal and chromosomal study. Recent Prog Horm Res 1968;24:321.
62. Giedd JN, Clasen LS, Wallace GL, et al. XXY (Klinefelter syndrome): a pediatric quantitative brain magnetic resonance imaging case-control study. Pediatrics 2007;119(1):e232-40.
63. Bruining H, Swaab H, Kas M, et al. Psychiatric characteristics in a self-selected sample of boys with Klinefelter syndrome. Pediatrics 2009;123(5):e865-70.
64. DeLisi LE, Maurizio AM, Svetina C, et al. Klinefelter's syndrome (XXY) as a genetic model for psychotic disorders. Am J Med Genet B Neuropsychiatr Genet 2005; 135(1):15-23.
65. Joshi PJ, Towbin KE. Psychosis in childhood and its management. Neuropsycho-pharmacology-5th generation of progress, an official publication of American College of Neuropsychopharmacology. Philadelphia (PA): Lippincott Williams & Wilkins; 2002. p. 613-22. Chapter 45.
66. Hall JG, Sybert VP, Williamson RA, et al. Turner's syndrome. West J Med 1982; 137:32-44.
67. Nielsen J, Wohlert M. Chromosome abnormalities found among 34910 newborn children: results from a 13-year incidence study in Aarhus, Denmark. Hum Genet 1991;87:81.
68. Rao E, Weiss B, Fukami M, et al. Pseudoautosomal deletions encompassing a novel homeobox gene cause growth failure in idiopathic short stature and Turner syndrome. Nat Genet 1997;16(1):54-63.
69. Ross JL, Scott C Jr, Marttila P, et al. Phenotypes associated with SHOX deficiency. J Clin Endocrinol Metab 2001;86(12):5674-80.
70. Ross JL, Kowal K, Quigley CA, et al. The phenotype of short stature homeobox gene (SHOX) deficiency in childhood: contrasting children with Leri-Weill dyschondrosteosis and Turner syndrome. J Pediatr 2005;147(4):499-507.
71. Rosenfeld GF, Tesch LG, Rodriguez-Rigau LJ, et al. Recommendations for diagnosis, treatment, and management of individuals with Turner syndrome. Endocrinologist 1994;4:351.
72. Siegel PT, Clopper R, Stabler B. The psychological consequences of Turner syndrome and review of the National Cooperative Growth Study psychological substudy. Pediatrics 1998;102(2 Pt 3):488-91.
73. Kesler SR. Turner syndrome. Child Adolesc Psychiatr Clin N Am 2007;16(3): 709-22.
74. Blinder BJ. Eating disorder specialist. Anorexia nervosa in association with medical disorder. Available at: http://www.ltspeed.com/bjblinder/anmeddis.htm. Accessed July 18, 2010.
75. Lippe BM. Turner syndrome. In: Sperling M, editor. Pediatric endocrinology. 3rd edition. Philadelphia: WB Saunders; 1996. p. 387.

Pharmacotherapy for Substance Abuse Disorders in Adolescence

Gabriel Kaplan, MD[a,b,*], Iliyan Ivanov, MD[c]

KEYWORDS

- Adolescence • Substance abuse • Withdrawal
- Dependence • Pharmacology

The public health effects of adolescent substance use disorders (SUD) reach beyond the immediate intoxicating effects of specific substances. SUD that begin in early adolescence are more difficult to treat, exhibit higher relapse rates, and have poorer outcomes.[1–4] Furthermore, SUD are strongly associated with major causes of youth mortality such as suicide, homicide, and motor-vehicle accidents. National data from the Youth Risk Behavior Survey (YRBS) conducted by US Centers for Disease Control (CDC) as well as local agencies illustrate the extent of the problem: during the 30 days before the survey, 41.8% of the participating high school students had drunk alcohol, 20.8% used marijuana, 28.3% rode in a car or other vehicle driven by someone who had been drinking alcohol, and 19.5% smoked cigarettes.[5] Moreover, during the 12 months before the survey, 2.1% of students had injected an illegal drug. Although these surveys do not make a distinction between drug use and abuse, they provide valuable information about early use patterns. Not all individuals who experiment with drugs and alcohol go on to develop SUD but early use is associated with increased risk for alcohol abuse and dependence, greater risk for alcohol-related injuries and violence, and increased risk for developing other drug disorders.[6–8] A recent epidemiologic study[9] of adolescents aged 13 to 17 years found that the lifetime prevalence for any substance disorder (based on *Diagnostic and statistical manual of mental disorders fourth edition (text revision)* [DSM-IV]) was 11.1%. Prevalence rates of 6.9% for alcohol dependence and 1.9% for illicit drug dependence were lower but

[a] Department of Psychiatry, Hoboken University Medical Center, 308 Willow Avenue, Hoboken, NJ 07030, USA
[b] Department of Psychiatry, University of Medicine and Dentistry of New Jersey, 65 Bergen Street, Newark, NJ 07107-3001, USA
[c] Department of Psychiatry, Mount Sinai Medical School, 1 Gustave L Levy Place, New York, NY 10029, USA
* Corresponding author. 535 Morris Avenue Springfield, NJ 07081.
E-mail address: drgkaplan@gmail.com

Pediatr Clin N Am 58 (2011) 243–258
doi:10.1016/j.pcl.2010.10.010
0031-3955/11/$ – see front matter © 2011 Elsevier Inc. All rights reserved.

pediatric.theclinics.com

these figures are nonetheless cause for concern. In general, legalized substances such as alcohol and tobacco are the most prevalent drugs of abuse among adolescents. This situation could be partially related to the perception that, because these drugs are legal, they may be less harmful. Among illicit drugs, marijuana is the most prevalent substance of abuse in adolescence. A worrisome trend is that prescription drugs are becoming increasingly abused. For instance, in the case of opioids, abuse of prescription narcotics has greatly surpassed the use of intravenous (IV) heroin. Other medications abused include stimulants and tranquilizers that adolescents obtain from classmates, friends, and family members who were prescribed these compounds for legitimate reasons.[10,11]

Standard treatment of adolescent SUD consists of a multipronged approach that includes 12-step programs as well as other psychosocial modalities addressing individual and family issues. Although biologic agents are a regular component of adult treatment, these agents have not been generally favored in youth, probably because of concerns regarding the risk/benefit ratio of medications in this population, lack of US Food and Drug Administration (FDA) approval, few available published data in adolescence, and because, for most individuals, experimentation does not usually lead to SUD. Although medications currently play a limited role in the treatment of youth beyond addressing short-term symptoms (ie, withdrawal), they may improve longer-term outcomes for some patients. Given the potential devastating consequences of SUD, it is important to become familiar with all potential available treatment options. The present article reviews the existing literature on the pharmacotherapy for adolescent SUD to inform clinicians considering the use of this modality for selected groups of patients.

DIAGNOSING ADOLESCENTS WITH SUBSTANCE ABUSE DISORDERS

DSM-IV[12] classifies substance-related diagnoses in 2 groups: (1) substance-induced disorders, including intoxication and withdrawal, which consist of physical and psychological symptoms that result from acute exposure to, or interruption of, a particular substance; and (2) disorders of substance use, which encompass abuse and dependence, and include chronic behavioral patterns with significant detrimental functional effects. Similarly to adults, adolescents are also slow to volunteer information about substance abuse problems, minimize the severity of symptoms, and resist seeking help and treatment. Therefore, providers frequently rely on indirect evidence to detect and identify substance abuse patterns. In order to gather collateral information, it is essential to establish a partnership with extended family members, with the caveat that, in many instances, parents of substance abusing adolescents are unaware or only partially aware of the activities that adolescents engage in during or after school. Warning signs of emerging drug abuse include physical findings such as weight loss, poor sleep, low energy, and deteriorating hygiene as well as changes in overall behavior patterns (ie, school truancy, disobeying house rules, fighting with parents, demands for financial allowances). Although none of these signs alone can prove the onset of substance abuse, the clustering of several signs should raise concern. Screening instruments/scales have been developed to assist in the early detection of substance abuse. For instance, the CRAFFT (car, relax, alone, forget, friends, trouble)[13] asks about situations related to any drug use and recommends further inquiry when responders answer "Yes" on 2 out of the 6 items. Assessing substance abuse risk factors is instrumental in prevention and can be done using scales such as the Drug Usage Screening Instrument and the Problem-oriented Screening Instrument for Teenagers. Results of such screens can be shared with the patient and family. When no problematic drug use is detected, the clinician may reinforce this positive behavior by complimenting the patient's ability to abstain from substances. In cases in which screening reveals drug use, the clinician can initially discuss the findings with the adolescent alone but in some circumstances may consider engaging the parents/caretakers, even if the adolescent objects.[14] When symptoms warrant treatment, the family must be involved and a more detailed assessment is necessary to determine the most appropriate substance abuse–specific level of care (ie, outpatient vs inpatient).

BIOLOGIC TREATMENTS

The American Academy of Child and Adolescent Psychiatry has provided extensive guidelines for psychosocial comprehensive and multimodal treatments,[15] the standard of care for adolescent SUD. Although comorbidity with psychiatric disorders is highly prevalent,[4] this review does not address medication coadministration strategies for dually diagnosed patients. The present article focuses solely on the small, but emergent, available literature on the pharmacotherapy for specific SUD. Biologic agents are recommended in diverse settings to achieve goals that vary according to the patient's level of acuity and the severity of the condition. For instance, treatments for substance-induced disorders are more likely to be conducted in a hospital or rehabilitation setting and, in severe cases, may require intensive medical interventions (eg, intubation, IV formulations, and continuous monitoring of vital signs) to quickly reverse the symptoms of intoxication and prevent or ameliorate withdrawal. In contrast, maintenance treatments for SUD attempt to improve maladaptive patterns in which the use of biologic agents is a helpful adjunct within the context of a comprehensive array of modalities (eg, group or supportive psychotherapy). Specific medications are recommended for treating various addictive disorders.

Alcohol

Treatment of acute intoxication and withdrawal

Alcohol intoxication rarely requires aggressive pharmacologic interventions unless ethanol plasma concentrations reach levels high enough to be potentially lethal. There are no specific antidotes for alcohol intoxication. The biochemical disturbances of intoxicated children 11 years of age and older resemble those of adults. Mild acidosis of a respiratory or metabolic origin and mild hypokalemia are common findings in young teenagers. Fluid replacement with glucose-containing fluids and follow-up are generally the only treatments needed for complete recovery.[16] In cases of coma and respiratory depression, patients are generally intubated to protect the airway. Alcohol withdrawal, particularly in its most severe form of delirium tremens, has a 6% mortality and requires timely and adequate pharmacologic interventions.[17] However, withdrawal develops late in the course of adolescent alcohol use and is an infrequent symptom among adolescents.[18] If present, the most prominent early manifestations of withdrawal include fine motor tremor, dysphoria, and autonomic instability manifested by increased heart rate and blood pressure. Benzodiazepines, which have affinity for the same γ-aminobutyric acid (GABA)-A2 receptor as alcohol, are the treatment of choice and the long-acting agents are preferred. These agents include chlordiazepoxide (Librium) and diazepam (Valium), which can be further supplemented with short-acting agents such as lorazepam (Ativan) especially if as-needed interventions are required. Treatment can be started on a schedule of divided doses (ie, Librium 50 mg 4 times a day, total daily dose of 200–300 mg based on the patient's weight, and a history of substance abuse and prior episodes of withdrawal) and is usually tapered off by decreasing the dose by 25% daily. The use of multivitamin preparations, particularly containing vitamin B complex, vitamin C, and ascorbic acid, is also advised. As noted earlier, acute alcohol withdrawal may present as a medical emergency and is best treated in a general medicine inpatient service. However, mild cases of withdrawal can be managed on an outpatient basis at specialized clinics.

Maintenance treatments

Three agents are approved by the FDA for the treatment of alcohol abuse in adults: disulfiram, naltrexone, and acamprosate. The use of these agents in adolescents has not been formally approved and information about efficacy and side effects is extrapolated mostly from adult data. A few adolescent studies have provided results generally concurring with those from adult trials.

Disulfiram (Antabuse) was serendipitously discovered in 1948 and its ability to produce unpleasant symptoms after alcohol intake led to the development of a preparation for the treatment of alcoholism. Disulfiram causes the irreversible inhibition of aldehyde dehydrogenase, an enzyme involved in the catabolism of ethanol. As a result, consuming alcohol while on disulfiram leads to the accumulation of acetaldehyde in the blood stream which produces a disulfiram-alcohol reaction. This reaction can occur as quickly as 5–10 minutes following the ingestion of alcohol and may last for 7 to 14 days after discontinuation. It is characterized by nausea, vomiting, flushing, and headache but may also progress to potentially more dangerous consequences related to dehydration and electrolyte imbalance secondary to vomiting. In severe cases, respiratory depression, cardiovascular collapse, acute heart failure, convulsions, loss of consciousness, and death can occur. The risk for such serious complications as well as the recent development of alternative alcohol treatment agents have resulted in decreased use of disulfiram. A report of two adolescent males described mixed results.[19] One patient experienced prolonged abstinence from alcohol but the other had poor compliance resulting in early relapse. A randomized study that recruited 26 adolescents[20] aged 16–19 years with chronic or episodic alcohol dependence, assigned patients to disulfiram or placebo. The mean cumulative abstinence duration was significantly greater in the disulfiram group and there was no difference in side effects between groups. Disulfiram is not a preferred agent for adolescents. Authors from both of the above studies advocate its judicious use only after a thorough medical and psychiatric evaluation, documentation of a serious alcohol use disorder, careful assessment for comorbid diagnoses, family involvement when possible, and securing of an informed consent that encompasses education about the nature and effects of disulfiram along with its potential interactions with other medications. The agent's dosing is 250 mg daily and requires baseline liver function testing and regular follow-up monitoring of enzymes to rule out hepatotoxicity.

Acamprosate (Campral) is a putative glutamate modulator believed to block glutamatergic excitatory receptors and to activate the inhibitory GABA-A receptors. Chronic alcohol intake is hypothesized to produce overexpression of N-methyl-D-aspartate (NMDA) receptors and to stimulate the release of glutamate, causing the amount of glutamate released in the synaptic cleft to increase with time. Acamprosate seems to counteract this type of glutamate excitatory effect and to restore in time the balance between the excitatory glutamatergic and the inhibitory GABA-ergic neurotransmission. However, these effects do not take place fast enough for acamprosate to improve acute withdrawal symptoms and it is not indicated for the treatment of delirium tremens. Furthermore, it does not cause alcohol aversion or produce a disulfiram-alcohol type of reaction. Acamprosate is mostly beneficial in reducing the frequency of relapse during early remission by decreasing the pleasant sensation associated with alcohol consumption. Otherwise, it has negligible effects on the central nervous system and its use has not been associated with the development of tolerance or dependence. The efficacy of acamprosate for abstinence in adults has been extensively studied.[21–23] A recent meta-analysis of unreported outcomes suggests that acamprosate has little effect on controlling consumption but could be helpful in supporting abstinence.[24] It has well-documented safety and is most commonly used in combination with nonpharmacologic therapeutic modalities.[23] Similarly to other agents, there is a dearth of clinical data for its use in youth. One double-blind, placebo-controlled study recruited 26 adolescents, aged 16 to 19 years, with chronic or episodic alcohol dependence, who were randomly assigned to acamprosate or placebo for 90 days. At the end of treatment, patients taking acamprosate were significantly more abstinent than placebo-treated patients.[25] Although the evidence is sparse, acamprosate may be an effective and well-tolerated pharmacologic adjunct to psychosocial treatment programs. Usual dose is 666 mg 3 times per day. No baseline or follow-up laboratory measures are needed for initiation and maintenance of treatment. Empirical evidence from adult studies suggests that the agent can be safely used for 6 to 12 months and possibly longer.[26]

Naltrexone (ReVia) is a partial opioid receptor antagonist FDA approved for the treatment of alcohol dependence and for the blockade of the effects of exogenously administered opioids. It is hypothesized that its antagonistic effect on the opioid receptors can also reduce the rewarding effects of alcohol. Several studies have documented the efficacy of naltrexone in alcohol relapse prevention, both alone[27] and in conjunction with psychosocial interventions.[28,29] Combination of naltrexone with other alcohol treatment agents (eg, acamprosate) has produced mixed results, with some investigators showing benefit[30] and others failing to find significant improvement.[31] The recommended dosage is 50 mg per day in a single dose. Naltrexone can produce hepatotoxicity[32] so periodic liver profile follow-up is advised. Long-term opioid therapy for chronic pain or heroin dependence is a contraindication because the drug could precipitate a severe withdrawal syndrome. It is also available in a depot preparation (Vivitrol) that showed efficacy in reducing heavy drinking and relapse among alcohol-dependent adults,[33] with an adverse-event profile that seemed milder than that of oral naltrexone. The only published report of naltrexone in adolescents involves 5 youth studied in an open-label format. It was found to be safe, well tolerated, and to reduce alcohol consumption and craving.[34]

The FDA-approved anticonvulsant agent topiramate (Topamax) has glutamatergic antagonist effects resulting in facilitation of GABA-A–mediated inhibition of mesocorticolimbic dopamine release, believed to be associated with craving for alcohol.[35] Although not FDA approved for the treatment of alcoholism in any age group, it has shown efficacy superior to placebo for alcohol relapse and is compatible with, or possibly superior to, approved agents like naltrexone.[36] Topiramate doses range between 100 mg to 300 mg daily in adults; no baseline laboratory work is required. Although no adolescent data have been published yet, an ongoing study scheduled for completion in December 2010 assessing the efficacy and tolerability of topiramate for the treatment of alcohol use disorders (alcohol abuse and dependence) in adolescents with bipolar disorder may provide guidance in the near future.

Stimulants and Cocaine

Natural and synthetic agents abused for their stimulant properties include cocaine, prescription agents for attention-deficit hyperactivity disorder (ie, amphetamines and methylphenidate), different forms of street/illegal amphetamines, and nicotine. From a neurobiological viewpoint, cocaine, amphetamines, and methylphenidate share similar neurophysiologic effects and are reviewed together in this article, whereas nicotine is reviewed separately.

Treatment of acute intoxication and withdrawal

DSM-IV outlines the same criteria for cocaine and amphetamine intoxication and withdrawal. Acute intoxication can present with pronounced cardiovascular symptoms that, in severe cases, may include acute myocardial infarction or brain insult. Unexpected cardiac events in young individuals, including chest pains and arrhythmias, should raise concerns about undiscovered stimulant drug abuse. Psychologically, stimulant intoxication can manifest as acute agitated or even psychotic state, and some individuals present with fully developed manic symptoms, including grandiosity, hyper-religiousness, reduced need for sleep, and hyperactivity. Other symptoms include papillary dilation, nausea and vomiting, weight loss, respiratory depression, confusion, seizures, dyskinesias, dystonias, and coma. Addressing the physiologic complications of the cocaine/stimulant intoxication should take priority and may necessitate treatments in the intensive care setting. The presentation of acute psychotic symptoms, such as hallucinations, delusions, and paranoia, is usually transient, and addressed by using sedatives and antipsychotics. Depression is a complication of cocaine/stimulant withdrawal and, in some cases, may be severe enough to produce suicidal behavior. Patients in acute abstinence from cocaine and other stimulants should be routinely assessed for suicidality, and psychiatric hospitalization should be initiated when warranted to assure safety.

Maintenance treatments

There are no FDA-approved agents for maintenance. Nevertheless, an expanding adult literature supports using agonistlike medications to treat stimulant abuse/dependence, although no studies have been done in youth. For instance, data suggest the use of a range of medications, from L-dopa/carbidopa to amphetamine preparations, depending on the severity of use.[37] A recent review on cocaine abuse concluded that, despite 20 years of extensive research, the development of medication to successfully combat cocaine addiction remains elusive.[38] Based on the known neurochemistry of cocaine, target compounds that have been studied include a D3 partial agonist compound, known as BP-897, and vanoxerine, a highly selective inhibitor of dopamine uptake. Other agents found effective (although non–FDA approved) in favoring abstinence in cocaine-abusing people include the antipsychotic aripiprazole and modafinil, approved for the treatment of narcolepsy.[39] Some placebo-controlled studies also reported effectiveness of topiramate and tiagabine, both approved as anticonvulsants, in increasing cocaine abstinence with no serious adverse events. Among agents that affect the activation of the GABA circuits, baclofen and valproic acid have shown promising preliminary results of efficacy compared with placebo in reducing cocaine use in volunteers[40] and chronic cocaine users.[41] An interesting experimental concept is binding cocaine to immunoglobulins to prevent its crossing of the blood-brain barrier.[39]

Cannabis

The endogenous cannabinoid system was discovered in the early 1990s and exerts action through specific receptors, CB(1) and CB(2), which are located predominantly in the brain and peripherally in adipose tissue, liver, skeletal muscle, and the gastrointestinal tract. These receptors mediate the multiple effects of marijuana that include reduced anxiety but also possibly impaired reality testing, hallucination, and paranoid delusion, and physiologic effects like increased appetitive drive, suppressed emetic reflex, and decreased pain sensitivity.

Treatment of acute intoxication and withdrawal

Although DSM identifies 4 signs/symptoms of cannabis intoxication (ie, conjunctival injection, increased appetite, dry mouth, and tachycardia), it sets no criteria for withdrawal. However, others describe a marijuana withdrawal syndrome that includes sleep disturbances, changes in appetite and weight, increased verbal and physical aggression, mood and sexual problems, and various physical signs such as headaches, sweating, chills, gastrointestinal disturbances, tremors, and muscle twitching.[42,43] Although intoxication and withdrawal are not life threatening per se, cannabis is not free of potentially dangerous complications, related to concomitant abuse with other drugs. For instance, cannabis suppression of the emetic reflex could lead to high alcohol levels because alcohol-induced vomiting is a mechanism that prevents further plasma-level escalation. Moreover, cannabis is sometimes mixed with phencyclidine, which may result in the development of a psychotic state. Adolescents may not be aware that such mixing took place and may unwittingly take substances that they would usually refuse. It is therefore important to order a full toxicology screen even if patients insist that they have used nothing else but marijuana. When intoxication and withdrawal are complicated by severe psychotic symptoms, a psychiatric hospitalization needs to be considered. Some preliminary data suggest that symptomatic treatments for sleep and mood symptoms during cannabis withdrawal also decrease the resumption of cannabis self-administration in adult volunteers. Of the several agents tested in treating cannabis withdrawal, only oral tetrahydrocannabinol and the antidepressant mirtazapine (Remeron) have shown some efficacy.[42] No data are available for the use of these agents in adolescents.

Maintenance treatments

There are no FDA-approved agents for the treatment of cannabis dependence. A recent review reported that, among the treatment agents evaluated to date, rimonabant (not available in the United States) and buspirone (Buspar) have shown promising results, whereas the use of oral tetrahydrocannabinol has failed to produce any clinically meaningful outcomes.[44] Psychotherapy has been shown to be most helpful in increasing the percentage of adolescents who remain abstinent from cannabis.[45]

Sedatives and Hypnotics

As noted earlier, there has been a significant increase in the abuse of prescription medications such as benzodiazepines.

Treatment of acute intoxication and withdrawal

Overdose with sedative/hypnotic agents may lead to life-threatening respiratory depression and require supportive treatment in intensive care settings. Priorities in management include assessment and establishment of effective ventilation and oxygenation, followed by hemodynamic support, and the administration of an antagonist. A specific antidote agent is available for benzodiazepines. Flumazenil, which competitively inhibits the activity of the GABA/benzodiazepine receptor complex and antagonizes the action of the benzodiazepines on the central nervous system, is indicated for the treatment of overdose in adults. Both short-acting (lorazepam) and long-acting benzodiazepine agents (chlordiazepoxide) are the treatment of choice for benzodiazepine withdrawal.[46] No specific antidote agents exist for the treatment of barbiturate intoxication and withdrawal. These symptoms are rarely seen in adolescents at present, and treatment follows general intensive care principles that can be consulted elsewhere.[47]

Maintenance treatments

No agents have been approved for the maintenance treatment of abuse and dependence of sedatives and hypnotics. Dependence is not frequently encountered in teenagers. The usual management approach involves tapering the dose of the abused agents over time and offering traditional services such as psychosocial support, group and individual psychotherapy, monitoring for possible withdrawal symptoms, and urine toxicology screening. These principles have been applied to both adult and adolescent patients.

Opioids

The 2009 Monitoring the Future[48] drug use survey included more than 46,000 8th-, 10th-, and 12th-grade students and showed that heroin use declined, with annual prevalence in all 3 grades fluctuating between 0.7% and 0.9% from 2005 to 2009. Heroin is perceived as dangerous and has high disapproval levels. However, the use of narcotics other than heroin has been increasing, holding steady at historically high levels since 2002 among 12th graders. Oxycodone (OxyContin) use increased for all grades from 2002 (when it was first measured) to 2009, although the trend lines have been irregular. Annual prevalence in 2009 was 2.0%, 5.1%, and 4.9% in grades 8, 10, and 12, respectively. However, use of hydrocodone (Vicodin) has remained fairly constant since 2002, although at considerably higher levels. In 2009, annual prevalence rates were 2.5%, 8.1%, and 9.7% in grades 8, 10, and 12. Despite these statistics, there are few studies addressing the use of pharmacotherapy, the gold standard of adult treatment, for youth opioid abuse disorders.

Acute intoxication and withdrawal

In the 5-year period from 2004 to 2008, there were marked increases in the number of medical emergencies that involved the nonmedical use of narcotic pain relievers and resulted in emergency department visits. For patients younger than 21 years, the increase was of 113%, reaching a total of 29,196 visits.[49] Regarding heroin, emergency room visits for 18 and 19 year olds increased more than 200% between 1995 and 2002.[50] The classic findings of an opioid overdose are miosis, respiratory depression, and central nervous system depression. Hypoxia from respiratory depression is the principal cause of most deaths. Other manifestations of opioid overdose can include bronchospasm, noncardiogenic pulmonary edema, peripheral vasodilation, orthostatic hypotension, dysrhythmias, dysphoria, mydriasis, seizures, nausea, vomiting, constipation, flushing, and pruritus. Most of the morbidity and mortality attributable to opiate use occurs after acute ingestion. In particular, hypoxia, anaphylaxis, pulmonary edema, acute respiratory acidosis, and aspiration pneumonitis are life-threatening complications demanding urgent attention. The specific agent of choice is naloxone (Narcan), a short-acting, nonselective, specific opioid receptor antagonist with high affinity for the μ-opioid receptor. The reversal effect of this agent manifests in a few minutes. If no response is apparent after slow administration (to avoid withdrawal) of IV naloxone 10 mg in divided doses, isolated opioid toxicity is considered unlikely. Because the duration of activity of naloxone is shorter than that of most opioids, the drug may need to be administered repeatedly.[51]

Opioid withdrawal produces craving, restlessness, muscle and bone pain, vomiting, insomnia, anxiety, yawning, lacrimation, rhinorrhea, diaphoresis, and mydriasis. Other signs that could start up to 3 days later include diarrhea, fever, chills, tremor, tachycardia, hypertension, and seizures. Withdrawal symptoms are uncomfortable but not life threatening. Symptoms peak between 48 and 72 hours after the last use, and then subside in a week. Detoxification is geared toward reducing or avoiding withdrawal. Treatment can take place with opioid agents, such as the full agonist methadone (not FDA approved in youth) and the partial agonist buprenorphine (available alone and combined with naloxone, FDA approved for ages 16 years and older). Alternatively, α2 adrenergic agents can be used, such as clonidine (not FDA approved for use in youth). The effectiveness of detoxification is assessed by evaluating symptom severity, duration of the withdrawal syndrome, and adherence to follow-up care. There are only 2 randomized controlled studies of detoxification in youth.[52] There is a reported a trial[53] of 152 patients aged 15 to 21 years who were randomized to 12 weeks of buprenorphine-naloxone maintenance compared with a 14-day buprenorphine taper. It concluded that continuing treatment with buprenorphine-naloxone improved the outcome compared with short-term detoxification. The direct medical costs that this cohort incurred were examined for 12 months, finding that extended buprenorphine treatment relative to brief detoxification was cost effective.[54] Another study compared the relative efficacy of buprenorphine with clonidine in the detoxification of 36 opioid-dependent adolescents. Combining buprenorphine with behavioral interventions was significantly more efficacious in the treatment of opioid-dependent adolescents than combining clonidine and behavioral interventions.[55] Methadone has been the most widely used agent in adults. Although few youth studies exist, data extrapolated from the adult literature offer additional guidance, although concerns about the potential cardiac side effects of methadone have increased. The recent availability of buprenorphine (Subutex) in the primary care setting has made it an appealing alternative and it is currently suggested as a safer alternative because of lower cardiac toxicity and reduced risk of overdose. Another advantage is that the combined buprenorphine/naloxone formulation (Suboxone) has reduced potential for abuse.[56] Clonidine seems to have worse detoxification outcomes relative to agonist replacement agents.[57]

Maintenance treatment
There are 2 approaches for maintenance: opioid agonist and opioid antagonist treatments.

Opioid agonist treatment In the United States, there are currently 3 FDA-approved medications for opioid dependence in adults: oral methadone, sublingual buprenorphine, and sublingual combination buprenorphine-naloxone. However, only the buprenorphine preparations are FDA approved for use in youngsters 16 years of age and older. Naloxone is added to buprenorphine to reduce the abuse potential of the preparation. Methadone is only available at tightly regulated treatment centers but recent regulations allow specially licensed physicians to prescribe buprenorphine in the office setting. According to the literature, adolescents are appropriate for opioid replacement treatment when they have failed 2 detoxification or rehabilitation attempts.[55] Although replacement is the gold standard for adults,[56] there is reluctance to start youth on it, perhaps explaining the paucity of research on its use in this population. In addition to the adolescent buprenorphine studies mentioned earlier, only 1 other randomized controlled agonist replacement study exists to date. This study compared the outcomes of 37 adolescents who were assigned either to methadone or levo-α-acetyl-methadol (no longer available in the United States because of cardiac concerns) for 16 weeks of treatment and concluded that both treatments had similar favorable outcomes.[58] However, other less rigorous studies also found favorable outcomes for replacement therapy in adolescents.[55]

Opioid antagonist treatment Naltrexone at an oral dose of 50 mg blocks the pharmacologic effects of 25 mg IV heroin for as long as 24 hours. Naltrexone, also mentioned in the alcohol section above, is considered an effective opioid dependence agent in many adult cases but it has not been widely utilized due to poor compliance. It is suggested that antagonist treatment may have better patient reception than agonist treatment in opioid-dependent youth who complete detoxification.[56] A recent case review of 16 adolescents treated with extended-release naltrexone showed promise.[59]

Tobacco

Cigarette smoking is a disorder that largely starts in adolescence. Ninety percent of adult smokers begin before the age of 18 years[60] and each day in the United States approximately 3900 young people between 12 and 17 years of age smoke their first cigarette. An estimated 1000 of these youth go on to become daily cigarette smokers. Factors associated with youth tobacco use include low socioeconomic status, use by peers or siblings, lack of skills to resist influences to tobacco use, parental smoking, accessibility, availability and price of tobacco products, low levels of academic achievement, low self-esteem, and aggressive behavior.[61] The significant long-term complications of smoking are well known. In the United States, chronic tobacco use results in an estimated 443,000 premature deaths and $193 billion in direct health care expenditures and productivity losses each year.[62] However, for adolescents, severe consequences can be noted earlier. Youth smoking is associated with the initiation of other addicting patterns, psychiatric illness, negative health effects, and decreased quality of life.[63] Cigarette use had begun to decline among US high school students in the late 1990s but the rate of decline slowed during 2003 to 2009.[64] In 2009, 19.5% of 9th to 12th graders admitted to current cigarette use. The Healthy People 2010 national health objective of reducing use to less than 16% has not been met.[65] Thus, as efforts to prevent the initiation of tobacco use seem to have stalled, treating current users has become even more imperative.

Treatment of withdrawal and maintenance

Acute nicotine intoxication is a rare occurrence,[66] unrelated to the use of tobacco, and not even listed in the DSM-IV. A brief outline of the posited mechanisms involved in tobacco addiction helps in understanding the therapeutic action of the agents used for treatment. Nicotine is the principal substance implicated in tobacco addiction and smoking is an efficient form of nicotine delivery. Following inhalation, nicotine enters the circulation through the lungs and crosses the blood-brain barrier within seconds. Although smokeless tobacco products do not deliver nicotine so quickly, systemic levels of nicotine are similar in users of smokeless tobacco and smokers of cigarettes.[67] Once it reaches the brain, nicotine binds to nicotinic cholinergic receptors, the same ones occupied during normal acetylcholine function. These receptors consist of several types of subunits of which the $\alpha 4\beta 2$ receptor subtype seems to be the principal mediator of nicotine dependence, although other subunits also mediate some effects. When these receptors are activated, calcium is allowed to enter into the neuron, resulting in the release of neurotransmitters such as dopamine. Nicotine mediates the release of dopamine in the ventral tegmental area of the midbrain and in the shell of the nucleus accumbens. These regions are well known for their role in pleasure and reward mechanisms. Nicotine also augments both glutamate and GABA release, transmitters that participate in a complex mechanism of receptor excitation and desensitization that contributes to reinforcement and withdrawal mechanisms.[68] In addition to nicotine, there are other substances that contribute to tobacco addiction. There is mounting evidence indicating that non-nicotinic components of tobacco smoke play a role by inhibiting monoamine oxidase, which leads to greater availability of dopamine.[69]

Among several reinforcing reasons, smokers report that smoking is pleasurable, improves concentration, and reduces stress, anger, and anxiety. Reaction time and problem solving also improve.[70] Smoke cessation results in nicotine withdrawal symptoms such as headache, nausea, constipation or diarrhea, decreasing heart rate and blood pressure, fatigue, drowsiness and insomnia, irritability, difficulty concentrating, anxiety, depression, increased hunger and caloric intake, increased pleasantness of the taste of sweets, and tobacco cravings. These symptoms peak at 48 hours and disappear within 6 months.[71] Nicotine addiction results from a combination of conditioned behavior with positive reinforcements, including enhancement of mood, and avoidance of withdrawal symptoms.[68] Research suggests that although a large number of adolescents express the desire to quit smoking, many also state that abstinence will be hard to achieve. Psychosocial treatments have been the main therapeutic modality for treating tobacco addiction in youth. Myriad psychotherapeutic approaches with documented efficacy exist.[63] However, in contrast with the adult population for which a significant body of research has shown the efficacy of pharmacotherapy,[72,73] results at the group level for the few studies conducted in the adolescent population have been less encouraging.[74] Reasons for this low documented efficacy may include small sample sizes, low dosages, adherence problems, and short-term trial duration. In addition, none of the available agents are FDA approved for use in youth younger than 18 years. However, according to US Department of Health guidelines regarding pharmacologic agents in adolescence,[73] "clinicians may consider their use when tobacco dependence is obvious." Furthermore, addiction experts[75] recommend that, "Behavior therapy in combination with the Transdermal Nicotine Patch should be the first line of treatment among adolescent daily smokers wanting to quit."

There are 7 agents currently approved by the FDA for smoking cessation in adults: 5 nicotine replacement therapies (NRTs), bupropion (Wellbutrin), and varenicline (Chantix). Clonidine and nortriptyline effectiveness has been documented[73] but they are not FDA approved for this indication and are not addressed here. A comprehensive review of adolescent pharmacotherapy trials and assessment procedures is available elsewhere.[63,75] Varenicline seems to be the most effective agent in adults,[72] but concerns regarding its potential psychiatric side effects may deter adolescent studies and, to date, there are no published effectiveness data regarding varenicline in youth. NRT and bupropion are used in conjunction with psychosocial treatments in adolescence.

NRT NRT products in the United States are available in 5 different formulations. A nicotine patch, the only long-acting formulation, can be obtained over the counter (OTC). The 4 other formulations are short acting. A nicotine chewing gum and a nicotine lozenge are available OTC, whereas a nicotine nasal spray and a nicotine vapor inhaler require a prescription. NRT stimulates nicotinic receptors in the ventral tegmental area of the brain and the consequent release of dopamine in the nucleus accumbens. This process results in a reduction in nicotine withdrawal symptoms in regular smokers who abstain from smoking. NRT may also provide a coping mechanism, making cigarettes less rewarding to smoke.[76] Adolescent data are available only for the patch and gum formulations. The patch is manufactured as 16- or 24-hour delivery systems. The 24-

hour delivery system is available in 7-, 14-, or 21-mg doses. For youth smoking a pack per day, the starting recommended dose is the 21-mg patch for at least 3 weeks, tapering gradually for 6 to 12 weeks.[75] Because the patch is not as effective for acute withdrawal symptoms, to minimize these it is recommended that the adolescent begins tapering the number of cigarettes smoked before using the patch. Smoking should stop once the patch is applied. Potential side effects are mild and include skin irritation, nausea, vomiting, sweating, and mood and sleep disturbances. Caution should be exercised in pregnancy and patients with cardiovascular illness.

Bupropion This agent is FDA approved for treating depression and exerts its main mechanism of action through dopamine reuptake inhibition, thereby possibly compensating for the decreased dopaminergic stimulation resulting from smoking cessation. Bupropion also attenuates the stimulant effects of nicotine on the nicotinic acetylcholine receptors.[77] Starting dose should be titrated according to weight and increased over time but it seems that better efficacy can be achieved by reaching doses of 300 mg per day.[78] Because the actions of bupropion are not immediate and do not increase smoking toxicity, the adolescent can continue to smoke during the titration period while being encouraged to decrease daily consumption of cigarettes. A quit day can be set 2 weeks after bupropion is started.[75] Commonly reported adverse events are insomnia, nausea, vomiting, and dizziness. There is a risk of seizures that, although low, seems to increase with higher doses. Bupropion carries the same black box suicide warning that is common to other antidepressants, so it is prudent to monitor the appearance of such ideation. The agent is contraindicated in seizure disorder, bulimia, or anorexia nervosa; and in situations in which there is already an increased risk of seizures, such as during abrupt discontinuation from alcohol or sedatives. Also, similarly to other antidepressants, it should not be used within 14 days of a monoamine oxidase inhibitor. Increased toxicity can occur if used concomitantly with other bupropion preparations approved for depression.

SUMMARY

Advances in the neurobiology of addiction and the related development of novel biologic agents that reduce cravings and minimize acute and latent withdrawal have revolutionized addiction medicine in adults. Even though these agents are not FDA approved in adolescence, extrapolating from the available adult evidence for safety and efficacy, pediatricians, family practitioners, and adolescent psychiatrists have recommend their use in some cases. The present article reviewed safety and efficacy data from adolescent studies that, in general, concur with findings from the adult literature. However, significantly more empirical and experimental data are needed for establishing adequate therapeutic parameters. As this article exclusively focused on the potential merits of biologic treatments for selected cases, in closing, it is again emphasized that psychotherapeutic modalities are a mandatory and essential component of the standard comprehensive approach to the treatment of adolescent addiction.

REFERENCES

1. Dawson DA. The link between family history and early onset alcoholism: earlier initiation of drinking or more rapid development of dependence? J Stud Alcohol 2000;61(5):637–46.
2. Dawson DA. Drinking patterns among individuals with and without DSM-IV alcohol use disorders. J Stud Alcohol 2000;61(1):111–20.

3. Pitkänen T, Lyyra A, Pulkkinen L. Age of onset of drinking and the use of alcohol in adulthood: a follow-up study from age 8–42 for females and males. Addiction 2005;100(5):652–61.
4. Bukstein OG, Brent DA, Kaminer Y. Comorbidity of substance abuse and other psychiatric disorders in adolescents. Am J Psychiatry 1989;146(9):1131–41.
5. Eaton DK, Kann L, Kinchen S, et al. Youth risk behavior surveillance - United States, 2009. MMWR Surveill Summ 2010;59(5):1–142.
6. DeWit D, Adlaf EM, Offord DR, et al. Age at first alcohol use: a risk factor for the development of alcohol disorders. Am J Psychiatry 2000;157(5):745–50.
7. Grant B, Dawson D. Age of onset of drug use and its association with DSM-IV drug abuse and dependence: results from the National Longitudinal Alcohol Epidemiologic Survey. J Subst Abuse 1998;10(2):163–73.
8. Hingson R, Heeren T, Jamanka A, et al. Age of drinking onset and unintentional injury involvement after drinking. JAMA 2000;284(12):1527–33.
9. Kessler R, Avenevoli S, Green J. National Comorbidity Survey Replication Adolescent Supplement (NCS-A): III. Concordance of DSM-IV/CIDI diagnoses with clinical reassessments. J Am Acad Child Adolesc Psychiatry 2009;48(4):386–99.
10. The Office of National Drug Control Policy Press Release 6/30/10. Available at: http://www.whitehousedrugpolicy.gov/news/press10/063010.html. Accessed August 10, 2010.
11. Ulbrich T. Prevalence of substance abuse in the adolescent population. 2010. Available at: www.uspharmacist.com/content/c/19742/. Accessed August 10, 2010.
12. DSM-IVTR. Diagnostic and statistical manual of mental disorders. Fourth edition (text revision). Washington (DC): American Psychiatric Association; 2000.
13. Knight J, Sherritt L, Shrier LA, et al. Validity of CRAFFT substance abuse screening test among adolescent clinic patients. Arch Pediatr Adolesc Med 2002;156:607–14.
14. Rae WA, Sullivan JR, Razo NP, et al. Adolescent health risk behavior: when do pediatric psychologists break confidentiality? J Pediatr Psychol 2002;27(6): 541–9.
15. Bukstein O, Bernet W, Arnold V, et al. Work group on quality issues. Practice parameter for the assessment and treatment of children and adolescents with substance use disorders. J Am Acad Child Adolesc Psychiatry 2005;44:609–21.
16. Lamminpaa A. Alcohol intoxication in childhood and adolescence. Alcohol Alcohol 1995;30(1):5–12.
17. Bayard M, McIntyre J, Hill KR, et al. Alcohol withdrawal syndrome. Am Fam Physician 2004;69(6):1443–50.
18. Clark DB. The natural history of adolescent alcohol use disorders. Addiction 2004;99(Suppl 2):5–22.
19. Myers W, Donahue J, Goldstein M. Disulfiram for alcohol use disorders in adolescents. J Am Acad Child Adolesc Psychiatry 1994;33(4):484–9.
20. Niederhofer H, Staffen W. Comparison of disulfiram and placebo in treatment of alcohol dependence of adolescents. Drug Alcohol Rev 2003;22(3):295–7.
21. Mason B. Treatment of alcohol-dependent outpatients with acamprosate: a clinical review. J Clin Psychiatry 2001;62(Suppl 20):42–8.
22. Anton RF, O'Malley SS, Ciraulo DA, et al. Combined pharmacotherapies and behavioral interventions for alcohol dependence: the COMBINE study: a randomized controlled trial. JAMA 2006;295(17):2003–17.
23. Kennedy W, Leloux M, Kutscher EC, et al. Acamprosate. Expert Opin Drug Metab Toxicol 2010;6(3):363–80.

24. Rosner S, Leucht S, Lehert P, et al. Acamprosate supports abstinence, naltrexone prevents excessive drinking: evidence from a meta-analysis with unreported outcomes. J Psychopharmacol 2008;22(1):11–23.
25. Niederhofer H, Staffen W. Acamprosate and its efficacy in treating alcohol dependent adolescents. Eur Child Adolesc Psychiatry 2003;12(3):144–8.
26. Annemans L, Vanoverbeke N, Tecco J, et al. Economic evaluation of Campral (acamprosate) compared to placebo in maintaining abstinence in alcohol-dependent patients. Eur Addict Res 2000;6(2):71–8.
27. Latt NC, Jurd S, Houseman J, et al. Naltrexone in alcohol dependence: a randomised controlled trial of effectiveness in a standard clinical setting. Med J Aust 2002;176(11):530–4.
28. Morris PL, Hopwood M, Whelan G, et al. Naltrexone for alcohol dependence: a randomized controlled trial. Addiction 2001;96(11):1565–73.
29. O'Malley SS, Rounsaville BJ, Farren C, et al. Initial and maintenance naltrexone treatment for alcohol dependence using primary care vs specialty care: a nested sequence of 3 randomized trials. Arch Intern Med 2003;163(14):1695–704.
30. Feeney GF, Connor JP, Young RM, et al. Combined acamprosate and naltrexone, with cognitive behavioural therapy is superior to either medication alone for alcohol abstinence: a single centres' experience with pharmacotherapy. Alcohol Alcohol 2006;41(3):321–7.
31. Anton RF, Swift RM. Current pharmacotherapies of alcoholism: a U.S. perspective. Am J Addict 2003;12(Suppl 1):S53–68.
32. Williams SH. Medications for treating alcohol dependence. Am Fam Physician 2005;72(9):1775–80.
33. Johnson BA. A synopsis of the pharmacological rationale, properties and therapeutic effects of depot preparations of naltrexone for treating alcohol dependence. Expert Opin Pharmacother 2006;7(8):1065–73.
34. Deas D, May MP, Randall C, et al. Naltrexone treatment of adolescent alcoholics: an open-label pilot study. J Child Adolesc Psychopharmacol 2005; 15(5):723–8.
35. Ait-Daoud N, Malcolm RJ Jr, Johnson BA. An overview of medications for the treatment of alcohol withdrawal and alcohol dependence with an emphasis on the use of older and newer anticonvulsants. Addict Behav 2006;31(9):1628–49.
36. Baltieri DA, Daro FR, Ribeiro PL, et al. Comparing topiramate with naltrexone in the treatment of alcohol dependence. Addiction 2008;103(12):2035–44.
37. Herin DV, Rush CR, Grabowski J. Agonist-like pharmacotherapy for stimulant dependence: preclinical, human laboratory, and clinical studies. Ann N Y Acad Sci 2010;1187:76–100.
38. Preti A. New developments in the pharmacotherapy of cocaine abuse. Addict Biol 2007;12(2):133–51.
39. Karila L, Gorelick D, Weinstein A, et al. New treatments for cocaine dependence: a focused review. Int J Neuropsychopharmacol 2008;11(3):425–38.
40. Haney M, Hart CL, Foltin RW. Effects of baclofen on cocaine self-administration: opioid- and nonopioid-dependent volunteers. Neuropsychopharmacology 2006; 31(8):1814–21.
41. Shoptaw S, Yang X, Rotheram-Fuller EJ, et al. Randomized placebo-controlled trial of baclofen for cocaine dependence: preliminary effects for individuals with chronic patterns of cocaine use. J Clin Psychiatry 2003;64(12):1440–8.
42. Benyamina A, Lecacheux M, Blecha L, et al. Pharmacotherapy and psychotherapy in cannabis withdrawal and dependence. Expert Rev Neurother 2008; 8(3):479–91.

43. Levin K, Copersino ML, Heishman SJ, et al. Cannabis withdrawal symptoms in non-treatment-seeking adult cannabis smokers. Drug Alcohol Depend 2010; 111(1–2):120–7.

44. Lee HK, Choi EB, Pak CS. The current status and future perspectives of studies of cannabinoid receptor 1 antagonists as anti-obesity agents. Curr Top Med Chem 2009;9(6):482–503.

45. Dennis M, Godley SH, Diamond G, et al. The cannabis youth treatment (CYT) Study: main findings from two randomized trials. J Subst Abuse Treat 2004; 27(3):197–213.

46. Grobin AC, Matthews DB, Devaud LL, et al. The role of GABA(A) receptors in the acute and chronic effects of ethanol. Psychopharmacology (Berl) 1998;139(1–2): 2–19.

47. Sellers EM. Alcohol, barbiturate and benzodiazepine withdrawal syndromes: clinical management. CMAJ 1988;139(2):113–20.

48. MTF. Monitoring the Future Survey. 2010. Available at: http://monitoringthefuture. org/. Accessed August 10, 2010.

49. DAWN. Available at: http://www.oas.samhsa.gov/2k10/DAWN016/OpioidED.htm. Accessed September 1, 2010.

50. Facts and Figures on Youth Heroin Use. 2010. Available at: http://www.adp. cahwnet.gov/FactSheets/FactshtYouth%20Heroin%202-07.pdf. Accessed August 11, 2010.

51. Forti R, Adam H. Opiate overdose. Pediatr Rev 2007;28:35–6.

52. Minozzi S, Amato L, Davoli M. Detoxification treatments for opiate dependent adolescents. Cochrane Database Syst Rev 2009;2:CD006749.

53. Woody GE, Poole SA, Subramaniam G, et al. Extended vs short-term buprenorphine-naloxone for treatment of opioid-addicted youth: a randomized trial. JAMA 2008;300(17):2003–11.

54. Polsky D, Glick HA, Yang J, et al. Cost-effectiveness of extended buprenorphine-naloxone treatment for opioid-dependent youth: data from a randomized trial. Addiction 2010;105(9):1616–24.

55. Simkin D, Grenoble S. Pharmacotherapies for adolescent substance use disorders. Child Adolesc Psychiatr Clin N Am 2010;19(3):591–608.

56. Stotts AL, Dodrill CL, Kosten TR. Opioid dependence treatment: options in pharmacotherapy. Expert Opin Pharmacother 2009;10(11):1727–40.

57. Lobmaier P, Gossop M, Waal H, et al. The pharmacological treatment of opioid addiction–a clinical perspective. Eur J Clin Pharmacol 2010;66(6): 537–45.

58. Lehmann W. The use of 1-alpha-acetyl-methadol (LAAM) as compared to methadone in the maintenance and detoxification of young heroin addicts [proceedings]. NIDA Res Monogr 1976;8:82–3.

59. Fishman M, Winstanley EL, Curran E, et al. Treatment of opioid dependence in adolescents and young adults with extended release naltrexone: preliminary case-series and feasibility. Addiction 2010;105(9):1669–76.

60. Rosen M, Maurer D. Reducing tobacco use in adolescents. Am Fam Physician 2008;77(4):483–90.

61. CDC. Youth and Tobacco Use. 2010. Available at: http://www.cdc.gov/tobacco/ data_statistics/fact_sheets/youth_data/tobacco_use/index.htm. Accessed July 2, 2010.

62. CDC. Smoking-attributable mortality, years of potential life lost, and productivity losses—United States, 2000–2004. MMWR Morb Mortal Wkly Rep 2008;57(45): 1226–8.

63. Schepis T, Rao U. Smoking cessation for adolescents: a review of pharmacological and psychosocial treatments. Curr Drug Abuse Rev 2008;1:142–54.
64. CDC. Cigarette use among high school students United States, 1991–2009. MMWR Morb Mortal Wkly Rep 2010;59(26):797–801.
65. HealthyPeople. 2010. Available at: http://www.healthypeople.gov/document/pdf/volume2/27tobacco.pdf. Accessed August 15, 2010.
66. Solarino B, Rosenbaum F, Riesselmann B, et al. Death due to ingestion of nicotine-containing solution: case report and review of the literature. Forensic Sci Int 2010;195(1–3):e19–22.
67. Benowitz N. Systemic absorption and effects of nicotine from smokeless tobacco. Adv Dent Res 1997;11:336.
68. Benowitz N. Nicotine addiction. N Engl J Med 2010;362:2295–303.
69. Lewis A, Miller J, Lea R. Monoamine oxidase and tobacco dependence. Neurotoxicology 2007;28:182–95.
70. Jones R, Benowitz N. Therapeutics for nicotine addiction. In: Davis KL, Charney D, Coyle JT, et al, editors. Neuropsychopharmacology—the fifth generation of progress. Philadelphia: Lippincott Williams & Wilkins; 2002. p. 1533–44.
71. Le Foll B, Goldberg S. Effects of nicotine in experimental animals and humans: an update on addictive properties. Handb Exp Pharmacol 2009;192:335–67.
72. Herman A, Sofuoglu M. Comparison of available treatments for tobacco addiction. Curr Psychiatry Rep 2010;12(5):433–40.
73. Fiore M, Jaén C, Baker T. Treating tobacco use and dependence: 2008 update. Clinical practice guideline. Rockville (MD): US Department of Health and Human Services, Public Health Service; 2008.
74. Sussman S, Sun P. Youth tobacco use cessation: 2008 update. Tob Induc Dis 2009;5:3.
75. Upadhyaya H, Deas D, Brady K. A practical clinical approach to the treatment of nicotine dependence in adolescents. J Am Acad Child Adolesc Psychiatry 2005; 44(9):942–6.
76. Molyneux A. ABC of smoking cessation. Nicotine replacement therapy. BMJ 2004;328:454–6.
77. Wilkes S. The use of bupropion SR in cigarette smoking cessation. Int J Chron Obstruct Pulmon Dis 2008;3(1):45–53.
78. Muramoto M, Leischow SJ, Sherrill D, et al. Randomized, double-blind, placebo-controlled trial of 2 dosages of sustained-release bupropion for adolescent smoking cessation. Arch Pediatr Adolesc Med 2007;161(11):1068–74.

Psychopharmacology of Tic Disorders in Children and Adolescents

Madeline A. Chadehumbe, MD[a],*,
Donald E. Greydanus, MD, Dr HC (ATHENS)[b],
Cynthia Feucht, PharmD, BCPS[c,d], Dilip R. Patel, MD, FSAM[b]

KEYWORDS

- Tics • Tourette syndrome • Children • Adolescents
- Pharmacology

Tics are patterned repetitive movements or vocalizations. They are classified as simple or complex. Simple motor tics are brief, sudden, repetitive movements involving only a few muscle groups, such as eye blinks, facial grimacing, shoulder or head jerks. Simple vocalization includes throat clearing, sniffing, barking, coughing, or grunting. Complex motor tics are coordinated patterns involving several muscle groups, such as facial grimacing with a head twist and shoulder shrug. They may seem purposeful, such as spinning and jumping. Complex vocal tics include uttering words or phrases, including coprolalia (uttering swearwords) or echolalia (repeating the words or phrases of others). Often tics are preceded by an urge or sensation in the affected muscles, commonly called a premonitory urge. Patients often describe the urge to complete the tic to get rid of this feeling. Tics are often exacerbated by anxiety or excitement and alleviated by calm and more focused activities such as playing an instrument or a video game. Tics may be present during sleep but often to a much less degree.

Typically, the onset is at school age, around 7 years, with a peak in the midteen years and a significant improvement in most by the late teens and early adulthood.

The authors have nothing to disclose.
[a] Division of Pediatric Neurology, Michigan State University, Helen DeVos Children's Hospital, Grand Rapids, 1300 Michigan Street, Suite 102, Grand Rapids, MI 49503, USA
[b] Department of Pediatrics and Human Development , Michigan State University College of Human Medicine, MSU/Kalamazoo Center for Medical Studies, 1000 Oakland Drive, Kalamazoo, MI 49009-1284, USA
[c] Borgess Ambulatory Care, 1701 Gull Road, Kalamazoo, MI 49048, USA
[d] Department of Pharmacy Practice, Ferris State University College of Pharmacy, Big Rapids, MI 49307, USA
* Corresponding author.
E-mail address: Madeline.Chadehumbe@devoschildrens.org

Pediatr Clin N Am 58 (2011) 259–272
doi:10.1016/j.pcl.2010.10.004
0031-3955/11/$ – see front matter © 2011 Elsevier Inc. All rights reserved.

About 10% of children have a progressive and disabling course that lasts into adult-hood. There is a strong male preponderance. The tics are often episodic and intermit-tent with a waxing and waning course; also, they change in location, severity, and frequency over time. Tics are the hallmark of Tourette syndrome (TS).[1] TS is a child-hood neuropsychiatric disorder characterized by motor and vocal (phonic) tics. It often has associated behavioral comorbidities such as obsessive-compulsive disorder (OCD) and attention-deficit/hyperactivity disorder (ADHD) in addition to other learning disorders. Tic disorders are genetic and thought to run in families, although a specific gene locus is yet to be found.[2]

TS was first described by a French neurologist (Gilles se la Tourette) and his student (Charcot) in 1885; they described 9 children with childhood-onset tics. It was not until the 1960s that treatment with neuroleptic medications was found favorable. This possibility also marks the shift of considering TS as a primarily psychogenic disorder to a neurologic disorder.

PATHOPHYSIOLOGY

The pathophysiology of tics is not completely understood, although the basal ganglia, in particular the caudate nucleus and the inferior prefrontal cortex, have been implicated.[1] Dysfunction within the cortico-striatal-thalamic-cortical circuits results in an inability to suppress unwanted movements, impulses, and behaviors. Multiple neurotransmitters are likely involved, given this large area of brain involvement. The role of dopamine has been studied in TS with specific interest. Functional neuroimag-ing studies suggest abnormalities in the dopaminergic systems located in the striatum and prefrontal cortex. Patients with TS have increased levels of dopamine receptors, suggesting increased uptake and release of dopamine.[3] The sensitivity to dopamine may explain the response of dopamine receptor blockers in patients with TS.

There is some speculation as to an immune-mediated pathogenesis such as that seen in pediatric autoimmune neuropsychiatric disorders associated with strepto-coccal infections. This hypothesis suggests an antecedent infection with group A β-hemolytic streptococci, leading to the formation of antineuronal antibodies that result in brain dysfunction. No current immune therapies are recommended in the treatment of TS.[4]

CLINICAL CONCEPTS

Tic criteria including criteria for TS have been developed by the American Psychiatry Association's *Diagnostic and Statistical Manual of Mental Disorders* (Fourth Edition, Text Revision).[5] TS causes marked distress or significant dysfunction in occupational, social, or other important areas of functioning; such dysfunction was thought to have a significant stigma with implications that could lead to discrimination within the work-force. There are many patients with TS who are not significantly impaired by this condition. It is important to recognize associated behavioral symptoms such as inat-tention, hyperactivity, impulsivity, obsessive-compulsive traits, learning disorders, and other school difficulties. Specific screening for mood-related disorders, such as depression and anxiety, are also helpful when evaluating and managing these patients.

Children and adolescents with tics or TS should otherwise have a completely normal neurologic examination; also, they should have a normal mental status examination. If the patient does not show any behavior of tics in the office, it is helpful to have the family videotape the tics to exclude other movement disorders such as myoclonus, chorea, tremor, and dystonia. A good developmental history is important to exclude underlying genetic disorders such as Down syndrome, fragile X syndrome, or autistic spectrum disorders. The physical examination (including a meticulous gait and tone assessment) should exclude dysmorphic features, neurocutaneous disorders, and signs of neurodegenerative disorders such as Kayser-Fleischer rings in the eyes diagnostic of Wilson disease, spasticity, and chorea suggestive of Huntington disease or associated disorders.

DIAGNOSTIC WORKUP

TS is a clinical diagnosis, and hence, no specific laboratory or genetic studies exist. Routine neuroimaging results in these patients will be normal and hence should be reserved only for patients with specific neurologic abnormalities.

TREATMENT

Tics often do not have any associated social or physical impairments, and hence, the greater majority of children with TS do not require any medication. Providing reassurance is encouraged, and education for families with written resources is helpful. Screening and addressing associated comorbidities are also important in the assessment and management of pediatric patients with tic disorders. The management of TS involves a multifaceted approach that includes the medical management of the frequent or disabling tics, medical and behavioral management of the coexisting behavioral symptoms, as well as educating and supporting the family. Often, a collaborative effort is needed, which includes the primary care physician, neurologist, psychiatrist, psychologist, family members, and school professionals.

Engaging classroom strategies that nurture self-esteem and self-correction is important in these patients. Behavioral counseling by an experienced psychologist is important, and beneficial behavioral techniques include conditioning techniques, competing response training, awareness training, habit reversal, relaxation training, biofeedback, and hypnosis. Often, parents and other care givers may benefit from behavioral management and discipline training with regard to the coexisting behavioral symptoms as well.

PHARMACOLOGIC TREATMENTS

Medical therapies are reserved only for tics that interfere with social interactions, school performance, or activities of daily living (ie, loss of self-esteem, peer difficulties, disruption of classroom setting, or musculoskeletal or physical discomfort). Unfortunately, there is no single medication that is helpful to all children and adolescents with tics, and conversely, no medication completely eliminates all symptoms of tic disorders. Rather, the goal of treatment is to control the tics such that the child or adolescent can encounter less embarrassment and discomfort from the tics. The treating physicians should be aware of the natural variability with waxing or waning of symptoms, placebo response, and strong influence of the environment, as well as other psychopathologies on outcome.

A comprehensive review of published studies with regard to pharmacologic therapies by Robertson[6] and Gilbert[7] highlight the limitations including small numbers in trials especially for children; few placebo-controlled trials; open-label trials, usually single-site studies; and the lack of pharmaceutical industry support that often funds larger trials.

According to the Tourette Syndrome Association's Medical Advisory Board guidelines (www.tsa-usa.org), evidence-based studies support the use of dopamine blocking agents such as haloperidol, pimozide, and risperidone for TS.[1,6,7] However, due to untoward side effects such as weight gain and sedation, often other agents are used first, as discussed later. A large randomized controlled trial supported the use of stimulants, specifically methylphenidate and clonidine, in children or adolescents with tics that have not worsened due to the stimulants.[8] Clinical experience supports the use of stimulants in children with tics, especially if comorbid ADHD is present.

Emphasis should be placed on treating coexisting behavioral symptoms such as ADHD, anxiety, and obsessive-compulsive traits. The general principles of treatment are outlined in **Box 1**. **Tables 1–4** provide information about the different treatment agents available for tic disorders.[8–13]

First line agents are the α_2-adrenergic agonists (clonidine and guanfacine, see **Table 1**), second line agents comprise nondopamine blocking agents (ie, atomoxetine, baclofen, and clonazepam; see **Table 2**), and third line agents include typical and atypical dopamine blockers (ie, haloperidol, pimozide, fluphenazine, risperidone, ziprasidone, and tetrabenazine; see **Tables 3** and **4**). Selective serotonin reuptake inhibitors (SSRIs) are useful in the management of anxiety and OCD, which are comorbid conditions of tic disorders. Topiramate is a useful agent if migraine headaches, obesity, or bipolar disorder is present. Less-common treatments of painful and intractable tics include Botox (botulinum toxin type A) administration and deep brain stimulation.[14,15] Selected comments on these agents are presented in the following sections.

Adrenergic Agonists (First Line Agents)

Clonidine

Clonidine is an α_2-adrenergic receptor agonist (ie, activates presynaptic receptors and reduces release of norepinephrine) (see **Table 1**). It is often used as a first line agent in children and adolescents with milder tics, especially with associated behaviors of ADHD, aggressive outbursts, insomnia, and easy frustration. A test dose of 0.05 mg is suggested; if no side effects are encountered, the dose can be increased gradually about every week by 0.05 mg to a up to a goal of 0.1–0.3 mg in 2 divided doses, with a maximum daily dose of 0.4 mg. The treatment response may not be noted for 2 to 6 weeks. Common side effects include drowsiness (which often improves spontaneously with time), dry mouth, dry eyes, postural hypotension, bradycardia, and headache. Clonidine use should be gradually tapered to avoid any rebound in tics, anxiety, or hypertension. Clonidine may be combined with stimulants.

Guanfacine

Guanfacine is a longer-acting α_2-adrenergic receptor agonist that is more selective for postsynaptic 2a receptors concentrated in the prefrontal cortex (see **Table 1**). It is less sedating than clonidine and hence often preferred. An initial doses of 0.5 mg at

---

Box 1
Basic principles of pharmacologic management of tic disorders

- Set realistic expectations at the start. Achieving a goal of modest tic suppression is realistic, and it is unlikely that complete abolishment will occur
- Address and treat significant comorbidities first
- Start at low doses, with gradual increments
- Evaluate frequently (at least monthly) for efficacy and side effects
- Use one drug at a time, as much as possible
- Seek specialist guidance once nonneuroleptic medications have failed

Table 1
First line treatment agents of tic disorders

	Clonidine	Guanfacine
Mechanism of action	α_2-adrenergic agonist	α_2-adrenergic agonist
Initial dose	0.05 mg daily Titrate by 0.05 mg increments every 3–7 d	0.5 mg daily Titrate every 3–14 d to an usual dose of 1.5–3.0 mg daily
Maximum dose	0.4 mg daily Give in divided doses	4 mg daily Give in 3 divided doses
Half-life	8–12 h	17 h
Drug interactions	Hypotensive agents Antidepressants with α_2-antagonist properties	Hypotensive agents Antidepressants with α_2-antagonist properties
Side effects	Sedation Dry mouth Headache/dizziness Constipation Orthostatic hypotension	Sedation Dry mouth Headache/dizziness Constipation
Precautions/warnings	Severe CV disease Caution in ESRD	Severe CV disease
Monitoring parameters	Blood pressure Heart rate	Blood pressure Heart rate
Comments	Discontinuation: titrate off to prevent withdrawal effects Taper over 1 wk to prevent rebound hypertension	More selective Less likely to have withdrawal effects

Abbreviations: CV, cardiovascular; ESRD, end-stage renal disease.
Data from Refs.[9–11]

Table 2
Second line treatment agents of tic disorders

	Atomoxetine	Baclofen	Clonazepam
Mechanism of action	Inhibits norepinephrine reuptake	Exact mechanism unknown Inhibits monosynaptic & polysynaptic reflexes at the spinal level	Binds to BZD receptor site on GABA complex and enhances GABA activity
Initial dose	0.5 mg/kg/d in 2 divided doses >70 kg: 40 mg/d	10–15 mg daily in 3 divided doses	0.5–12.0 mg daily Divided doses
Maximum dose	1.8 mg/kg/d Maximum: 100 mg/d Maximum: 80 mg/d if receiving potent CYP2D6 inhibitor	60–80 mg daily in 3 divided doses	Same as above
Half-life	5–21 h Longer in CYP2D6 poor metabolizers	2.5–4.0 h	22–33 h
Drug interactions	CYP2D6 substrate MAO inhibitors (avoid concurrent use) Sympathomimetic agents CYP2D6 inhibitors/inducers	CNS depressants	CYP3A4 substrate CYP3A4 inhibitors/inducers CNS depressants
Side effects	Hypertension Tachycardia Insomnia Decreased appetite Headache Early morning awakenings Allergic reactions Severe liver injury (rare)	Hypotension Sedation Fatigue Dizziness Headache Rash Nausea/constipation	Ataxia Sedation Depression Concentration decreased Dizziness Change in behavior Physical dependence Psychological dependence

Precautions/ warnings	Increased risk of suicidal ideation Avoid in patients with cardiac disease Use in hepatic dysfunction Use in CYP2D6 poor metabolizers	Patients with Seizure d/o Impaired renal function Peptic ulcer disease Psychotic d/o	Patients with Impaired hepatic & renal function Chronic respiratory disease
Monitoring parameters	ECG at baseline BP & HR	None noted	CBC LFTs
Comments	Cardiovascular assessment recommended before initiation Two divided doses: morning & late afternoon/early evening Active metabolite with equal potency	Avoid abrupt withdrawal Dose-related side effects may be minimized by slow titration Take with food or milk	Avoid abrupt discontinuation Gradually taper C-IV restriction

Abbreviations: BP, blood pressure; BZD, benzodiazepine; CBC, complete blood cell count; CNS, central nervous system; C-IV, controlled substance class IV; d/o, disorder; HR, heart rate; LFTs, liver function tests; MAO, monoamine oxidase.

Data from Refs.[9–11]

Table 3
Third line treatment agents of tic disorders: typical antipsychotics

	Haloperidol	Pimozide	Fluphenazine
Mechanism of action	Dopamine (D_2), alpha-adrenergic, and 5-HT_2 blockade	Dopamine (D_2), alpha-adrenergic, and 5-HT_2 blockade	Dopamine (D_2), H_1, alpha-adrenergic, and 5-HT_2 blockade
Initial dose	0.25–0.5 mg daily	0.05 mg/kg daily at bedtime (maximum 1 mg)	1 mg at bedtime
Maximum dose	0.05–0.075 mg/kg/d 2–3 divided doses	0.2 mg/kg daily, not to exceed 10 mg daily	4 mg daily in divided doses
Half-life	12–38 h	Approximately 66 h	Approximately 33 h
Drug interactions	CYP3A4 substrate & CYP2D6 inhibitor QTc prolonging agents (such as quinolones, antiarrhythmic agents) Potent CYP inducers Lithium	CYP1A2 & CYP3A4 substrate, weak CYP inhibitor QTc prolonging agents (CI) CYP1A2 & CYP3A4 inducers/inhibitors Potent CYP3A4 inhibitors are CI (macrolides, azoles, sertraline, protease inhibitors) Lithium St John's wort Grapefruit juice	CYP2D6 substrate, weak CYP inhibitor Moderate to potent CYP2D6 inhibitors ↑ effect (paroxetine, fluoxetine) CYP2D6 inducers Lithium Antacids QTc prolonging agents
Side effects	Hypo/hypertension Tachycardia QTc prolongation Sedation Agitation Depression EPS/NMS ↑ Prolactin levels Lower seizure threshold	Sedation Behavioral changes Dizziness Hypotension QTc prolongation ACH symptoms EPS/NMS ↑ Prolactin levels Lower seizure threshold	Sedation Hypotension Tachycardia Photosensitivity Behavior changes EPS/NMS ↑ Prolactin levels Lower seizure threshold

Precautions/ warnings	Use in patients with CV disease Seizure disorder Prolonged QT interval Hepatic/renal dysfunction	Use in patients with CV disease Seizure disorder Prolonged QT interval/arrhythmias (CI) Hepatic/renal dysfunction	Use in patients with CV disease Seizure disorder Hepatic disease (CI) Renal dysfunction Subcortical brain damage (CI)
Monitoring parameters	BP/HR CBC/LFTs Electrolyte levels	ECG (baseline & periodically) BP/HR Electrolyte levels	BP/HR CBC/LFTs
Comments	On d/c, taper dosage to prevent withdrawal dyskinesias EPS risk ↑ with dose & duration ↓ Propensity for ACH effects	On d/c, taper dosage to prevent withdrawal dyskinesias Moderate propensity to cause ACH effects	Lower propensity for ACH effects Do not mix oral concentrate with caffeine products or apple juice Greater risk for EPS

Abbreviations: ACH, anticholinergic; BP, blood pressure; CBC, complete blood cell count; CI, contraindicated; CV, cardiovascular; d/c, discontinue; HR, heart rate; LFTs, liver function tests; ↓, decreased; ↑, increased.
Data from Refs.[9-12]

Table 4
Third line treatment agents of tic disorders: atypical and monoamine depleting agent

	Risperidone	Ziprasidone	Tetrabenazine
Mechanism of action	Dopamine (D_2) & 5-HT_2 antagonists; H_1 & alpha-adrenergic blocker (low to moderate)	Dopamine (D_2 & D_3), α_1-adrenergic, H_1, and multiple 5-HT receptors	Monoamine-depleting agent & blocks dopamine receptors
Initial dose	0.25–0.5 mg at bedtime Gradually titrate at weekly intervals	5 mg at bedtime Gradually titrate to effective dose	6.25 mg twice daily Gradually titrate to effective dose
Maximum dose	4 mg daily in divided doses	40 mg daily in divided doses	2D6 (PM) or receiving potent 2D6 inhibitor: 25 mg/dose & 50 mg daily (adult) 2D6 (EM): 37.5 mg/dose & 100 mg daily (adult)
Half-life	20 h	7 h	4–8 h
Drug interactions	CYP2D6 (major) & CYP3A4 (minor) substrate & weak inhibitor CYP2D6 & CYP3A4 inhibitors & inducers Grapefruit juice St John's wort	CYP3A4 & CYP1A2 (minor) substrate CYP3A4 & CYP1A2 inhibitors & inducers QTc prolonging agents Grapefruit juice St John's wort	CYP2D6 substrate CYP2D6 inhibitors & inducers MAO inhibitors (CI) Reserpine (CI) Dopamine blockers
Side effects	Sedation Fatigue Dizziness Gastrointestinal upset OSH Weight gain ↑ Prolactin levels EPS/NMS	Sedation Dizziness Nausea OSH Rash QTc prolongation ↑ Prolactin levels EPS/NMS	Depression Fatigue Sedation/insomnia Anxiety Nausea Parkinsonism ↑ Prolactin levels

Warnings/precautions	CV disease Renal & hepatic dysfunction Seizure disorder	CV disease Arrhythmias (CI) Prolonged QT interval/QTc prolonging agents (CI) Seizure disorder	Depression Suicidal ideations or untreated/inadequately treated depression (CI) Liver disease (CI) Use of potent CYP2D6 inhibitors
Monitoring parameters	BP & HR Weight/BMI LFTs/lipid profile Fasting blood glucose level	ECG BP & HR Electrolyte levels Lipid profile Fasting blood glucose level	BP & HR
Comments	Affects other 5-HT receptors Less risk for ACH side effects Available in oral solution & ODT Do not mix oral solution with cola or tea	Less risk for ACH side effects d/c if QTc interval >500 msec Administer with food Less risk for weight gain	Approved for Huntington chorea Recommend CYP2D6 gentoyping at baseline

Abbreviations: ACH, anticholinergic; BMI, body mass index; BP, blood pressure; CI, contraindicated; CV, cardiovascular; d/c, discontinue; EM, extensive metabolizer; HR, heart rate; LFTs, liver function tests; MAO, monoamine oxidase; ODT, oral disintegrating tablet; OSH, orthostatic hypotension; PM, poor metabolizer; ↓, decreased; ↑, increased.

Data from Refs.[9–13]

bedtime are suggested with gradual increases up to a goal of 1.0 to 3.0 mg/d in 2 to 3 divided doses; a maximum dose of 2 mg twice daily is may be administered. Side effects include drowsiness, fatigue, and headache.

Nondopamine Receptor Blocking Medications (Second Line Agents)

Atomoxetine
Atomoxetine is useful if ADHD is a comorbidity.[16] An initial dose of 0.5 mg/kg/d is administered in 2 divided doses (see **Table 2**). A maximum daily dose of 1.8 mg/kg/d or up to 100 mg/d is used, and side effects are nausea, vomiting, fatigue, abdominal pain, decreased appetite, and insomnia.

Baclofen
Baclofen is a γ-aminobutyric acid (GABA) analogue and inhibits monosynaptic and polysynaptic reflexes at the spinal cord level. An initial daily dose of 10 to 15 mg in 3 divided doses is preferred, with a maximum dose of 60 to 80 mg daily in divided doses. A single placebo-controlled crossover study showed that baclofen at doses of 20 mg given 3 times a day statistically improved the overall well-being of patients without reducing motor or vocal tic burden.[17] Side effects include sedation, dizziness, headache, fatigue, hypotension, nausea, and constipation. Abrupt discontinuation of drug use should be avoided because of the risk of seizures and/or hallucinations.

Clonazepam
This is a benzodiazepine receptor antagonist that binds to benzodiazepine sites on a GABA receptor complex and enhances the inhibitory activity of GABA. Clonazepam is widely used for tic suppression, especially when anxiety is a strong comorbid condition. Doses of 0.5 to 12 mg daily have been used. Side effects include drowsiness, dizziness, ataxia, decreased concentration, depression, and behavior change. It is associated with physical and psychological dependence.

Dopamine Receptor Blocking Agents (Third Line Agents)

Haloperidol
This is a typical neuroleptic, and its mechanism of action includes being a dopamine (D_2) blocker, an alpha-adrenergic blocker, and a 5-HT (5-hydroxytryptamine/serotonin) 2 antagonist (see **Tables 3** and **4**).[18] Its initial dose is 0.25 to 0.5 mg daily, with gradual weekly titration; its maximum dose is 0.050 to 0.075 mg/kg/d in 2 to 3 divided doses. Side effects include sedation, hypotension, hypertension, agitation/restlessness, extrapyramidal symptoms (EPS), withdrawal dyskinesias, depression, increased prolactin levels, QTc prolongation, decreased seizure threshold, and risk for neuroleptic malignant syndrome (NMS).

Pimozide
This is a typical diphenylbutylpiperidine derivative, and its mechanism of action includes being a dopamine (D_2) blocker, an alpha-adrenergic blocker, and a 5-HT$_2$ antagonist.[19–23] In 2 studies, pimozide was found to be either equal to or more effective than haloperidol at suppressing tics with fewer side effects.[19,20] Its initial dose is 0.05 mg/kg daily at bedtime, and it should be titrated slowly at 1- to 2-week intervals. Its maximum dose is 0.2 mg/kg daily and should not to exceed 10 mg daily. Electrocardiography (ECG) should be performed before starting this medication. It cannot be administered with macrolide antibiotics and azole antifungals because of the increased incidence of cardiac arrhythmias and long QT syndrome. Side effects include QTc prolongation, sedation, anticholinergic symptoms, elevated prolactin levels, behavioral changes, EPS, and NMS.

ECG is recommended to rule out cardiac conduction abnormalities.

Fluphenazine

It is a dopamine (D_2) blocker, histamine (H_1) blocker, alpha-adrenergic antagonist, and 5-HT_2 antagonist. The initial dose is 1 mg at bedtime, which is gradually increased at weekly increments; the maximum dose is 4 mg in divided doses. Side effects include sedation, behavioral changes, hypotension, tachycardia, photosensitivity, EPS, NMS, and elevated prolactin levels. It has less risk for anticholinergic side effects.

Risperidone

This is a benzisoxazole derivative whose mechanism of action includes being a dopamine (D_2) and 5-HT_2 antagonist; there are also H_1 and alpha-adrenergic blocker mechanisms that are low to moderate in effect. Risperidone affects other serotonin receptors. It is an atypical neuroleptic that is probably superior to the typical neuroleptics.[16,21] Its administration should be considered with comorbid OCD. Its initial dose is 0.25 to 0.50 mg at bedtime with gradual titrations at weekly intervals; the maximum dose is 4 mg daily in divided doses. Side effects include sedation, weight gain, orthostatic hypotension, fatigue, gastrointestinal upset, elevated prolactin levels, EPS (dose dependent), and NMS.

Ziprasidone

It is an atypical neuroleptic with a mechanism of action including being a dopamine (D_2 and D_3), α_1-adrenergic, and H_1 antagonists; it also affects other 5-HT receptors. Its initial dose is 5 mg at bedtime, with gradual titration at weekly intervals. The maximum dose is 40 mg daily in divided doses. Side effects include sedation, dizziness, orthostatic hypotension, nausea, rash, QTc prolongation, elevated prolactin levels, EPS, and NMS. ECG is recommended to rule out cardiac conduction abnormalities.

Tetrabenazine

This is a benzoquinolizine derivative that depletes catecholamines presynaptically and blocks dopamine receptors postsynaptically. Its initial dose is 6.25 mg twice daily, with gradual titration. Maximum daily dose in adults is 50 mg daily for CYP (cytochrome P450) 2D6 poor metabolizers or those receiving potent CYP2D6 inhibitors. Maximum daily dose in adults is 100 mg if they are CYP2D6 extensive metabolizers. Side effects include depression, fatigue, sedation, insomnia, nausea, parkinsonism, and elevated prolactin levels. It is recommended that CYP2D6 genotyping be performed at baseline.

SUMMARY

Tics in children and adolescents are a common occurrence; however, a small proportion of these disorders require pharmacologic interventions. Several limitations exist with the use of pharmacologic interventions, and hence, a more ideal multifaceted approach is suggested with emphasis on nonpharmacologic management for improved functioning, adaptation, and comorbidities. Mutual and realistic goals ensure a trustful and successful relationship between the clinician and patient.

Several pharmacologic agents are available but with limited data to support their use; thus, an individualized plan is recommended with the goal of limiting side effects of the drug and managing comorbid conditions as a priority before addressing the tics specifically.[24,25] Several local and national advocacy and resource organizations exist for family and provider support, such as the Tourette Syndrome Association.

REFERENCES

1. Jankovic J. Tourette's syndrome. N Engl J Med 2001;345:1184–92.
2. Alsobrook JP 2nd, Pauls DL. The genetics of Tourette syndrome. Neurol Clin 1997;15(2):381–93.

3. Bohlhalter S, Goldfine A, Matteson S, et al. Neural correlates of tic generation in Tourette syndrome: an event-related functional MRI study. Brain 2006;129: 2029–37.
4. Singer HS, Hong JJ, Yoon DY, et al. Serum autoantibodies do not differentiate PANDAS and Tourette syndrome from controls. Neurology 2005;65(11):1701–7.
5. American Psychiatric Association. DSM-IV-TR. Washington, DC: American Psychiatric Association; 2000.
6. Robertson NM. Tourette syndrome, associated conditions and the complexities of treatment. Brain 2000;123(3):425–62.
7. Gilbert DL. Treatment of children and adolescents with tics and Tourette syndrome. J Child Neurol 2006;21:690–700.
8. Tourette Syndrome Study Group. Treatment of ADHD in children with tics: a randomized controlled trial. Neurology 2002;58:527–36.
9. Pediatric Lexi-Drugs, Lexi-Comp, Inc. 2010.
10. Lexi-Drugs, Lexi-Comp, Inc. 2010.
11. Facts and Comparisons. Drug information full monographs. Wolters Kluwer Health, Incorporated. Available at: http://0-online.factsandcomparisons.com.libcat.ferris. edu/index.aspx. Accessed September 16, 2010.
12. Haddad P, Sharma S. Adverse effects of atypical antipsychotics, differential risk and clinical implications. CNS Drugs 2007;21(1):911–36.
13. Xenazine [package insert]. Mississauga (Canada): Bioavail Laboratories, Institute; revised September, 2009.
14. Allen AJ, Kurlan RM, Gilbert DL, et al. Atomoxetine treatment in children and adolescents with ADHD and comorbid tic disorders. Neurology 2005;65:1941–9.
15. Singer HS, Wendlandt J, Krieger M, et al. Baclofen treatment in Tourette syndrome: a double-blind, placebo-controlled, crossover trial. Neurology 2001; 56:599–604.
16. Gilbert D, Singer HS. Commentary. "Risperidone was as effective as pimozide for Tourette's disorder." Evid Based Ment Health 2001;4:75.
17. Gilbert DL, Dure L, Sethuraman G, et al. Tic reduction with pergolide in a randomized controlled trial in children. Neurology 2003;60:606–11.
18. Chapel JL, Brown N, Jenkins RL. Tourette's disease. Symptomatic relief with haloperidol. Am J Psychiatry 1964;121:608–10.
19. Gilbert DL, Batterson JR, Sethuraman G, et al. Tic reduction with risperidone vs. pimozide in a randomized, double-blind, crossover trial. J Am Acad Child Adolesc Psychiatry 2004;43:206–14.
20. Bruggeman R, van der Linden C, Buitelaar JK, et al. Risperidone versus pimozide in Tourettes's disorder: a comparative double-blind parallel-group study. J Clin Psychiatry 2001;62:50–6.
21. Ratzoni G, Gothelf D, Brand-Golthelf A, et al. Weight gain associated with olanzapine and risperidone in adolescent patients: a comparative prospective study. J Am Acad Child Adolesc Psychiatry 2002;41:337–43.
22. Marras C, Andrews D, Sime E, et al. Botulinum toxin for simple motor tics: a randomized, double-blind controlled clinical trial. Neurology 2001;56(5):605–10.
23. Visser-Vanderwalle V, Ackermans L, van der Linden C, et al. Deep brain stimulation in Gilles de la Tourettes's syndrome. Neurosurgery 2006;58(3):E590.
24. Greydanus DE, Calles J, Patel DR. Pediatric and adolescent psychopharmacology: a practical manual for pediatricians. Cambridge (England): Cambridge University Press; 2008. p. 223–40.
25. Greydanus DE, Patel DR, Olipra D. Tic disorders in children and adolescents: current concepts. Int J Child Adolesc Health 2010;3(2):50–60.

Pharmacology of Sleep Disorders in Children and Adolescents

Bantu Chhangani, MD[a],*,
Donald E. Greydanus, MD, Dr HC (ATHENS)[b], Dilip R. Patel, MD, FSAM[b],
Cynthia Feucht, PharmD, BCPS[c,d]

KEYWORDS

- Pediatric sleep disorders • Medications • Narcolepsy
- Restless legs syndrome • Obstructive sleep apnea • Insomnia

---

There is a high prevalence of sleep disorders in children and an apparent increasing need for pharmacologic management. However, because of the paucity of data available with regards to dosing, efficacy, tolerability, and safety profiles of medications as well as a lack of adequate well-designed clinical trials, medications are currently not approved in the pediatric population by the US Food and Drug Administration (FDA). No pharmacologic guidelines have been developed for the specific sleep disorders or the different pediatric age ranges. Additional research is needed for evidence-based pediatric sleep pharmacotherapy. This article reviews the various pediatric sleep disorders and the pharmacologic therapeutic options that are available.

INSOMNIA

Pediatric insomnia is defined as repeated difficulty with sleep initiation, duration, consolidation, or quality that occurs despite age-appropriate time and opportunity for sleep and results in daytime functional impairment for the child and/or the family.[1,2] It is a common problem and one of the most frequently reported parental concerns in

---

Funding support: This work did not have any funding support.
Financial disclosures: The authors have nothing to disclose.
a Sleep Medicine, Saint Mary's Neuroscience Program, Saint Mary's Neuroscience Institute, 220 Cherry Street South East, 1000 Oakland Drive, Kalamazoo, MI 49503, USA
b Department of Pediatrics and Human Development, Michigan State University College of Human Medicine, MSU/Kalamazoo Center for Medical Studies, 1000 Oakland Drive, Kalamazoo, MI 49009-1284, USA
c Borgess Ambulatory Care, 1701 Gull Road, Kalamazoo, MI 49048, USA
d Department of Pharmacy Practice, Ferris State University College of Pharmacy, Big Rapids, MI 49307, USA
* Corresponding author.
E-mail address: bantuchhangani@yahoo.com

Pediatr Clin N Am 58 (2011) 273–291
doi:10.1016/j.pcl.2010.11.003
0031-3955/11/$ – see front matter © 2011 Elsevier Inc. All rights reserved.

pediatric practices.[3] Prevalence rates range from 1% to 6% in the otherwise healthy pediatric population to as high as 50% to 75% in children and adolescents with psychiatric and neurodevelopmental disorders. Although most of the sleep disturbances are usually short-lived, emerging data indicate these can persist and become chronic.[4–7]

Several studies have shown the profound adverse consequences of pediatric insomnia, which affect not only the children and adolescents concerned but also their families. A few commonly reported daytime consequences in children include hyperactivity, poor memory, learning difficulties, impulsive behaviors, and an increase in accidental injuries. Parents of sleepless children are also more likely to have depressed mood, poor daytime performance, and increased stress levels. These symptoms have been shown to improve with the treatment of the pediatric insomnia.[8–10] Given the high prevalence and chronicity within select populations and negative consequences of pediatric insomnia, effective management of this condition is becoming increasingly necessary.

Two main therapeutic approaches are generally used: cognitive-behavioral therapy and pharmacologic therapy. Whereas the efficacy of cognitive-behavioral therapy or behavioral therapy alone is relatively well established, there is a paucity of evidence-based data for use of pharmacologic therapy within the pediatric population.[2,11,12] Despite this, it appears that the rate for the use of medications by physicians for the treatment of pediatric insomnia in an outpatient setting in the United States is increasing, which is concerning given the lack of information regarding specific guidelines for dosing regimens, efficacy, and safety profiles of these medications.[13] The medications currently used are not approved by the FDA for the different pediatric age ranges nor for the specific sleep disorder, leading to off-label use. Some of the commonly used medications include melatonin, antihistamines, and α_2 adrenergic agonists among others.

Melatonin

Melatonin (N-acetyl-5-methoxytryptamine) is a hormone synthesized and secreted predominantly by the pineal gland. In a survey of 3424 community-based pediatricians, melatonin ranked as the third most frequently used medication after antihistamines and α_2 agonists.[14] It is synthesized from its precursor tryptophan, and the secretion from the pineal gland is regulated by the suprachiasmatic nucleus in the hypothalamus. Levels of endogenous melatonin are usually high at nighttime and decrease during the habitual wake-up time, suggesting that it may play a cardinal role in the control of the sleep-wake cycle in humans. Exogenous melatonin is hepatically metabolized, has a half-life of 30 to 50 minutes, and onset of action is typically within 30 to 60 minutes. Although dosing guidelines have not been established, exogenous melatonin doses of 0.3 mg typically produce physiologic nocturnal levels of 50 to 200 pcg/mL.[15]

Studies have reported a reduction in the latency to sleep onset as well as an increase in sleep maintenance and total sleep time, with doses ranging from 0.5 to 10 mg. Melatonin has both chronobiotic and weak hypnotic properties and its use has been suggested to be most effective in blind children, children with attention-deficit/hyperactivity disorder (ADHD), and autistic spectrum disorder or insomnia caused by circadian disorders such as circadian rhythm disorder-delayed sleep phase type.[16–18] Although melatonin is generally well tolerated, long-term effects of chronic use are unknown. Potential side effects may include disturbances of the central nervous system (CNS) and lowering of seizure threshold, along with rare reports of gynecomastia and autoimmune hepatitis. The National Sleep Foundation has urged avoidance of the use of melatonin in patients with immune disorders, or in patients taking immunosuppressants or corticosteroids.[19–21] The FDA does not regulate the safety, purity, or efficacy of commercially available preparations of melatonin; one preparation may differ significantly from the other and results can thus vary.

Melatonin Agonists

Ramelteon is a melatonin agonist that acts by binding to the melatonin receptors MT_1 and MT_2 in the suprachiasmatic nucleus.[22] It is approved by the FDA for the treatment of insomnia in adults and is the only prescription sedative-hypnotic medication that is not a scheduled substance with the US Drug Enforcement Administration. Ramelteon has been shown to reduce latency to sleep onset, increase total sleep time, and result in reports of subjective benefit, although changes in sleep may increase slowly over weeks of nightly use.[23] It can be used for sleep initiation problems and is not associated with next-day hangover effect/residual sedation, rebound insomnia, or withdrawal. Side effects such as headache are rare.[24] Ramelteon has a half-life of up to 5 hours because of an active metabolite. The adult dose is 8 mg daily 30 minutes before bedtime, and patients should avoid a fatty meal before administration.[25] Ramelteon is primarily metabolized by cytochrome (CYP) 1A2 and should be used with caution when administered with other medications that inhibit this substrate (eg, fluvoxamine).[25] Ramelteon is currently not approved for use in children and adolescents.

Antihistamines

In pediatric practices, antihistamines are generally used in the treatment of allergies, and are often an active ingredient of many over-the-counter (OTC) cold and allergy preparations. However, despite the lack of randomized controlled trials showing the efficacy of antihistamines as hypnotic medications in children, antihistamines have increasingly become one of the more popular choices of pediatricians and parents and are currently the most commonly used medications to treat sleep disturbances in children.[26] Diphenhydramine is a lipophilic, first-generation antihistamine that causes sedation by easily crossing the blood-brain barrier and competitively blocking the histamine (H_1) receptors. It is rapidly absorbed from the gastrointestinal system, undergoes extensive first-pass metabolism, and is hepatically metabolized. The peak sedative effect occurs 1 to 3 hours after administration and typically lasts 4 to 7 hours. Pediatric dosing ranges from 1 mg/kg up to 50 mg per day.[15]

Diphenhydramine reduces the latency to sleep onset but overall, an improvement in parental satisfaction or reduction in nighttime awakenings has not been shown when compared with placebo.[27] Side effects are anticholinergic in nature and include dry mouth, urinary retention, daytime drowsiness, hypotension, and tachycardia. Children have also been reported to experience paradoxic excitation, and tolerance to antihistamines, which can result in the administration of higher doses and greater risk of side effects.[28] Seizures, cardiac arrhythmias, rhabdomyolysis, and respiratory insufficiency are more serious but rare consequences reported predominantly in overdose situations.[29]

Chloral Hydrate

Chloral hydrate was commonly used as a sedative hypnotic in children but lost its popularity because of the significant side-effect profile, including respiratory compromise and the potential hangover effect that can occur because of the long half-lives of its active metabolite, trichloroethanol.[15,30] Chloral hydrate results in a reduction in latency to sleep onset, and hypnotic doses in children range from 25 to 50 mg/kg/dose (maximal dose 1 g) at bedtime. Maximal effect is typically seen within 30 to 60 minutes and lasts approximately 4 to 8 hours.[15]

Side effects can range from drowsiness, malaise, paradoxic excitement, nausea, vomiting, and gastric distress to depression of the CNS, arrhythmias, and respiratory compromise. Chloral hydrate should thus be used cautiously or avoided in children with sleep-disordered breathing, gastritis/esophagitis, severe cardiac disease, hepatic and renal dysfunction, and patients with porphyria or on stimulant medications.[15] Tolerance is also a concern, and used chronically (>2 weeks) chloral hydrate can become habit forming. Withdrawal symptoms, including seizures and delirium, may occur if discontinued abruptly after prolonged use.[31,32] The American Academy of Pediatrics recommends limiting the use of chloral hydrate to short-term sedation.[33]

Benzodiazepines

This class of sleep-promoting medications acts by binding to several γ-aminobutyric acid (GABA) type A receptor subtypes. Medications include temazepam, estazolam, triazolam, quazepam, flurazepam, and clonazepam.[25,34] They reduce the latency to sleep onset, the number of arousals or awakenings that occur between sleep-stage transitions, and increase total sleep time. Benzodiazepines have also been associated with an alteration in sleep structure including an increase in stage N2 sleep as well as rapid eye movement (REM) latency.[25] They have anxiolytic and anticonvulsant properties. Potential side effects include residual daytime sedation, memory impairment, behavioral disinhibition, and dependence with prolonged use.[35]

Benzodiazepines are not commonly used in the treatment of pediatric insomnia. Clonazepam is the possible exception in the treatment of disorders of partial arousal in children and adolescents when frequent and disruptive to the patient and family, predominantly because of its ability to increase the arousal threshold and suppress slow-wave sleep. The administered dose of clonazepam ranges from 0.25 mg to 0.5 mg at bedtime, although dosing guidelines have not been established. It has a prolonged half-life of 22 to 33 hours, onset of effect in 20 to 60 minutes, and levels typically peak within 1 to 4 hours of administration. Clonazepam is hepatically metabolized by CYP 3A4, and concomitant medications that inhibit or induce this substrate may affect the concentrations of clonazepam (**Tables 1** and **2**).[15]

Selective benzodiazepine receptor agonists

This class of medications includes zolpidem, zaleplon, and eszopiclone. Despite being known as benzodiazepine receptor agonists, these medications differ in their chemical structure from the benzodiazepines and bind more selectively to the benzodiazepine-1 receptor site.[36] They thus lack the anxiolytic, anticonvulsant, and muscle-relaxing properties of the traditional benzodiazepines associated with binding at the benzodiazepine-2 receptor.[36] They are not known to alter the sleep architecture and are less likely to result in rebound insomnia or hangover effects. Studies have shown a decrease in the latency to sleep onset and the number of awakenings during the night as well as an improvement in the sleep duration and quality.[35]

Zaleplon has a half-life of 1 to 2 hours, zolpidem, 2 to 3 hours, and eszopiclone, 5 to 7 hours. They typically reach peak values between 30 and 60 minutes and are hepatically metabolized.[37,38] Zolpidem and eszopiclone are major substrates for CYP 3A4 and have the potential for drug interactions. In adults zolpidem immediate release is considered for difficulty with sleep initiation and the controlled release can be used for difficulty with sleep onset and/or sleep maintenance. Zaleplon may be considered for sleep initiation problems and can also be used for the reinitiation of sleep during awakenings in the middle of the night because of its short half-life.[39] Eszopiclone can be considered for difficulty in initiating and maintaining sleep throughout the night.

Table 1
Medications used for the treatment of insomnia

Medication Class	Medication	FDA Approved	Schedule
Melatonin agonist	Ramelteon (Rozerem)	Yes	Prescription (noncontrolled)
Antihistamines	Diphenhydramine (Benadryl)	Yes	OTC
	Doxylamine (Unisom)	Yes	Often found in combination with analgesic
Nonbarbiturate hypnotic	Chloral hydrate (Somnote)	Yes	C-IV
Benzodiazepines	Temazepam (Restoril)	Yes	C-IV
	Triazolam (Halcion)	Yes	
	Flurazepam (Dalmane)	Yes	
	Estazolam (Prosom)	Yes	
	Quazepam (Doral)	Yes	
	Clonazepam (Klonopin)	No	
	Lorazepam (Ativan)	No	
Nonbenzodiazepines	Zolpidem (Ambien)	Yes	C-IV
	Zalepon (Sonata)	Yes	
	Eszopiclone (Lunesta)	Yes	
α_2 agonists	Clonidine (Catapres)	No	Prescription (noncontrolled)
Antidepressants	Amitriptyline (Elavil)	No	Prescription (noncontrolled)
	Nortriptyline (Pamelor)	No	
	Doxepin (Sinequan)	No	
	Trazodone (Desyrel)	No	
	Mirtazapine (Remeron)	No	
Herbal supplements	Melatonin	No	Dietary supplements
	Kava-kava	No	Not FDA regulated
	Valerian	No	
	Lavender	No	
	Chamomile	No	

Abbreviation: C-IV, controlled substance schedule IV.
Data from Refs.[15,25,36,101]

Eszopiclone is currently approved by the FDA for the treatment of chronic insomnia in adults because of evidence for long-term safety with no development of tolerance or dependence.[40] Typical adult dosages are zolpidem immediate release 5 to 10 mg, zolpidem extended release 12.5 mg, zaleplon 5 to 10 mg, and eszopiclone 1 to 3 mg. However, the use of these medications in children is considered off-label because they are currently not approved by the FDA. Dosing guidelines are not available for the pediatric population. Although these drugs are generally well tolerated, potential side effects can include excess sedation, dizziness, amnesia, parasomnias, complex sleep behaviors (eg, sleepwalking, sleep-related eating disorders, sleep-driving) and worsening of untreated sleep-disordered breathing. Eszopiclone has also been noted to have an unpleasant metallic taste.[25] Tolerance, dependence, and rebound effects are less common than benzodiazepines.[41]

Centrally Acting α_2 Agonists

Clonidine and guanfacine are both centrally acting α_2 receptor agonists indicated for the treatment of hypertension in the adult population. However, despite the lack of randomized clinical trials, these medications (particularly clonidine) are widely used

Table 2
Characteristics of FDA-approved medications for the treatment of insomnia

Medication	Adult Initial Dose	Onset of Action	Sleep Latency	Total Sleep Time	Delta Sleep
Melatonin agonists					
Ramelteon	8 mg	30 min	Decreased	Increased	No effect
Antihistamines					
Diphenhydramine	0.5 mg/kg/dose (pediatric)	1–3 h	Decreased	Increased	N/A
Doxylamine	25 mg	N/A			
Nonbarbiturate hypnotic					
Chloral hydrate	25–50 mg/kg/dose (pediatric)	10–20 min	Decreased	Increased	No effect
Benzodiazepines					
Temazepam	7.5–15 mg	30–60 min	Decreased	Increased	Decreased
Triazolam	0.125–0.25 mg	15–30 min			
Estazolam	1 mg	60 min			
Clonazepam	0.25–0.5 mg (pediatric)	20–60 min			
Nonbenzodiazepines					
Zolpidem	5–10 mg	30 min	Decreased	Increased	Increased
Zaleplon	5–10 mg	20 min		Increased or no effect	
Eszopiclone	1–2 mg	30 min		Increased	

Abbreviation: N/A, not available.
Data from Refs. [15,25,36,102]

as soporifics in the pediatric population because of their sedating properties.[26] Clonidine use has also been reported for the management of sleep disturbances in children with ADHD.[42] It has a half-life of 8 to 12 hours in children, and plasma levels typically peak between 2 and 4 hours, with an onset of action within an hour.[15] As with other medications used in the treatment of pediatric insomnia, optimum soporific dosing guidelines have not been established, but clonidine is typically administered at a starting dose of 0.05 mg at bedtime and increased in increments of 0.05 mg every 3 to 4 days (usual maximum 0.3–0.4 mg/d) depending on efficacy.[15,43]

Effects on sleep include a reduced latency to sleep onset and REM sleep suppression. Clonidine has a narrow therapeutic index, and side effects include hypotension, bradycardia, dry mouth, irritability, and dysphoria. Tolerance can also develop over time, leading to an increase in dosage and the potential for adverse effects. A dramatic increase in clonidine overdoses has recently been reported.[44] Rebound hypertension and REM rebound can occur with abrupt discontinuation. Therefore, when discontinuing this medication, a gradual taper of over 1 week should be recommended to patients.

Antidepressants

Commonly used medications in this class include amitriptyline, trazodone, and doxepin. These antidepressants are sedating because of their anticholinergic or antihistaminergic activity and despite only a few randomized controlled and open-label trials in adults and no data in the pediatric population, they continue to be a popular choice amongst both adult and pediatric providers because of familiarity with the medications. However, the use of sedating antidepressants for the treatment of insomnia is not approved by the FDA. Tolerance can develop, resulting in the need for higher doses, and common side effects include hangover effect, dry mouth, dizziness, confusion, and constipation. Tricyclic antidepressants are also associated with cardiovascular toxicity (eg, tachycardia, orthostatic hypotension, and conduction abnormalities) and death can occur from overdosage.[45,46]

Herbal Supplements

There are few data with regards to efficacy and safety profile of herbal supplements in children. Adult studies have at best shown either a lack of beneficial effect[47] or safety concerns like severe hepatotoxicity with certain herbal supplements like kava-kava.[48]

RESTLESS LEGS SYNDROME

Restless legs syndrome (RLS) is a neurologic sensorimotor disorder characterized by unpleasant paresthesias that occur primarily in the lower extremities and are accompanied by a strong and nearly irresistible urge to move. The paresthesias may include numbness, tingling, and aching and can also be experienced, albeit less commonly, in other parts of the body, including the arms and the trunk. These symptoms are brought on during periods of inactivity and display a circadian pattern such that the paresthesias are worse in the evening and night in those with normal circadian rhythm activity. A complete or partial improvement is usually seen with movement for as long as the movement continues.[49]

The 4 essential criteria for the diagnosis of RLS can be summarized in the pneumonic URGE, explained as U: urge to move the legs because of unpleasant sensations; R: worsening during periods of rest; G: gets better with movement; and E: worse in the evenings. To make a diagnosis of RLS in the pediatric population (aged 2–12 years), it is essential that in addition to meeting all 4 of these criteria, the child should be able to describe the unpleasant sensations in their own words.[49,50] If the child is unable to do so, but does meet the 4 criteria, a diagnosis of RLS can be made if 2 of the following 3 criteria are also present: sleep disturbance appropriate for age, a biologic parent or sibling who has RLS, or a periodic limb movement in sleep index of greater than 5/h on polysomnography.

The adult diagnostic criteria can be used for adolescents (ie, older than 12 years).[49,50] Patients with RLS may experience 2 types of leg movements: voluntary and involuntary. The former are movements that are made to obtain relief from the unpleasant paresthesias, such as walking the floor or stretching. The involuntary leg movements are repetitive movements over which the patient has minimal control. These movements may occur during sleep (periodic limb movements in sleep) or while awake (periodic limb movements during wakefulness). Periodic limb movements in sleep are a common feature on polysomnography in about 80% of patients with RLS although they may also exist on their own.[51]

Although originally believed to be a disorder of adults, RLS has been increasingly described in the pediatric population, with an estimated prevalence rate of 1.9% in school-aged children and 2% in adolescents, with no gender differences reported. These prevalence rates are higher than that of diabetes or epilepsy.[52] Patients with RLS can have a prolonged latency to sleep and disrupted nocturnal sleep and other adverse consequences affecting mood, behavior, and quality of life.[53] There is increasing evidence suggesting a relationship of RLS with ADHD,[54] conduct disorder,[55] depression/anxiety, and parasomnias.[56]

The management of children and adolescents with RLS is challenging and there are currently no specific recommendations made by the American Academy of Sleep Medicine.[57] Children with mild or infrequent symptoms of RLS may be managed conservatively with nonpharmacologic therapy. The aim is to eliminate or reduce factors that may exacerbate the symptoms of RLS, including caffeine, alcohol, nicotine, selective serotonin reuptake inhibitors, dopamine antagonists, and antihistamines. Adherence to good sleep hygiene and avoidance of sleep deprivation is essential as a worsening of symptoms has been noted with drowsiness. Massaging the affected areas, application of hot/cold packs, and engaging in moderate exercise may also be beneficial.[58]

Commonly used classes of medications in the treatment of adult RLS include iron supplementation, dopaminergic agents, benzodiazepines, anticonvulsants, and opioids. Pharmacologic therapy for significant RLS in children is more challenging because of the limited data available with regards to efficacy and safety profile of these medications. Medications should be used in conjunction with nonpharmacologic therapy and started only after carefully considering the benefits of the medication compared with potential risks.

Dopaminergic Medications

Studies have suggested that hypofunction of the dopaminergic system may play a role in the pathophysiology of RLS. The improvement noted in clinical symptoms with dopaminergic medications further supports this finding.[59,60] Dopaminergic agents are currently considered to be first-line therapy in adult patients with RLS[61,62] and medications in this class that have been found to be effective include carbidopa/levodopa, and the nonergot dopamine agonists ropinirole and pramiprexole. The last two are FDA-approved medications for the treatment of moderate to severe primary RLS in adults. The rare but serious consequences including the development of pleuropulmonary fibrosis[63] and cardiac valvulopathy[64] limit the use of ergot dopaminergic agents such as pergolide and bromocriptine.

Although there are currently no FDA-approved medications for the treatment of RLS in children, published reports have emerged suggesting the efficacy of dopaminergic agents in children with RLS.[65–67] However, there are no dosing guidelines currently available. Most providers usually start with the lowest dose and then adjust according to clinical symptoms. Potential side effects include nausea, vomiting, hallucinations, excessive daytime sleepiness, rebound, and augmentation. Augmentation is the development of RLS symptoms during the afternoon or early evening (ie, earlier in the day than noted prior to starting the medication) and is treated by either reducing the dose or switching to another dopaminergic medication. Administration of an earlier dose of the same dopaminergic agent should be avoided because this may lead to further exacerbation of augmentation symptoms. Although reported more commonly with levodopa/carbidopa, augmentation can also occur with the dopamine agonists.[68] Rebound phenomenon is the appearance of symptoms of RLS usually in the early morning compatible with the half-life of the medication.

Iron

Therapy with iron is based on increasing evidence that iron deficiency may play a role in the pathophysiology of RLS and periodic limb movements of sleep. Iron is a cofactor for tyrosine hydroxylase, the rate-limiting enzyme in dopamine synthesis, and has been found to be low in the substantia nigra, cerebrospinal fluid (CSF), and serum of adult patients with RLS.[69,70] Although the studies are not so robust in children, there is emerging evidence that low iron levels may also exist in children with RLS and period limb movements of sleep. Such children may benefit from iron therapy (3 mg/kg/d of elemental iron) to maintain serum ferritin levels greater than 50 ng/mL.[71,72] Absorption of iron is enhanced when combined with vitamin C and reduced with calcium, and the latter should be avoided at least 1 to 2 hours before or after iron administration. Patients on iron replacement should have regular follow-up appointments to assess for clinical improvement. The serum ferritin levels should also be monitored periodically to prevent iron overload. Medication doses may be adjusted according to clinical relevance and pertinent laboratory data.

Miscellaneous

Although the other medication classes have not yet been adequately studied, clona-zepam, clonidine, and gabapentin[73] are often used by providers to treat RLS in children (**Table 3**).

OBSTRUCTIVE SLEEP APNEA SYNDROME

Obstructive sleep apnea is a sleep-related disorder characterized by intermittent episodes of complete or partial upper-airway obstruction, resulting in gas exchange abnormalities (hypoxia and hypercapnea) and fragmented sleep. It is a common disorder, with a high prevalence rate of 2% to 5% when compared with other child-hood conditions such as sickle cell anemia and diabetes.[74,75] Pediatric obstructive sleep apnea can occur at any age, but because most cases are caused by adenoton-sillar hypertrophy, the highest prevalence is observed to be between the ages of 2 and 6 years, coinciding with peak adenotonsillar hypertrophy relative to upper-airway size.[76,77]

The diagnosis of pediatric obstructive sleep apnea begins with a detailed history and physical examination followed by a diagnostic nocturnal polysomnogram, which continues to be the gold standard. The *International classification of sleep disorders second edition* (ICSD-2) diagnostic criteria for pediatric obstructive sleep apnea

Table 3
Dopaminergic agents used in the treatment of RLS

	Carbidopa/levodopa	Ropinirole	Pramipexole
Brand name	Sinemet	Requip	Mirapex
Formulations	Immediate release Extended release Generic available: IR and CR Oral disintegrating	Immediate release Extended release Generic available: IR only	IR No generic available
Initial dose (adult)	25/100 mg IR 30–60 min before bedtime	0.25 mg IR 1–3 h before bedtime	0.125 mg 2–3 h before bedtime
Warnings	Augmentation (more common with levodopa) Rebound (more common with levodopa) Compulsive behaviors (eg, hypersexuality, binge eating)		
Adverse effects	Gastrointestinal (nausea, vomiting, constipation) Anorexia Headaches/dizziness Daytime sedation Hypotension Dry mouth Peripheral edema Nasal congestion Abnormal dreams		

Abbreviations: CR, controlled release; IR, immediate release.
Data from Refs.[15,103,104]

require caregiver report of snoring, labored or obstructed breathing noted during sleep, and the observation of either diaphoresis, neck hyperextension during sleep, morning headaches, paradoxic inward rib-cage motion during inspiration, slow rate of growth, excessive daytime sleepiness/hyperactivity, or secondary enuresis. One or more scoreable respiratory events per hour on polysomnography in conjunction with the relevant history are required to make the diagnosis.[1] Commonly reported nocturnal symptoms include snoring, apneic episodes, enuresis, perspiration, restlessness, unusual sleeping positions, and parasomnias.[78] Daytime symptoms may include hyperactivity, learning deficits, inattention and less commonly hypersomnolence.[79]

Physical examination findings may be completely unremarkable or may include tonsillar hypertrophy, obesity, failure to thrive, craniofacial anomalies such as high-arched palate, retrognathia, and midface hypoplasia.[80] Several studies have shown profound adverse consequences of pediatric obstructive sleep apnea if left untreated, including neurobehavioral deficits such as inattention and hyperactivity[81] and cardiovascular complications such as cor pulmonale and hypertension.[82,83]

Pharmacologic therapy for obstructive sleep apnea is limited, and no medications are currently approved for use in the treatment of pediatric obstructive sleep apnea. Adenotonsillectomy remains the most frequently used treatment of pediatric obstructive sleep apnea, with resolution of the obstructive sleep apnea in 75% to 100% of otherwise healthy children.[84] Nasal continuous positive airway pressure is usually reserved for patients who have residual sleep apnea after surgery, are not surgical candidates, or based on patient and parental preference.[85] The concept of using pharmacologic agents for the treatment of pediatric obstructive sleep apnea is an attractive one when compared with the potential complications of surgery or the discomfort of wearing a nasal positive airway pressure interface device.

Oxygen

Oxygen has limited use as the sole therapeutic intervention for children and adolescents with obstructive sleep apnea. It is usually reserved for patients who cannot tolerate nasal continuous positive airway pressure, have significant residual sleep apnea despite adenotonsillectomy and/or refuse tracheostomy. The major limitation of using oxygen as a sole therapeutic intervention is that although its use may result in higher oxygen saturations, it has no effect on apnea duration, frequency, or arousals from sleep.[86] It also has not been reported to improve daytime symptoms, including excessive daytime fatigue/sleepiness. Hypercapnea can occur with the use of supplemental oxygen, and children on supplemental oxygen need to be monitored carefully.[86]

Nasal Steroids and Leukotriene Receptor Antagonists

Nasal steroids and leukotriene receptor antagonists have been investigated as potential pharmacologic interventions in the treatment of pediatric obstructive sleep apnea based on the rationale that nasal congestion and allergic rhinitis can narrow the size of the nasal airways, thus contributing to the severity of the apnea. Also, the presence of nasal and oropharyngeal mucosal inflammation noted in adult patients with obstructive sleep apnea raises the possibility that nasal steroids and leukotriene inhibitors could be used as an alternative to adenotonsillectomy in mild cases of pediatric sleep apnea.

Brouillette and colleagues[87] conducted a 6-week randomized, triple-blind, placebo-controlled, parallel-group trial of nasal fluticasone propionate versus placebo in 25 children aged 1 to 10 years. Although the study concluded that nasal fluticasone decreased the number of mixed and obstructive apneas and hypopneas, the post-treatment apnea hypopnea index remained high, and no improvement was noted symptomatically.[87]

Other studies have assessed the effect of 4 weeks and 6 weeks of intranasal budesonide, and these have shown an improvement, although with incomplete resolution of the apneas and hypopneas such that the posttreatment apnea hypopnea index still remained within the pathologic range.[88,89] Goldbart and colleagues[90] found that 16 weeks of therapy with daily montelukast resulted in significant reductions in adenoid size and respiratory-related sleep disturbances. These investigators concluded that therapy with a leukotriene receptor antagonist appeared to be associated with improved breathing during sleep but emphasized the need for further double-blind, placebo-controlled trials.

In summary, intranasal steroids cannot be advocated as the sole therapeutic intervention because of the incomplete resolution of apneas and hypopneas in the studies mentioned earlier as well as the lack of long-term trials assessing safety of these medications. Intranasal steroids and leukotriene modifiers may thus be considered as a bridge in mild to moderate cases of pediatric sleep apnea until surgery or nasal positive airway pressure is available.

NARCOLEPSY

Narcolepsy is a chronic neurologic disorder characterized by instability of the sleep-wake cycle believed to be related to deficiency of the hypothalamic hypocretin system such that elements of sleep intrude into wakefulness and vice versa.[91] It is an uncommon disorder, with a prevalence of 0.02% to 0.18% and an equal male-to-female predominance. The prevalence increases to about 40 times in first-degree relatives. Although the peak age of onset is usually in the second decade of life, there is frequently a 10- to 15-year delay in diagnosis from the time of onset of symptoms.[1]

Several studies have reported a reduction or absence of hypocretin in patients with narcolepsy and cataplexy. Because hypocretin is the hypothalamic neuropeptide that plays an important role in regulating wake-promoting mechanisms, its absence leads to abnormalities of the transition between wakefulness, REM sleep, and non-REM sleep. Most of the symptoms of narcolepsy, including sleep paralysis, hypnogogic hallucinations, and cataplexy, are caused by inappropriate intrusions of REM sleep into wakefulness. Ninety percent of patients who have narcolepsy with cataplexy have been found to have undetectable CSF levels of hypocretin. These levels are normal in patients who have narcolepsy but no cataplexy, suggesting a different pathophysiology for these patients.[92,93] Genetic, immunologic, and environmental factors have also been implicated.

The tetrad of narcolepsy symptoms includes excessive daytime sleepiness, cataplexy, sleep paralysis, and hypnapompic/hypnogogic hallucinations. Other features also commonly reported in patients with narcolepsy are disrupted sleep, repeated nighttime awakenings, terrifying dreams, and sleep initiation as well as maintenance problems. Children with narcolepsy may be inappropriately diagnosed as having ADHD because of behavioral problems, poor school performance, and inattentiveness. The hallmark feature found in 100% of patients is excessive daytime sleepiness, although the only feature that is specific to narcolepsy is cataplexy. This condition is the abrupt and reversible loss of muscle tone elicited by emotions like laughter and anger. The patient is usually fully conscious during these episodes, which typically last from a few seconds to minutes. Cataplexy may be misdiagnosed as epilepsy.[1]

In adults the diagnosis is usually made by clinical assessment and diagnostic testing, including nocturnal polysomnography and multiple sleep latency testing.[94] Rarely, cerebrospinal hypocretin level may be measured. The diagnosis in prebubertal children is more challenging, especially because there are few normative diagnostic testing data in this age population.[95] Narcolepsy when left untreated can lead to significant functional impairment.

The current mainstays of therapy are behavioral therapy and pharmacological therapy.[96] The former includes educating the patients, parents, and teachers about the nature of the disorder and extensively counseling them on the importance of maintaining adequate sleep hygiene and adhering to a structured sleep schedule. Patients should be given the opportunity to take short 20-minute naps at least twice a day and sleep deprivation should be avoided because it can worsen the narcolepsy symptoms.[97] Patients may also benefit from joining narcolepsy support groups.

The goal of pharmacologic therapy is to treat the excessive daytime sleepiness and cataplexy to the extent that patients can lead normal lives. There are no double-blind, placebo-controlled trials specifically for children with narcolepsy. Medication use is usually lifelong, and patients need to be carefully monitored for the development of side effects.

Medications Used for the Treatment of Excessive Daytime Sleepiness

Modafinil is a nonamphetamine wakefulness-promoting medication and is considered as first-line therapy for the treatment of excessive daytime sleepiness in narcoleptic adults. Although the mode of action is not completely clear it is believed to be related to dopaminergic signaling.[98] Modafinil has been studied in children with ADHD[98–100] and can be started at 100 mg daily preferably given before 2 PM to avoid nocturnal sleep disruption. The dose may be titrated up to 200 to 400 mg in divided doses. The advantage of this medication is its long half-life, which enables it to be administered as a single morning dose, the good control of sleepiness, and relative lack of illicit use. Potential side effects include headache, nausea, and dry mouth. An alternative form of contraception should be recommended to women of child-bearing age who are using oral contraception, because modafinil can reduce the effectiveness of oral contraception.

Methylphenidate is a CNS stimulant, which acts by blocking the reuptake of norepinephrine and dopamine by the presynaptic neurons, thus increasing the concentration of these neurotransmitters in the extraneuronal space. It is a potent wakefulness-promoting medication but is considered second line because of its sympathomimetic side effects and potential for dependency. Patients taking this medication should have their weight, blood pressure, and pulse monitored carefully and should be informed about side effects, including psychosis, arrhythmias, anorexia, and sudden death. Starting doses for ADHD are 0.3 mg/kg/dose with titration weekly as clinically relevant.

Amphetamines are another class of CNS stimulants that improve daytime alertness but just like methylphenidate are considered second line in the treatment of narcolepsy due to the potential side effects. These side effects include hypertension, psychosis, sudden death, and addiction. Patients on this medication need to be monitored closely. Typical starting doses are 5 mg administered twice a day, with the last dose before 3 PM.

Medications Used for the Treatment of Cataplexy

Commonly used medications for the treatment of cataplexy include REM suppressing sleep medications such as tricyclic antidepressants, selective serotonin reuptake inhibitors, and noradrenergic reuptake inhibitors. These medications act by inhibiting reuptake of norepinephrine and serotonin by the presynaptic neurons, increasing the levels of these neurotransmitters in the neuronal space. These neurotransmitters in turn inhibit the brainstem circuits that generate REM sleep and hence reduce cataplexy or other REM-related phenomena. Care must be taken to avoid abrupt discontinuation of these medications as this may lead to rebound cataplexy.

γ-Hydroxybutyrate (GHB) is a metabolite of GABA and acts by binding specifically to $GABA_B$ and GHB receptors. It is approved by the FDA for the treatment of narcolepsy with cataplexy in adults. It also improves the quality of nocturnal sleep and daytime alertness. GHB is a liquid and is given in 2 separate doses with the first at bedtime and the second 2.5–4 hours later because of its short half-life. There are no dosing guidelines for the various pediatric age ranges. Potential side effects include nausea, deep sedation leading to coma and death in overdoses, and a significant potential for abuse.

SUMMARY

Pediatric sleep disorders are highly prevalent and there is evidence showing the development of adverse consequences when these disorders are not adequately treated. There is a need for more research to develop evidence-based pharmacologic guidelines for the specific sleep disorders, taking into account the different pediatric age ranges. Currently, there are no FDA-approved medications for the treatment of these disorders.

ACKNOWLEDGMENTS

The authors would like to acknowledge the editorial assistance of James Wyatt, PhD DABSM.

REFERENCES

1. American Academy of Sleep Medicine. The international classification of sleep disorders. 2nd edition. Westchester (IL): American Academy of Sleep Medicine; 2005. p. 58–66, 125–32.
2. Mindell J, Emslie G, Blumer J, et al. Pharmacologic management of insomnia in children and adolescents: consensus statement. Pediatrics 2006;117:e1223–32.
3. Mindell J, Owens J. A clinical guide to pediatric sleep: diagnosis and management of sleep problems in children and adolescents. Philadelphia: Lippincott Williams and Wilkins; 2003. p. 1–10.
4. Sadeh A, Raviv A, Gruber R. Sleep patterns and sleep disruptions in school-age children. Dev Psychol 2000;36(3):291–301.
5. Quine L. Sleep problems in primary school children: comparison between mainstream and special school children. Child Care Health Dev 2001;27(3):201–21.
6. Stores G. Sleep–wake function in children with neurodevelopmental and psychiatric disorders. Semin Pediatr Neurol 2001;8(4):188–97.
7. Katari S, Swanson MS, Trevathan GD. Persistence of sleep disturbances in preschool children. J Pediatr 1987;110:642–6.
8. Roberts RE, Roberts CR, Duong HT. Chronic insomnia and its negative consequences for health and functioning of adolescents: a 12-month prospective study. J Adolesc Health 2008;42(3):294–302.
9. Wiggs L, Stores G. Behavioral treatment for sleep problems in children with severe intellectual disabilities and daytime challenging behavior: effect on mothers and fathers. Br J Health Psychol 2001;6(Pt 3):257–69.
10. Mindell JA, Durand VM. Treatment of childhood sleep disorders: generalization across disorders and effects on family members. J Pediatr Psychol 1993;18: 731–50.
11. Kuhn BR, Eliott AJ. Treatment efficacy in behavioral pediatric sleep medicine. J Psychosom Res 2003;54:587–97.
12. Mindell JA. Empirically supported treatments in pediatric psychology: bedtime refusal and night waking in young children. J Pediatr Psychol 1999;24:465–81.
13. Stojanovski SD, Rasu RS, Balkrishnan R, et al. Trends in medication prescribing for pediatric sleep difficulties in the US outpatient settings. Sleep 2007;30: 1013–7.
14. Owens JA, Rosen CL, Mindell JA. Medication use in the treatment of pediatric insomnia: results of a survey of community-based pediatricians. Pediatrics 2003;111:e628–35.
15. Pediatric Lexi-Drugs: Lexi-Comp, Inc. 2010.
16. Weiss MD, Wasdell MB, Bomben MM, et al. Sleep hygiene and melatonin treatment for children and adolescents with ADHD and initial insomnia. J Am Acad Child Adolesc Psychiatry 2006;45(5):512–9.
17. Giannotti F, Cortesi F, Cerquiglini A, et al. An open-label study of controlled release melatonin in the treatment of sleep disorders in children with autism. J Autism Dev Disord 2006;36(6):741–52.
18. Sack RL, Brandes RW, Kendall AR, et al. Entrainment of free-running circadian rhythms by melatonin in blind people. N Engl J Med 2000;343(15):1070–7.
19. Luboshitzky R, Lavi S, Thuma I, et al. Increased nocturnal melatonin secretion in male patients with hypogonadotropic hypogonadism and delayed puberty. J Clin Endocrinol Metab 1995;80(7):2144–8.
20. Sheldon SH. Pro-convulsant effects of oral melatonin in neurologically disabled children [letter]. Lancet 1998;351(9111):1254.

21. Sutherland ER, Martin RJ, Ellison MC, et al. Immunomodulatory effects of melatonin in asthma. Am J Respir Crit Care Med 2002;166(8):1055–61.
22. Turek FW, Gillette MU. Melatonin, sleep and circadian rhythms: rationale for the development of specific melatonin agonists. Sleep Med 2004;5(6):523–32.
23. Erman M, Seiden D, Zammit G, et al. An efficacy, safety and dose-response study of ramelteon in patients with chronic primary insomnia. Sleep Med 2006;7(1):17–24.
24. Griffiths RR, Johnson MW. Relative abuse liability of hypnotic drugs: a conceptual framework and algorithm for differentiating among compounds. J Clin Psychiatry 2005;66(Suppl 9):31–41.
25. Passarella S, Duong M. Diagnosis and treatment of insomnia. Am J Health Syst Pharm 2008;65:927–34.
26. Schnoes CJ, Kuhn BR, Workman EF, et al. Pediatric prescribing practices for clonidine and other pharmacologic agents for children with sleep disturbance. Clin Pediatr (Phila) 2006;45(3):229–38.
27. Merenstein D, Diener-West M, Halbower AC, et al. The trial of infant response to diphenhydramine: the TIRED study–a randomized, controlled, patient-oriented trial. Arch Pediatr Adolesc Med 2006;160(7):707–12.
28. Richardson GS, Roehrs TA, Rosenthal L, et al. Tolerance to daytime sedative effects of H1 antihistamines. J Clin Psychopharmacol 2002;22(5):511–5.
29. Dinndorf PA, McCabe MA, Frierdich S. Risk of abuse of diphenhydramine in children and adolescents with chronic illnesses. J Pediatr 1998;133:293–5.
30. Malvija S, Voepel-Lewis T, Tait AR. Adverse events and risk factors associated with the sedation of children by nonanesthesiologists. Anesth Anal 1997;85:1207–13.
31. Reed MD, Findling RL. Overview of current management of sleep disturbances in children: pharmacotherapy. Curr Ther Res Clin Exp 2002;63(Suppl B):B18–37.
32. Sheldon SH. Insomnia in children. Curr Treat Options Neurol 2001;3:37–50.
33. American Academy of Pediatrics Committee on Drugs and Committee on Environmental Health: use of chloral hydrate for sedation in children. Pediatrics 1993;92:471–3.
34. Lieberman JA. Update on the safety considerations in the management of insomnia with hypnotics: incorporating modified-release formulations into primary care. Prim Care Companion J Clin Psychiatry 2007;9(1):25–31.
35. Buscemi N, Vandermeer B, Friesen C, et al. The efficacy and safety of drug treatments for chronic insomnia in adults. A meta-analysis of RCTs. J Gen Intern Med 2007;22(9):1335–50.
36. Wagner J, Wagner M, Hening W. Beyond benzodiazepines: alternative pharmacologic agents for the treatment of insomnia. Ann Pharmacother 1998;32: 680–91.
37. Salva P, Costa J. Clinical pharmacokinetics and pharmacodynamics of zolpidem. Therapeutic implications. Clin Pharmacokinet 1995;29:142–53.
38. Mohler H, Fritschy JM, Rudolph U. A new benzodiazepine pharmacology. J Pharmacol Exp Ther 2002;300(1):2–8.
39. Zammit GK, Corser B, Doghramji K, et al. Sleep and residual sedation after administration of zaleplon, zolpidem and placebo during experimental middle of the night awakenings. J Clin Sleep Med 2006;2:417–23.
40. Najib J. Eszopiclone, a nonbenzodiazepine sedative-hypnotic agent for the treatment of transient and chronic insomnia. Clin Ther 2006;28:491–516.
41. Stahl SM. Essential psychopharmacology: the prescriber's guide. Cambridge (UK): Cambridge University Press; 2006. Physician's desk reference. 61st edition. Montvale (NJ): Thomson Healthcare Inc; 2007.

42. Prince JB, Wilens TE, Biederman J, et al. Clonidine for sleep disturbances associated with attention-deficit hyperactivity disorder: a system chart review of 62 cases. J Am Acad Child Adolesc Psychiatry 1996;35:599–605.

43. Ingrassia A, Turk J. The use of clonidine for severe and intractable sleep problems in children with neurodevelopmental disorders–a case series. Eur Child Adolesc Psychiatry 2005;14:34–40.

44. Kappagoda C, Schell DN, Hanson RM, et al. Clonidine over-dose in childhood: implications of increased prescribing. J Paediatr Child Health 1998;34:508–12.

45. Walsh JK, Erman M, Erwin CL, et al. Subjective hypnotic efficacy of trazodone and zolpidem in DSM-III-R primary insomnia. Hum Psychopharmacol 1998;13:191.

46. Drug Facts and Comparisons (database on the Internet). Indianapolis (IN); Facts and comparisons 4.0. 2010. Amitriptyline chloride (about 3 screens). Available at: http://0-online.factsandcomparisons.com.libcat.ferris.edu/MonoDisp.aspx?monoID=fandc-hcp13106&quick=338751/5&search=338751/5isstemmed=true. Accessed August 24, 2010.

47. Balderer G, Borbely A. Effect of valerian on human sleep. Psychopharmacology 1985;87I:406–9.

48. From the Centers for Disease Control and Prevention. Hepatic toxicity possibly associated with kava-containing products–United States, Germany and Switzerland, 1999–2002. JAMA 2003;289:36–7.

49. American Academy of Sleep Medicine. The international classification of sleep disorders: diagnostic and coding manual. 2nd edition. Westchester (IL): American Academy of Sleep Medicine; 2005. p. 114–6, 137.

50. Allen RP, Pichietti D, Hening WA, et al. Restless legs syndrome diagnosis and epidemiology workshop at the National Institutes of Health. Sleep Med 2003; 4:101–19.

51. Montplaisir J, Boucher S, Poirier G, et al. Clinical polysomnographic and genetic characteristics of restless legs syndrome: a study of 133 patients diagnosed with new standard criteria. Mov Disord 1997;12:61–5.

52. Picchiette D, Allen RP, Walters AS, et al. Restless legs syndrome: prevalence and impact in children and adolescents. The Peds REST Study. Pediatrics 2007;120(2):253–6.

53. Abetz L, Allen R, Follet A, et al. Evaluating the quality of life of patients with restless legs syndrome. Clin Ther 2004;26:925–35.

54. Chervin RD, Archbold KH, Dillon JE, et al. Associations between symptoms of inattention, hyperactivity, restless legs, and periodic leg movements. Sleep 2002;25:213–8.

55. Chervin RD, Dillon JF, Archbold KH, et al. Conduct problems and symptoms of sleep disorders in children. J Am Acad Child Adolesc Psychiatry 2003;42: 201–8.

56. Picchietti DL, Stevens HE. Early manifestations of restless legs syndrome in children and adolescence. Sleep Med 2008;9(7):770–81.

57. Chesson AL Jr, Anderson WM, Littner M, et al. Practice parameters for the treatment of restless legs syndrome and period limb movement disorder. An American Academy of Sleep Medicine Report. Standards of Practice Committee of the American Academy of Sleep Medicine. Sleep 1999;33:961–8.

58. Pichietti MA, Pichietti DL. Restless legs syndrome and periodic limb movement disorder in children and adolescents. Semin Pediatr Neurol 2008;15:91–9.

59. Brodeur C, Montplaisir J, Godbout R, et al. Treatment of restless legs syndrome and periodic movements during sleep with L-dopa: a double-blind, controlled study. Neurology 1988;38:1845–8.

60. Montplaisir J, Nicolas A, Denesle R, et al. Restless legs syndrome improved by pramipexole: a double-blind randomized trial. Neurology 1999;52:938–43.
61. Hening WA, Allen RP, Earley CJ, et al. An update on the dopaminergic treatment of restless legs syndrome and periodic limb movement disorder. Sleep 2004;27: 560–83.
62. Akpinar S. Restless legs syndrome treatment with dopaminergic drugs. Clin Neuropharmacol 1987;10(1):67–79.
63. Danoff SK, Grasso ME, Terry PB, et al. Pleuropulmonary disease due to pergolide use of restless legs syndrome. Chest 2001;120(1):313–6.
64. Schade R, Andersohn F, Suissa S, et al. Dopamine agonists and the risk of cardiac valve regurgitation. N Engl J Med 2007;356(1):29–38.
65. Walters AS, Mandelbaum DE, Lewin DS, et al. Dopaminergic therapy in children with restless legs/periodic limb movements in sleep and ADHD. Dopaminergic Study Group. Pediatr Neurol 2000;22(3):182–6.
66. Konofal E, Arnulf I, Lecendreux M, et al. Ropinirole in children with attention-deficit hyperactivity disorder and restless legs syndrome. Pediatr Neurol 2005;32:350–1.
67. Kotagal S, Silber MH. Childhood-onset restless legs syndrome. Ann Neurol 2004;56:803–7.
68. Allen RP, Earley CJ. Augmentation of the restless legs syndrome with carbidopa/ levodopa. Sleep 1996;19:205–13.
69. Earley CJ, Connor JR, Beard JL, et al. Abnormalities in CSF concentrations of ferritin and transferring in restless legs syndrome. Neurology 2000;54:1698–700.
70. Allen RP, Barker PB, Wehrl F, et al. MRI measurement of brain iron in patients with restless legs syndrome. Neurology 2001;56:263–5.
71. Kryger MH, Otake K, Foerster J. Low body stores of iron and restless legs syndrome: a correctable cause of insomnia in adolescents and teenagers. Sleep Med 2002;3:127–32.
72. Simakajornboon N, Gozal D, Vlasic V, et al. Periodic limb movements in sleep and iron status in children. Sleep 2003;26:735–8.
73. Garcia-Borreguero D, Larrosa O, de la Liave Y, et al. Treatment of restless legs syndrome with gabapentin: a double-blind, cross-over study. Neurology 2002; 59:1573–9.
74. Newacheck PW, Taylor WR. Childhood chronic illness: prevalence, severity and impact. Am J Public Health 1992;82(3):364–71.
75. Gislason T, Benediktsdottir B. Snoring, apneic episodes, and nocturnal hypoxemia among children 6 months to 6 years old. An epidemiologic study of lower limit of prevalence. Chest 1995;107:963–6.
76. Fujioka M, Young LW, Girdany BR. Radiographic evaluation of adenoidal size in children: adenoidal naso-pharyngeal ratio. Am J Roentgenol 1979;133:401–4.
77. Marcus CL. Sleep-disordered breathing in children. Am J Respir Crit Care Med 2001;164(1).16–30.
78. Goodwin JL, Kaemingk KL, Fregosi RF, et al. Parasomnias and sleep disordered breathing in Caucasian and Hispanic children–the Tucson children's assessment of sleep apnea study. BMC Med 2004;2(1):14.
79. Blunden S, Lushington K, Kennedy D. Cognitive and behavioral performance in children with sleep-related obstructive breathing disorders. Sleep Med Rev 2001;5(6):447–61.
80. Redline S, Tishler PV, Schluchter M, et al. Risk factors for sleep-disordered breathing in children: associations with obesity, race and respiratory problems. Am J Respir Crit Care Med 1999;159(5 Pt 1):1527–32.

81. O'Brien LM, Mervis CB, Holbrook CR, et al. Neurobehavioral correlates of sleep-disordered breathing in children. J Sleep Res 2004;13(2):165–72.

82. Marcus CL, Greene MG, Carroll JL. Blood pressure in children with obstructive sleep apnea. Am J Respir Crit Care Med 1998;157(4 Pt 1):1098–103.

83. Tal A, Lieberman A, Margulis G, et al. Ventricular dysfunction in children with obstructive sleep apnea: a radionuclide assessment. Pediatr Pulmonol 1988; 4:139–43.

84. Section on Pediatric Pulmonology. Clinical practice guideline: diagnosis and management of childhood obstructive sleep apnea syndrome. Pediatrics 2002;109(4):704–12.

85. Massa F, Gonsalez S, Laverty A, et al. The use of nasal continuous positive airway pressure to treat obstructive sleep apnea. Arch Dis Child 2002;87(5): 438–43.

86. Marcus CL, Carroll JL, Bamford O, et al. Supplemental oxygen during sleep in children with sleep-disordered breathing. Am J Respir Crit Care Med 1995; 152(4 Pt 1):1297–301.

87. Brouillette RT, Manoukian JJ, Ducharme FM, et al. Efficacy of fluticasone nasal spray for pediatric obstructive sleep apnea. J Pediatr 2001;138(6):838–44.

88. Mansfield LE, Diaz G, Posey CR, et al. Sleep disordered breathing and daytime quality of life in children with allergic rhinitis during treatment with intranasal budesonide. Ann Allergy Asthma Immunol 2004;92(2):240–4.

89. Alexopoulos EI, Kaditis AG, Kalampouka E, et al. Nasal corticosteroids for children with snoring. Pediatr Pulmonol 2004;38(2):161–7.

90. Goldbart AD, Goldman JL, Veling MC, et al. Leukotriene modifier therapy for mild sleep-disordered breathing in children. Am J Respir Crit Care Med 2005; 172:364–70.

91. Taheri S, Zeitzer JM, Mignot E. The role of hypocretins (orexins) in sleep regulation and narcolepsy. Annu Rev Neurosci 2002;25:283–313.

92. Challamel MJ, Mazzola ME, Nevimalova S, et al. Narcolepsy in children. Sleep 1994;17:S17–20.

93. Mignot E, Lammers GJ, Ripley B, et al. The role of cerebrospinal fluid hypocretin measurement in the diagnosis of narcolepsy and other hypersomnias. Arch Neurol 2002;59(10):1553–62.

94. Mignot E, Lin L, Finn L, et al. Correlates of sleep onset REM periods during the multiple sleep latency test in community adults. Brain 2006;129:1609–23.

95. Guilleminault C, Pelayo R. Narcolepsy in prepubertal children. Ann Neurol 1998; 43:135–42.

96. Morgenthaler TI, Kapur VK, Brown T, et al. Practice parameters for the treatment of narcolepsy and other hypersomnias of central origin. Sleep 2007;30(12): 1705–11.

97. Rogers AE, Aldrich MS, Lin X. A comparison of three different sleep schedules for reducing daytime sleepiness in narcolepsy. Sleep 2001;24(4):385–91.

98. Wisor JP, Nishino S, Sora I, et al. Dopaminergic role in stimulant-induced wakefulness. J Neurosci 2001;21(5):1787–94.

99. Swanson JM, Greenhill LL, Lopez FA, et al. Modafinil film-coated tablets in children and adolescents with attention-deficit hyperactivity disorder: results of a randomized, double-blind, placebo-controlled, fixed-dose study followed by abrupt discontinuation. J Clin Psychiatry 2006;67:137–47.

100. Meoli A, Rosen C, Kristo D, et al. Oral nonprescription treatment for insomnia: an evaluation of products with limited evidence. J Clin Sleep Med 2005;1(2): 173–87.

101. Wheatley D. Medicinal plants for insomnia: a review of their pharmacology, efficacy and tolerability. J Psychopharmacol 2005;19(1):414–21.
102. Morin A, Jarvis C, Lynch A. Therapeutic options for sleep-maintenance and sleep-onset insomnia. Pharmacotherapy 2007;27(1):89–110.
103. Ryan M, Slevin J. Restless legs syndrome. Am J Health Syst Pharm 2006;63: 1599–612.
104. Satija P, Ondo W. Restless legs syndrome; pathophysiology, diagnosis and treatment. CNS Drugs 2008;22(6):497–518.

Index

Note: Page numbers of article titles are in **boldface** type.

A

Abacavir, pharmacogenetics of, 17
Absorption, of drugs, 11–12
Acamprosate, for alcohol abuse, 246–247
Acarbose, for obesity, 143
Acetylcholine, as neurotransmitter, 26
Active transport, of drugs, 12
Addison disease, 229–230
Adenotonsillectomy, for sleep apnea, 282
ADHD. *See* Attention-deficit hyperactivity disorder.
Adrenal disorders, 229–232
Aggression, **73–84**
    anxiety disorders with, 78–79
    attention-deficit hyperactivity disorder with, 75–76
    autistic spectrum disorders with, 86–91, 195
    cognitive-adaptive disabilities with, 198
    conduct disorder with, 76–77
    fragile X syndrome with, 192–193
    intermittent explosive disorder with, 80–81
    mood disorders with, 77–78
    neurofibromatosis with, 196
    oppositional defiant disorder with, 76
    prevention of, 74
    provocation of, 73–74
    schizophrenia with, 79
    statistics on, 73
    Tourette syndrome with, 79–80
    treatment of, 86–91
    tuberous sclerosis complex with, 199
Agonists, in neurotransmission, 26
Agoraphobia, 224
Alcohol
    abuse of, 245–247
    prenatal exposure to, 193–194, 198
Allosteric modulation, in neurotransmission, 25
Alpha-agonists
    for aggression, 89–90
    for autistic spectrum disorders, 89–90
    for insomnia, 277–279
Alternative medicine. *See* Herbal medicines.
Alzheimer dementia, 191–192
Amino acids, as neurotransmitters, 24–25

Pediatr Clin N Am 58 (2011) 293–314
doi:10.1016/S0031-3955(10)00224-5
0031-3955/11/$ – see front matter © 2011 Elsevier Inc. All rights reserved.

U

Moving?

Make sure your subscription moves with you!

To notify us of your new address, find your **Clinics Account Number** (located on your mailing label above your name), and contact customer service at:

Email: journalscustomerservice-usa@elsevier.com

800-654-2452 (subscribers in the U.S. & Canada)
314-447-8871 (subscribers outside of the U.S. & Canada)

Fax number: 314-447-8029

**Elsevier Health Sciences Division
Subscription Customer Service
3251 Riverport Lane
Maryland Heights, MO 63043**

*To ensure uninterrupted delivery of your subscription, please notify us at least 4 weeks in advance of move.

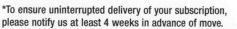

Moving?

Printed and bound by CPI Group (UK) Ltd, Croydon, CR0 4YY

03/10/2024

01040452-0015